New Developments in Medical Research

Palliative Care

The Role and Importance of Research in Promoting Palliative Care Practices

Reports from Developed Countries

Volume II

NEW DEVELOPMENTS IN MEDICAL RESEARCH

Additional books and e-books in this series can be found on Nova's website under the Series tab.

NEW DEVELOPMENTS IN MEDICAL RESEARCH

PALLIATIVE CARE

THE ROLE AND IMPORTANCE OF RESEARCH IN PROMOTING PALLIATIVE CARE PRACTICES

REPORTS FROM DEVELOPED COUNTRIES

VOLUME II

MICHAEL SILBERMANN
EDITOR

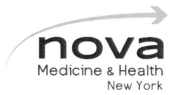

Copyright © 2019 by Nova Science Publishers, Inc.

All rights reserved. No part of this book may be reproduced, stored in a retrieval system or transmitted in any form or by any means: electronic, electrostatic, magnetic, tape, mechanical photocopying, recording or otherwise without the written permission of the Publisher.

We have partnered with Copyright Clearance Center to make it easy for you to obtain permissions to reuse content from this publication. Simply navigate to this publication's page on Nova's website and locate the "Get Permission" button below the title description. This button is linked directly to the title's permission page on copyright.com. Alternatively, you can visit copyright.com and search by title, ISBN, or ISSN.

For further questions about using the service on copyright.com, please contact:
Copyright Clearance Center
Phone: +1-(978) 750-8400   Fax: +1-(978) 750-4470   E-mail: info@copyright.com.

NOTICE TO THE READER

The Publisher has taken reasonable care in the preparation of this book, but makes no expressed or implied warranty of any kind and assumes no responsibility for any errors or omissions. No liability is assumed for incidental or consequential damages in connection with or arising out of information contained in this book. The Publisher shall not be liable for any special, consequential, or exemplary damages resulting, in whole or in part, from the readers' use of, or reliance upon, this material. Any parts of this book based on government reports are so indicated and copyright is claimed for those parts to the extent applicable to compilations of such works.

Independent verification should be sought for any data, advice or recommendations contained in this book. In addition, no responsibility is assumed by the Publisher for any injury and/or damage to persons or property arising from any methods, products, instructions, ideas or otherwise contained in this publication.

This publication is designed to provide accurate and authoritative information with regard to the subject matter covered herein. It is sold with the clear understanding that the Publisher is not engaged in rendering legal or any other professional services. If legal or any other expert assistance is required, the services of a competent person should be sought. FROM A DECLARATION OF PARTICIPANTS JOINTLY ADOPTED BY A COMMITTEE OF THE AMERICAN BAR ASSOCIATION AND A COMMITTEE OF PUBLISHERS.

Additional color graphics may be available in the e-book version of this book.

Library of Congress Cataloging-in-Publication Data

ISBN: 978-1-53616-199-1

Published by Nova Science Publishers, Inc. † New York

This volume is dedicated to the founders of the Middle East Cancer Consortium (MECC), Richard Klausner, MD, former director of the National Cancer Institute at the National Institutes of Health, USA, and to Ephraim Sneh, MD, former Minister of Health, State of Israel, who were so catalytic in MECC's odyssey and success, and to whom I owe so much.

CONTENTS

Preface		xi
Acknowledgments		xix
Introductory Remarks		xxi
Part I	**North America**	1
Chapter 1	End-of-Life Care in Persons with Severe and Persistent Mental Illness: A Review of the Research Outcomes *Phyllis Whitehead, Senaida Keating, Shereen Gamaluddin and Kye Y. Kim*	3
Chapter 2	Beyond Quality of Life: An Approach to Complexity *Lodovico Balducci*	13
Chapter 3	Using Evidence to Improve Palliative Care Practice *Regina M. Fink and Jeannine M. Brant*	25
Chapter 4	Research Tools and Approaches to Reduce the Suffering of Cancer Patients in Developing Countries *Lidia Schapira and Karl Lorenz*	47
Chapter 5	Integrating Palliative Care in Non-Oncologic Patient Populations: The Case for Renal Supportive Care *Emily Lu and Craig D. Blinderman*	57
Chapter 6	Palliative Care Research: Increasing the Awareness, Delivery and Quality of Palliative Care *Egidio Del Fabbro and J. Brian Cassel*	83
Part II	**Western Europe**	95
Chapter 7	Strategies for the Promotion of Home Palliative Care – What Is Still to Be Learned and How? *Manuel Luís Capelas, Sílvia Patrícia Coelho, and Tânia Sofia Afonso*	97

Chapter 8	Coping with Death Competence in Pediatric Nurses *Amparo Oliver, Laura Galiana, Noemí Sansó and Juan Manuel Gavala*	113
Chapter 9	The Need for a Research Oriented Psycho-Oncology in Palliative Care *Simone Cheli*	123
Chapter 10	Palliative Care Service Provision and Outcomes in Low and Middle Income Countries *Kennedy Nkhoma, Ping Guo, Eve Namisango and Richard Harding*	133
Chapter 11	Global Palliative Care Development Research *Stephen R. Connor*	157
Chapter 12	Research Methods in Palliative Care *Paz Fernández Ortega and Julio C. de la Torre-Montero*	167
Chapter 13	Early Intervention of Palliative Care: An Innovative, Effective and Efficient Model of Care to Meet the Challenge of the Phenomena of Disease Chronication and Demographic Transition in the 21st Century: What Is the Situation in France? *Rana Istambouly*	175
Part III	**Eastern Europe**	189
Chapter 14	Medical Research in Palliative Medicine in Poland: The Bottom-Up versus the Top-Down Approach *Zbigniew (Ben) Zylicz and Aleksandra Kotlińska-Lemieszek*	191
Part IV	**Middle East**	199
Chapter 15	Early Palliative Care (EPC) Trials for Patients with Advanced Incurable Cancer: What Have We Learned and How Can We Improve Future Trials and Patients' Care *Haris Charalambous and Angelos P. Kassianos*	201
Chapter 16	The Role and Importance of Research in Promoting Pharmacological Management of Cancer Related Pain *Elon Eisenberg*	227
Chapter 17	Research on What 'Meaning' Really Means for Cancer Patients Near the End of Life: Findings from a Mixed Methods Study *Adi Ivzori Erel, Lee Greenblatt-Kimron and Miri Cohen*	239
Chapter 18	Importance and Effect of Research Findings on the Outcome of Clinical Practice of Palliative Care *Azar Naveen Saleem and Azza Adel Hassan*	265

Chapter 19	The Importance of Palliative Care Research in a Clinical Setting: Identifying Barriers and Implementation Strategies *Tahani H. Al Dweikat*	275
Chapter 20	Promoting Research and Practices in Palliative Care in an Islamic Middle-Income Country: Oman as an Example *Zakiya Al Lamki*	283
Part V	**Far East**	**305**
Chapter 21	Palliative Care Nursing in Japan: Practice and Research *Tomoko Majima and Tomoko Otsuka*	307
Part VI	**Oceania**	**317**
Chapter 22	The Role and Importance of Research in Promoting Palliative Care Practice: Methods and Outcomes *Paul A. Glare*	319

Countries Represented in this Volume	335
About the Editor	337
List of Contributors	339
Index	347
Related Nova Publications	361

PREFACE

OVERVIEW

Palliative care is a healthcare specialty that is both a philosophy of care and an organized, highly-structured system for delivering care. It improves healthcare quality in three domains: Relief of physical and emotional suffering; Improvement of patient-physician communication; Assurance of coordinated continuity of care across multiple Healthcare settings - hospital, home, hospice and long-term care.

All over the globe, palliative care - the forefront of patient-centered care - affirms life by supporting patients' and family's goals for the future, including their hopes for cure or life prolongation as well as comfort and control. Comprehensive palliative care services integrate the expertise of a team which typically includes physicians, nurses, social workers, chaplains, pharmacists and others; but unfortunately such teams are still lacking in most parts of the world.

Essential to an evidence-based approach to palliative care is well-designed research. Palliative care provides a rich and challenging set of research questions, and as research in this setting focuses on patients who are approaching an expected death, there are many medically, ethically and psychosocially complex issues to consider. Among the challenges that are unique or significant in palliative care in a research setting are:

> Difficulty with recruiting and retaining participants whose health is declining.
> Problems with building collaborative research teams and conducting research across the range of settings in which palliative care is provided.
> Difficulty with how best to measure effectiveness and cost-effectiveness of treatments and services in the midst of the inevitable deterioration of a dying patient.
> Challenges of engaging clinicians in a sector where there has not traditionally been a research culture.
> The predominance of investigator-led over pharmaceutical company-led research which limits financing opportunities for researchers.[2]

These genuine difficulties are valid even in high-income countries, but much more so in most emerging countries globally.

In palliative care research, many important activities involve the careful collection and analysis of data. These activities involve many of the same general principles of good research, such as:

> Defining the question to answer
> Determining the appropriate methods to be used
> Introducing measures to minimize bias
> Feeding the results back to those involved.

In addition to audit, service evaluation, questionnaires or surveys may also be utilized.[2]

Although many treatments currently exist to manage symptoms and complications of advanced cancer, there continues to be a paucity of well-designed prospective clinical trials examining state-of-the-art practices, impeding the further development of evidence-based guidelines. The current situation is much more complicated while investigators design palliative care trials. Such challenges include ethical issues in conducting clinical trials, barriers to collaborative research across specialties, and unclear standards for the types of best-care practices that should be employed as part of such trials. Therefore, as long as the randomized controlled trial is the standard by which effectiveness is judged, fields such as palliative care, where interventions have not been proven by this test, is at risk of being relegated to second-class status in the medical hierarchy.[3]

Optimal care of patients with advanced illness requires a commitment to base treatment approaches on scientific fact rather than anecdotal experience.[3] The nature of palliative care is a holistic one, being managed by a multidisciplinary team. Considering the interactive involvement of cancer suffering, research involving the psychosocial aspects and palliative care (emotional reactions, interactive emotions, coping strategies, spirituality) is a basic task in trying to alleviate the suffering of patients and their families. However, to analyze the psychological aspects in cancer patients we face significant barriers:

1. Psychological issues are subjective; variables or constructs are complex and difficult to operationalize.
2. Psychological variables are difficult to measure.
3. Patients are fragile, their condition (both physical and psychological) is mediated by the progress of the disease and the presence of impending death.
4. Health professionals have limited time to conduct assessments or research.
5. There is a lack of validated clinical tools.

The causes for emotional distress associated with suffering are multiple - changing with time, with the progress of the disease and with faith. This implies the need to assess the patient's condition holistically and continuously. At the end of life, threats develop at both the mind and body level, and therefore suffering entails physical, emotional, and environmental changes, and responses are oriented toward the recovery of homeostasis.[4]

A recent review of end-of-life care in the UK expressed serious concerns about the lack of research in this field and the underuse of existing research. Thus, funding leading-edge needs-led research is essential for improving palliative care across all disease areas, including programs evaluating the effectiveness and impact of healthcare treatment and services. This approach is especially suitable for palliative care (where and when its emphasis is on the patient and family first, rather than their disease) which intends to meet the needs identified by patients [5] rather than on emphasizing their disease.

The benefit of involving patients early in research planning will facilitate reaching models of care while taking into account patients' needs. A greater evidence base will also develop good models of practice, particularly in supporting generalists' work. Adopting an international collaborative approach to research, involving both developed and underdeveloped countries, is becoming increasingly important to address priorities in end-of-life care.[5]

To date, in large portions of the globe, practicing clinicians fail to identify patients who need specialty palliative care, thus leading to inefficient and inadequate care. Identifying such patients automatically, using electronic health records, could both enrich enrollment in palliative care trials and promote patient-centered allocation of the limited resources in specialty palliative care. This would eventually result in better clinician documentation of uncontrolled symptoms and psychosocial distress.[6]

Since palliative care offers various services that may have different effects on patients, an understanding of how different types of palliative care clinicians contribute to outcomes is needed, and how such relationships are modified by the way in which institutional culture provides primary palliative care—that is, palliative care delivered by patients' primary clinicians. In view of the insurmountable shortage of palliative care physicians, especially in the community, nonphysicians such as trained nurses who can deliver equivalent or even better care are essential in order to maximize value.[6] Therefore, experimental evidence for outpatient and home-based palliative care is highly needed and should be of the same quality as for inpatient services.[7]

Several studies have supported the concept that "early" palliative care improves outcomes for patients with cancer. Research is needed to determine what constitutes "early" and how such definitions differ by illness and care setting. In addition, evidence is also needed to guide the optimal duration of these services. Even if we succeed in determining the best timing and duration of palliative care, the challenge of how best to promote effective service delivery will remain.

One research challenge in thriving for high-value specialty palliative care is to aim toward simple interventions that could go a long way toward optimizing the implementation of specialty palliative care.[6] Unlike other areas of medicine, the knowledge base to support the basic elements of palliative care clinical practice is small and inadequate in developing countries.

In order to improve the current situation, especially in the developing world, there is a need to develop:

1. A cadre of palliative care experts
2. Research networks and multi-site studies which will contribute to the goal of bringing an evidence-based approach to palliative care practice.

Women all over the world will have to shoulder a significantly larger caregiving burden of as a direct result of their governments' attempts to push palliative care into the community.

Consequently, further research is required to explore the complex construction of gender and family caregiving, in an end-of-life context, which is currently limited.

As societies age, there will be a greater demand for palliative care in the context of old age, as well as an ageing pool of family carers. These societal changes mean that even women aged 80 and older provide a significant portion of unpaid family caregiving. Of interest is the finding that this experience negatively affects women more than men, as women are at a greater risk of stress, anxiety and depression than men who provide care.[8]

Differences in the construction of gender across societies and cultures have led to the common perception of gender and how, consequently, people conduct themselves and explain their actions and behavior - features that are still evident in many countries.

The above study has highlighted several significant implications for future research.[8]

First, it revealed how important gender is to the experience of end-of-life caregiving, including:

1. why people accept the role
2. The nature of the care they provide
3. Health-related outcomes for carers

Therefore, gender must be included as a category of analysis when conducting further research related to palliative care. Moreover, the research should also allude to the issue of ethnicity – the degree to which gender intersects with other identity-defining characteristics. Accordingly, future research should take into account that gender is a malleable product of particular socio-cultural contexts and influenced heavily by the distribution of power within societies. In this way, the palliative care process can be seen to reflect dominant cultural expectations which relegate women to the private sphere and devalue their labor – a process which is exacerbated for older adults because of undercurrents of ageism in society. In sum, there is an urgent need for more gender analysis to fill this significant gap in palliative care literature in both developed and developing countries.[8]

DILEMMAS AND BARRIERS

Palliative care researchers must confront distinctive ethical dilemmas and barriers that extend far beyond those of standard research trials. While many ethical issues are not unique to patients facing life's end; they are often magnified in this population, compounding the potential ethical issues present in all clinical research trials. These include the vulnerability of the population from which study subjects are recruited, high rates of mental incapacity and emotional distress. Methodological challenges include the high incidence of the loss of follow-up information due to physical and mental incapacity and death, the biases introduced by the need for surrogate respondents, and the difficulty of determining appropriate outcomes and methods for assessing those outcomes.[3]

Despite the challenges alluded to above, the effectiveness of palliative interventions - regardless of the country's income - must nevertheless be assessed with the same vigor that is employed in assessing other medical interventions. In addition, designing palliative care research with methodological precision must account for the diversity of ethnic, cultural and religious backgrounds that patients bring with them into their experience of life-limiting illness. The patients' experience is shaped in large by the cultural milieu in which they reside.[3]

The lack of high-quality clinical research in palliative care relative to other non-palliative clinical conditions suggests a clear opportunity to advance the science and improve the quality of care for patients afflicted with cancer. Without such advancements in research methods, policies and procedures, the field of palliative care risks a future where clinical practices are ill-informed. As with all cancer therapies, the gold standard continues to be the randomized prospective clinical trial.[3] Research in palliative care, especially in developing countries, has been dogged by recruitment problems.

Conducting research with palliative populations is necessary to ensure the development of evidence-based policies and services which reflect and respond to the needs of this vulnerable and often underserved population in both developed and developing countries. It is only through actively engaging in research with the palliative population that we can develop evidence-based policies, protocols and treatments to maximize their quality of life as they approach the end of their lives.[9]

To positively influence clinical practice in palliative care, healthcare professionals need access to "best available evidence" and acquiring evidence from this client group presents a great challenge. There is a clear need for the urgent development of evidence-based guidelines to aid in the education, diagnosis and management of the physio-psycho complaints of cancer patients - in developed and even more so in developing countries - especially close to the end of life.[9]

Why is research required in hospice care?

1. To provide evidence-based treatment and care
2. To test and improve complex interventions
3. To create a culture of inquiry
4. To best understand the changing needs of the communities that hospices serve.[10]

In Ireland, as an example of a developed country, the following list of priorities was declared to take precedence for research and palliative care:

1. Best ways of providing palliative care outside of "working hours"
2. Best ways of providing palliative care in the patient's home
3. Best ways of providing pain symptom relief
4. Explaining the dying process compassionately and honestly, and determining the best person to communicate this information
5. Advance care planning
6. Advance care planning continuity for patients at end of life
7. Support of children and young people
8. What kind of training do the caregivers need?

SUMMARY

Not long ago "palliative care" was synonymous with end-of-life cancer care, but today it is no longer specific to terminal cancer. Recent research projects supported by the American Cancer Society investigate measures for effective control of pain, other symptoms, and of side effects for those who have been affected by cancer. As the number of cancer survivors - especially in developed countries - continues to grow, finding ways to help them live well will become increasingly important. Special emphasis is given to identifying the needs of long-term survivors and designing programs and interventions to improve their quality of life.[12]

Research into palliative and end-of-life care touches on hugely important issues that will affect the lives of so many of us in the developing world: challenges of an aging population, range of diseases that people die from where palliative care is poorly provided, the need to give support to patients and their carers (especially where care is given at home or other non-hospital settings) and the need for improved symptom management.[13]

Michael Silbermann, DMD, PhD
Haifa, Israel

REFERENCES

[1] *The national Palliative Care Research Center: Curing suffering through palliative care research.* 2018. http://www.npcrc.org/content/15/About-Palliative-Care.aspx# tabs-2453.

[2] Getting started in palliative care research. *CARESEARCH*. Palliative care knowledge network. 2018. https://www.caresearch.com.au/caresearch/tabid/2631/Default.aspx.

[3] Krouse, R.S., Rosenfeld, K.E., Grant, M., Aziz, N., Byock, I., Sloan, J., Casarett, D., Palliative care research: Issues and opportunities. *Cancer Epidemiology, Biomarkers & Prevention* 13:337-339, 2004. http://cebp.aacrjournals.org/content/13/3/337.

[4] Limonero, J.T., Gil-Moncayo, F. Importance of psychological research in palliative care: Barriers in its development. *Palliative Medicine and Hospice Care Open J* 1:1-3, 2014. doi:10.17140/PM-MCOJ-1-101.

[5] Higginson, I.J. Research challenges in palliative and end of life care. *BMJ Support & Palliative Care.* 6:2-4, 2016. doi:10.1136/bmjspcare-2015-001091.

[6] Courtright, K.R., Cassel, T.B., Halpern, S.D. A research agenda for high-value palliative care. *Ann. Inter. Med.* 168:71-72, 2018. doi:10.7326/M17-2614.

[7] Kavalieratos, D., Corbelli, J., Zhang, D., Dionne-Odom, J.N., Ernccoff, N.C., Hanmer, J. et al. Association between palliative care and patient and caregiver outcomes: A systematic review and meta-analysis. *JAMA* 316:2014-2114, 2016.

[8] Morgan, T., Williams, L.A., Trussardi, G., Gott, M. Gender and family caregiving at the end-of-life in the context of old age; A systematic review. *Pall. Med.* 30:616-624, 2016. doi:10.1177/0269216315625857.

[9] Reid, J., Scott, D., Porter, S. Challenges in palliative care research: Experience from a randomized controlled trial in refractory cancer cachexia. *Palliative Medicine and Hospice Care Open J.* 1:e1-e3, 2015. doi:10.17140/PMHJCO7-1-e001.

[10] Payne, S., Preston, N., Turner, M., Rolls, L. *Research in palliative care: Can hospices afford not to be involved?* International Observatory of End of Life Care & Lancaster University, Oct. 2013. www.helpthehospices.org.uk/commission.

[11] *Top 10 Palliative Care Research Priorities List* – All Ireland Institute for Hospice and Palliative Care, 2018. http://aiihpc.org/research/launch-of-top-10-palliative-care-research-priorities/top-10-palliative-care-research-priorities-list/

[12] *Palliative Care Research* – American Cancer Society 2018. https://www.cancer.org/research/ we-conduct-cancer-research/ behavioral-research-center/ palliative-care-research.html.

[13] Walshe, C., Palliative care: Why I moved from nursing to research. *The Guardian,* Feb. 2014. https://www.theguardian.com/higher-education-network/blog/2014/fb/21/ nursing-palliative-care-research-lancaster-university-academic-careers.

ACKNOWLEDGMENTS

In 1996 I accepted the position of Executive Director of the Middle East Cancer Consortium (MECC). Our first assignment was to create a cancer registry network in the Middle East in order to establish the scope of cancer in this part of the world. We were surprised to learn that about 70% of all cancer patients in the region see a physician only when the cancer has already reached stage III or IV, which for most patients was too late for a curative treatment. Since these patients suffered from "total pain" throughout the trajectory of the illness, we understood that the only alternative left was palliation, be it in the hospital and/or the community. Realizing this grave situation, the Consortium decided to embark on regional training programs for professionals (physicians, nurses, social workers, art therapists and spiritual counselors) who 15 years ago lacked the understanding and objectives of palliative care in cancer patients. After visiting most of the cancer centers in the region, I decided to head to New York and spend some time at Calvary Hospital in the Bronx (Robert Brescia), the largest palliative care hospital in the United States. At Calvary, along with our close association with the American Society of Clinical Oncology (ASCO) (Thomas Smith), the American Oncology Nursing Society (ONS) (Jeannine Brant), I learned a great deal about how care should be delivered, especially at the terminal stage of the disease.

Sitting on the airplane on the way home, however, it struck me that it was unfortunate that we still lack essential information, based on solid research, in order to have our practice on evidence-based data that can only be achieved via systematic, well-designed research in the different countries. Joe Harford, from the National Cancer Institute (NCI) in Bethesda, MD, provided me with excellent guidance and mentorship. As a result, our teams published many peer-reviewed papers and books that were published by NOVA and Springer. I was astonished to learn that, to date, the issue of research in palliative care had not been sufficiently explored. I'm thankful that NOVA offered us the opportunity to provide a global perspective on these matters. We hope that this book will be a useful resource for those who wish to further develop and promote palliative care services in their own countries. The authors, most of whom report from developing countries, provide, in their respective chapters, valuable information on the current situation vis-à-vis research activities in their countries, taking into consideration the current underfunding and resource constraints. As a result of the creation of this book, we will find together (scientists from developed and developing countries) satisfactory solutions.

We would have no book without the exceptional contributions of each and every author. Thank you all. The patients and their families around the world have been the inspiration for, and the recipients of, palliative care programs and were the reason for publishing this book.

Special thanks to Genoveba Breitstein, my right hand assistant since the creation of MECC, despite being busy in her own life. I am blessed by her guidance, advice and friendship.

Michael Silbermann

INTRODUCTORY REMARKS

Following years of personal involvement in promoting palliative care, firstly throughout the Middle East, and more recently in other regions worldwide, I have come to realize that priorities for palliative care interventions are basically similar in various parts of the world. While starting and focusing on training in pain management, it became apparent that regardless of cultural, religious or ethnic background the majority of cancer patients are concerned with emotional-mental issues more than their physical suffering.

While visiting the King Hussein Cancer Center in Amman, Jordan, I met a 38-year-old Jordanian woman who was at a stage IV breast cancer with metastases in her spine. I asked her why she waited so long before going to a doctor. Her answer was: "I realized that I have cancer, and I accepted the fact that this disease is involved with bad pains, but that is not what bothers me. What really concerns me is the question who will take care of my three children after my death".

In a recent survey in Lebanon which involved breast cancer patients, women were asked to prioritize the matters that bothered them throughout their disease trajectory. The issue of pain was categorized only at the 5th place, while the leading factors for their suffering were emotional matters. In other countries I was told that physicians are utilizing non-pharmacological modalities to control pains, and that with great success. These responses, which came out in Middle East countries, appear to represent feelings in other parts of the world as well, most of which are developing countries.

However, while visiting a large hospital in a Western country, I experienced the following: A patient was admitted at a terminal stage after being treated in another well-known hospital for his cancer. At admission, the patient was screaming because of extreme pain, and it was impossible to communicate with him. Following an injection of a potent pain killer he relaxed, let the nurse clean him, and lay quietly in his bed. The attending physician then told me: "Now we can start with our palliative care".

In two books that I edited recently:

1. *Cancer Care in Countries and Societies in Transition.* Springer, New York, 2016
2. *Palliative Care: Perspectives, Practices and Impact on Quality of Life. A Global View.* NOVA, New York, 2017

clinicians and scientists from 30 countries expressed their experiences and views on topics focusing on clinical issues. These publications add to the vast and rich literature dealing with both the development and integration of palliative care in mainstream clinical care.

My personal idea concerning a possible unique contribution of a new book is to further emphasize the importance of solid research in order to be able to come up with evidence-based protocols and recommendations for healthcare professionals dealing with palliative care wherever they are. The translation of research data into practical terms is essential and will grant this relatively new subspecialty the status that it so rightfully deserves.

One of the complaints that I repeatedly receive refers to severe problems in communication between the patient and his physician and/or caregivers among his family members. Of course one should not generalize things, but yes, this issue is still a relevant problem worldwide. Having served as a former dean of a medical school in a world renowned university, I know that the curriculum is lacking these items of medical education, while emphasis nowadays goes mainly to molecular genetics and related topics. Even residents do not always receive systematic, well-organized courses, but get rather pieces of information on an optional basis. Let me reiterate that the current situation is universal, but by no means is this so in all hospitals, especially not in North America, Australia and the United Kingdom.

How to overcome such conflicts which constitute a serious dilemma should be an topic for discussion in the new book. This could involve issues related to the different approaches to different age groups from childhood to senescence.

I hope that this short introduction will assist you in formalizing our contribution to the new book. A tentative deadline for submission would be mid-year 2018.

Part I. North America

In: Palliative Care
Editor: Michael Silbermann

ISBN: 978-1-53616-199-1
© 2019 Nova Science Publishers, Inc.

Chapter 1

END-OF-LIFE CARE IN PERSONS WITH SEVERE AND PERSISTENT MENTAL ILLNESS: A REVIEW OF THE RESEARCH OUTCOMES

Phyllis Whitehead[1], Senaida Keating[1], Shereen Gamaluddin[1] and Kye Y. Kim[2*]

[1]Department of Internal Medicine, Carilion Clinic
and Virginia Tech Carilion School of Medicine, Roanoke, VA, US
[2]Department of Psychiatry and Behavioral Medicine, Carilion Clinic
and Virginia Tech Carilion School of Medicine, Roanoke, VA, US

ABSTRACT

The National Care Institute defines palliative care as care given to improve the quality of life of patients who have a serious or chronic disease, such as cancer. The goal of palliative care is to prevent or treat, as early as possible, the symptoms and side effects of the disease and its treatment, in addition to the related psychological, social, and spiritual problems. Many healthcare clinicians overlook the importance of integrating palliative care into the care of patients with a severe and persistent mental illness (SPMI). Common diagnoses include schizophrenia, bipolar affective disorder, major depression or a personality disorder. Research shows that patients who have battled SPMIs have a much higher mortality rate than the average person. Other studies have shown that people diagnosed with mental illness are upwards of 3.5 times less likely to have access to palliative care when compared to the general population. This vulnerable population is underserved, dying prematurely and without adequate symptom management. It is clear SPMI patients can appropriately choose palliative care but accessibility is being denied to due lack of knowledge and understanding by healthcare clinicians. More research is needed for this vulnerable population and palliative care.

Keywords: severe and persistent mental illness, palliative care, end of life, premature death

---

[*] Corresponding Author's E-mail: kykim@carilionclinic.org

BACKGROUND/INTRODUCTION

The National Care Institute defines palliative care as care given to improve the quality of life of patients who have a serious or life-limiting disease, such as cancer. The goal of palliative care is to prevent or treat, as early as possible, the symptoms and side effects of the disease and its treatment, in addition to the related psychological, social, and spiritual problems. The goal may not be to cure but to support both the patient and his loved ones. Palliative care is also called comfort care, supportive care, and symptom management. (Ferrell et al., 2018)

For many patients as well as providers, palliative care is often viewed as end-of-life (EOL) care, a term typically reserved for hospice care. Hospice is defined as care focused on symptom management and quality of life for patients with a life expectancy of six months or less and who decide to forgo life prolonging interventions. Patients must decide between seeking additional quantity of life with additional treatments versus quality of life by accepting the possibility of the likeliness of reduction in the quantity of life. Medicare, Medicaid and commercial insurances provide a Hospice Benefit for patients who choose to elect this type of care/coverage. (Ferrell et al., 2018)

In contrast, palliative care does not have a defined life expectancy limit. Palliative care supports patients with life-limiting diseases until the patient succumbs to the disease and may be provided along with traditional life prolonging interventions such as chemotherapy, dialysis, etc. (Hunnicutt, Tjia, & Lapane, 2017)

A decision to accept palliative care can be a challenging decision for any patient. Unfortunately, many healthcare clinicians overlook the importance of integrating palliative care into the care plan of patients with a severe and persistent mental illness (SPMI). It is important to note those patients with SPMI and a serious or life limiting diseases are capable of selecting palliative care. The ability and desire to select palliative care does not differ significantly than with those patients without SPMI. However, there is a disparity of access between the general population and patients with SPMI. (Elie et al., 2018)

PALLIATIVE CARE NEED IN PERSONS WITH SPMI COMPARED TO THE GENERAL POPULATION

SPMI has been defined as a prolonged and recurrent mental illness affecting people over the age of eighteen years. Most commonly they have a diagnosis of schizophrenia, bipolar affective disorder, major depression or a personality disorder. (Woods, Willison, Kington, & Gavin, 2008) Approximately 6% of the population suffers from SPMI. (Shalev, Brewster, Arbuckle, & Levenson, 2017) A study in the 2015 edition of the Schizophrenia Bulletin notes that patients that have battled SPMIs have a much higher mortality rate than the average person, sometimes dying as much as 10 to 20 years sooner than people in the same age bracket in the general population. In addition, studies have shown that patients with SPMI have an increased risk of debilitating physical conditions and certain cancers compared with the general population. (Elie et al., 2018)

Patients with schizophrenia, for example, have a similar incidence of most cancers to the general population, but these patients have up to two-fold the risk of dying of their disease due to under-detection and under-treatment. (Shalev et al., 2017) According to the World Health Organization (WHO), although suicide is important cause of death, the vast majority of these deaths are due to chronic physical medical conditions such as cardiovascular, respiratory and infectious diseases, diabetes, and hypertension.(Center for Health Statistics, 2012; Public & Concern, 2012; Trachsel, Irwin, Biller-Andorno, Hoff, & Riese, 2016) Excess mortality from chronic diseases is multi-factorial, increased substance use and its medical sequelae, decreased engagement with preventative health care, and poor access to medical care all contribute. (Shalev et al., 2017)

PALLIATIVE CARE DESIRES FOR PATIENTS WITH SPMI COMPARED TO THE GENERAL POPULATION

A recent Canadian study (Elie et al., 2018) demonstrated that in most cases, patients with SPMI have a similar desire for palliative care as those patients who are not diagnosed with SPMI. In this study, researchers provided a two question questionnaire based upon an imaginary scenarios for EOL preferences to 106 patients with SPMI and 95 chronically medically ill (CMI), used as the control group. (Elie et al., 2018) The results are similar to other studies in which the research showed similar desires in EOL care between persons with SPMI and the non-SPMI general population. Elie found similarities in the desire for quality of life, including control of pain and other symptoms, control over levels of intervention to avoid prolonging of the dying phase, and control over maintaining meaningful relationships. (Bussmann et al., 2015; PJ, MEG, & JC, 2004) These studies support the assumption that patients with SPMI possess the capacity to rationalize the benefits of palliative care.

PALLIATIVE CARE UTILIZATION FOR PATIENTS WITH SPMI

Research demonstrates that patients with SPMI are more likely to qualify for palliative care services and actually desire these treatment and interventions. Other studies have shown that people diagnosed with mental illness are upwards of 3.5 times less likely to have access to palliative care when compared to the general population. (Butler & O'Brien, 2017) In short, data suggest that the provision of palliative care to SPMI patients is dramatically lacking. In a large cohort study of schizophrenia patients with a prognosis of 6 months or less to live, these patients were found to access palliative care at rates approximately half that of the control group without schizophrenia. Such lack of access to palliative care directly affects the management of EOL symptoms. Patients with schizophrenia in the same study received significantly less opioid analgesia than those in the control group. (Shalev et al., 2017)

LITERATURE

The literature on the EOL care of people with a pre-existing mental illness is scarce. Multiple studies have demonstrated that there is lack of research on palliative care and SPMI and advocate for research to better understand care of SPMI patients at EOL.(Ellison, Russinova, Lyass, & Rogers, 2008; Foti, 2003; Picot, Glaetzer, & Myhill, 2015)

Psychiatric advance directives (PADs) provide an invaluable mechanism for SPMI adults to document their future care preferences including EOL interventions. Unfortunately studies have found poor completion rates of these invaluable documents. (Easter, Swanson, Robertson, Moser, & Swartz, 2017) There are many challenges related to completing these advance directives (ADs) that include patient factors, decisional factors and historical legal precedents. (Olsen, 2016) More research is needed to examine the benefit of PADs and AMDs for SPMI patients as well exploring the challenges related to the implementation of these documents. (Olsen, 2017)

DEFICITS/CONCERNS/SPECIAL CONSIDERATIONS

Having palliative care conversations regarding goals and care preferences are difficult within the context of a standard population. Discussions about EOL care, completed advance directives, and tools to assess competence of EOL choices are lacking in all patients regardless of diagnosis (PJ, MEG, & JC, 2004). The added complexity of SPMI amplifies the difficulty and the deficits surrounding the issues even more. Those with SPMI are part of a vulnerable population that is often disengaged from the medical community. The lack of integration of mental and medical health services is significant and impacts patient's care access as well as continuity. This is compounded by the stereotype that those with SPMI as less adherent to medical recommendations and more likely to be violent. (Irwin, Henderson, Knight, & Pirl, 2014) Stereotypes such as this lead to social stigma and even self-stigma as those with SPMI begin to believe the stereotypes as true. (Hinshaw & Stier, 2008) Stereotypes and stigma consequently shape how those with SPMI relate to and experience their illness. (Rüsch, Angermeyer, & Corrigan, 2005) These experiences, shape expectations and desires at EOL. (Woods, Willison, Kington, & Gavin, 2008)

Persons with SPMI die earlier than the general population (World Health Organization). Often suicide and homicide are blamed as the primary reasons for earlier deaths. While they are associated with higher rate ratios, the majority of premature deaths in this population are in fact due to physical illnesses; specifically cardiovascular disease, respiratory illness, and cancer. Other factors which increase the risk of physical illness include substance use, unhealthy lifestyles, unstable living situations, and medication side effects. (Lawrence & Kisely, 2010)

Personal behaviors such a cigarette smoking, for example, may increase cancer mortality in SPMI. However, additional factors such as missed cancer screening opportunities, later presentation with more advanced disease, and less treatment opportunities can be related to external factors. (Irwin et al., 2014)

The confines and organization or disorganization of the medical system itself contributes to this health disparity. At the provider level the effects of stigma as well as time and resource constraints can affect physician attitudes. Providers may even disregard physical complaints and attribute them as psychosomatic. (Leucht, Burkard, Henderson, Maj, & Sartorius, 2007) Within healthcare, mental health is often considered distinct and a separate entity. Even at a very concrete, visible level there is often physical separation of medical and mental health care facilities. This fosters poor communication and a lack of ownership by providers for the physical health of patients. This absence of integration between medicine and psychiatry contributes to a gap in care for those with SPMI. (Druss, 2007) Irwin et al. describes a Canadian study where in the last 6 months of life individuals with schizophrenia were twice as likely to be in a nursing facility. However, they were less likely to be given a palliative care referral or be have pain treated with opioids compared with matched controls.

A system with a more integrated care model can change the trajectory for those with SMI living with chronic or terminal illness. The Veterans Administration (VA) is given as an example of an integrated care model. Within the VA system there is more of a continuum of care. Patients with schizophrenia and cancer were found to have longer hospice stays and more documented Do Not Resuscitate orders compared to controls without SPMI. (Irwin et al., 2014; Trachsel, Irwin, Biller-Andorno, Hoff, & Riese, 2016)

Gaining access to care, and maintaining access and continuity is clearly a challenge. If a patient with SPMI were able to be successful in navigating personal barriers as well as the medical system, the next factor that often comes into play is capacity and ability to participate in decision making. Individuals with SPMI are often excluded from making decisions about EOL care preferences. In part due to provider concerns about their emotional fragility as well as concerns regarding competence. Individuals with SPMI have demonstrated interest in EOL care discussions and the ability to articulate their preferences. (Elie et al., 2018) Though it is true it can be more difficult to assess choices if complicated by depression or psychosis, particularly as the decision making becomes more complex.

Decision making capacity relies on the patient being considered able to understand, have insight, reason, evaluate, and making then communicate a choice. (Sjostrand et al., 2015) Psychiatric disorders such as psychosis and mania can affect ability to have decision making capacity. Capacity to make treatment decisions can also fluctuate over the course of mental illness.(Foti, Bartels, Van Citters, Merriman, & Fletcher, 2005) It needs to be clear, however, those with SPMI can still retain their ability to make decisions. Providers own bias needs to be taken into consideration. It has been shown if a patient with psychiatric illness makes a choice felt to be medically unsound they are often thought to be lacking decision making ability. However, in those without somatic illness that capacity is generally not questioned. (Sjostrand et al., 2015)

While providers may have a difficult time assessing patient's ability to make decision, unfortunately family members or surrogate decision makers are not much more help. In general they have often have not discussed the wishes of a patient with SPMI in the context of a terminal condition. (Harman, 2017)

EVIDENCE-BASED STRATEGIES TO IMPROVE CARE

Improved access to mental health services is critical to address the disparity and higher mortality rates for people with SPMI. (Butler & O'Brien, 2017) Length of waiting time between reporting symptoms and diagnosis and reduced access to treatment are related factors for higher mortality rate for those with SPMI. Evidence based education strategies are needed to correct the assumptions of health professionals that persons diagnosed with SPMI are incapable of making informed medical decisions.

Recognition of the poor coordination and lack of integration should be a priority for healthcare institutions to prevent persons with SPMI "falling through the cracks." Programs to enhance healthcare infrastructures need to be designed to correct the delay and duplication of care. (Butler & O'Brien, 2017) Acknowledgement of the stigma associated with mental illness needs to be another strategy to improve care. Persons with SPMI are vulnerable and need to be given special attention at EOL. (Butler & O'Brien, 2017; Cholbi, 2013) Clinical guidelines and best practices standards should be developed to improve access to palliative care. (Butler & O'Brien, 2017)

Additionally national health strategies should to be developed to address the special needs of people with SPMI. Governmental focus fostering plans to tear down the fragmentation of healthcare systems and enhance collaboration of providers are critical. Task forces between mental health and palliative care clinicians should be considered to increase knowledge and awareness (Taylor et al., 2012; Trachsel et al., 2016)

Healthcare providers should learn about SPMI and work on therapeutic relationships. They should develop skills to address the challenges such as improving medical history taking competencies, using active listening, providing more interpersonal supports, advocating on behalf of these individual, and developing more tolerance to noncompliance of SPMI patients.(Woods et al., 2008) Mental health workshops for palliative care clinicians may enhance awareness and confidence in dealing with patients with SPMI by simply learning how to conduct a comprehensive mental state examination. (Taylor et al., 2012) Additionally, mental health clinicians would have the opportunity to gain important clinical experience in palliative care. (Taylor et al., 2012)

Palliative psychiatry is a growing field and may improve the quality of life of patients and their loved ones facing SPMI. (Trachsel et al., 2016)

IMPLICATIONS/FUTURE RESEARCH FOCUSES

More research is needed in all areas of SPMI and palliative care. Studies examining what define a good death while maintaining the patients' perspectives of quality care are crucial. (Harman, 2017; Meier et al., 2016) Well designed quantitative and qualitative studies are needed to understand successful dying for SPMI patients. Diverse studies should be included to compare similarities and differences in themes such as age cohorts, mental health diagnoses, palliative care accessibility, and place of care and death. (Meier et al., 2016) These factors are essential to fully understanding the care preferences of individuals with SPMI. (Woods et al., 2008) Future studies should assess the effect of prominent psychiatric and cognitive symptoms on medical decision making capacity at EOL. (Elie et al., 2018; Trachsel, 2017)

A fuller understanding of palliative care is required for individuals with SPMI. (Butler & O'Brien, 2017) More effort needs to be devoted in the area of disease prevention and earlier diagnosis of physical illness. Furthermore, studying the perceptions of palliative care specialists may gain a better understanding of their experiences for caring for these patients while improving patient outcomes. (Butler & O'Brien, 2017; Westmoreland & Mehler, 2016)

More research is needed to examine the impact of palliative psychiatry on improving quality of life for persons with SPMI. Collaborative initiatives and community based programs should be examined to determine the effectiveness of co-managing persons with SPMI and serious conditions. (Foti, 2003; Picot et al., 2015; Shalev et al., 2017)

CONCLUSION

Palliative care is lacking in caring for individuals with SPMI at EOL. This vulnerable population is underserved, dying prematurely and without adequate symptom management. It is clear SPMI patients can appropriately choose palliative care but accessibility is being denied to due lack of knowledge and understanding by healthcare professionals.

Healthcare organizations need to be restructured promoting quality care for individuals with SPMI and serious illnesses/diseases. It is deplorable to accept the current standard of care for these patients. Barriers must be torn down and redesigned. Strategies must be employed to alter how we care for individuals with SPMI at EOL. Healthcare professionals must be educated on SPMI and palliative care.

Funding and research are needed to focus on improving knowledge in caring for SPMI and seriously ill patients. With improved knowledge and tolerance will come improved outcomes and prognoses for these most vulnerable individuals. We encourage mental health professionals to pay attention to this vulnerable population in terms of more palliative medicine research.

REFERENCES

Butler, H. & O'Brien, A. J. (2017). Access to specialist palliative care services by people with severe and persistent mental illness: A retrospective cohort study. *International Journal of Mental Health Nursing*. https://doi.org/10.1111/inm.12360.

Center for Health Statistics, N. (2012). Vital and Health Statistics Series 10, Number 252, January 2012. *U.S. Department of Health and Human Services*, *10*(252). Retrieved from https://www.cdc.gov/nchs/data/series/sr_10/sr10_252.pdf.

Cholbi, M. J. (2013). The terminal, the futile, and the psychiatrically disordered. *International Journal of Law and Psychiatry*, *36*(5–6), 498–505. https://doi.org/10.1016/j.ijlp.2013.06.011.

Easter, M. M., Swanson, J. W., Robertson, A. G., Moser, L. L. & Swartz, M. S. (2017). Facilitation of Psychiatric Advance Directives by Peers and Clinicians on Assertive Community Treatment Teams. *Psychiatric Services*, *68*(7), 717–723. https://doi.org/10.1176/appi.ps.201600423.

Elie, D., Marino, A., Torres-Platas, S. G., Noohi, S., Semeniuk, T., Segal, M. & Rej, S. (2018). End-of-Life Care Preferences in Patients with Severe and Persistent Mental Illness and Chronic Medical Conditions: A Comparative Cross-Sectional Study. *American Journal of Geriatric Psychiatry*, *26*(1), 89–97. https://doi.org/10.1016/j.jagp.2017.09.018.

Ellison, M. L., Russinova, Z., Lyass, A. & Rogers, E. S. (2008). Professionals and managers with severe mental illnesses: Findings from a national survey. *Journal of Nervous and Mental Disease*, *196*(3), 179–189. https://doi.org/10.1097/NMD.0b013e318166303c.

Ferrell, B. R., Temel, J. S., Temin, S., Alesi, E. R., Balboni, T. A., Basch, E. M. & Smith, T. J. (2018). *Integration of Palliative Care Into Standard Oncology Care : American Society of Clinical Oncology Clinical Practice Guideline Update*, 35(1). https://doi.org/10.1200/JCO.2016.70.1474.

Foti, M. E. (2003). End-of-Life Care Persons with Serious Mental Illness End-of-Life Care for Persons with Serious Mental Illness. *Journal of Palliative Medicine*, 6(4), 137–147.

Harman, S. M. (2017). Psychiatric and Palliative Care in the Intensive Care Unit. *Critical Care Clinics*, 33(3), 735–743. https://doi.org/10.1016/j.ccc.2017.03.010.

Hunnicutt, J. N., Tjia, J. & Lapane, K. L. (2017). Hospice Use and Pain Management in Elderly Nursing Home Residents With Cancer. *Journal of Pain and Symptom Management*, 53(3), 561–570. https://doi.org/10.1016/j.jpainsymman.2016.10.369.

Meier, E. A., Gallegos, J. V., Montross-Thomas, L. P., Depp, C. A., Irwin, S. A. & Jeste, D. V. (2016). Defining a Good Death (Successful Dying): Literature Review and a Call for Research and Public Dialogue. *American Journal of Geriatric Psychiatry*, 24(4), 261–271. https://doi.org/10.1016/j.jagp.2016.01.135.

Olsen, D. P. (2016). Ethically Relevant Differences in Advance Directives for Psychiatric and End-of-Life Care. *Journal of the American Psychiatric Nurses Association*, 22(1), 52–59. https://doi.org/10.1177/1078390316629958.

Olsen, D. P. (2017). Increasing the use of psychiatric advance directives. *Nursing Ethics*, 24(3), 265–267. https://doi.org/10.1177/0969733017708881.

Picot, S. A., Glaetzer, K. M. & Myhill, K. J. (2015). Coordinating end of life care for individuals with a mental illness--A nurse practitioner collaboration. *Collegian (Royal College of Nursing, Australia)*, 22(1), 143–149. Retrieved from http://0-ovidsp.ovid.com.lib.exeter.ac.uk/ovidweb.cgi?T=JS&PAGE=reference&D=medl&NEWS=N&AN=26285419.

Public, A. G. & Concern, H. (2012). *Depression*, 6–8. Retrieved from http://www.who.int/mediacentre/factsheets/fs396/en/.

Shalev, D., Brewster, K., Arbuckle, M. R. & Levenson, J. A. (2017). A staggered edge: End-of-life care in patients with severe mental illness. *General Hospital Psychiatry*, 44(2017), 1–3. https://doi.org/10.1016/j.genhosppsych.2016.10.004.

Taylor, J., Swetenham, K., Myhill, K., Picot, S., Glaetzer, K. & Loon, A. Van. (2012). *for Cross-Training Palliative Care and Mental Health Clinicians*, 18(6).

Trachsel, M. (2017). Title: The Ethical Importance of Assessing End-of-Life Care Preferences in Patients with Severe and Persistent Mental Illness. *The American Journal of Geriatric Psychiatry*, 26(1), 98–99. https://doi.org/10.1016/j.jagp.2017.09.026.

Trachsel, M., Irwin, S. A., Biller-Andorno, N., Hoff, P. & Riese, F. (2016). Palliative psychiatry for severe persistent mental illness as a new approach to psychiatry? Definition, scope, benefits, and risks. *BMC Psychiatry*, 16(1), 1–7. https://doi.org/10.1186/s12888-016-0970-y.

Westmoreland, P. & Mehler, P. S. (2016). Caring for Patients with Severe and Enduring Eating Disorders (SEED): Certification, Harm Reduction, Palliative Care, and the Question of Futility. *Journal of Psychiatric Practice*, 22(4), 313–320. https://doi.org/10.1097/PRA.0000000000000160.

Woods, A., Willison, K., Kington, C. & Gavin, A. (2008). Palliative care for people with severe persistent mental illness: a review of the literature. *Can J Psychiatry*, 53(11), 725–736. https://doi.org/10.1177/070674370805301104.

BIOGRAPHICAL SKETCHES

Phyllis Whitehead, PhD, APRN/CNS, ACHPN, RN-BC

Dr. Phyllis Whitehead is the clinical nurse specialist with the Carilion Roanoke Memorial Hospital Palliative Care Service and Associate Professor at the Virginia Tech Carilion School of Medicine. She is a clinical ethics consultant and initiated the Moral Distress Consult Service at CRMH. She is certified in pain management and as an advanced practice hospice and palliative care nurse. Dr. Whitehead has done numerous presentations on pain and symptom management, opioid induced sedation, moral distress, and patients' end of life preferences locally, regionally, nationally and internationally. Her research interests include moral distress and improving communication with seriously ill patients. She has been a co-lead of the NACNS Pain Task Force and the Access to Care Workgroup and recently appointed as co-lead of the Virginia Action Coalition. She is a graduate of Radford University where she earned her BSN and MSN and earned her doctorate degree at Virginia Tech.

Senaida Keating, MD

Dr. Senaida Keating is a geriatrician with Carilion Roanoke Memorial Hospital Center for Healthy Aging and is the Medical Director of Springtree Health and Rehabilitation Center in Roanoke, VA. She also practices Hospitalist/Internal Medicine at the Carilion Roanoke Memorial Hospital and the Salem VA Medical Center. She is an Associate Professor at the Virginia Tech Carilion School of Medicine, and she serves on Geriatric Fellowship Program Evaluation Committee there as well. She is a coauthor of the chapter "Palliative Care for Persons with Serious Mental Illness" in Palliative Care, Perspectives, Practices, and impact on Quality of Life, a Global View published in 2017. She completed her Internal Medicine Residency Program at Virginia Tech Carilion School of Medicine/Roanoke Memorial Hospital as well as Fellowships in Geriatric, and Palliative and Hospice Medicine. She is board certified in Internal, Geriatric, and Palliative and Hospice Medicine, respectively.

Shereen Gamaluddin, MD

Dr. Shereen Gamaluddin is a palliative attending with the Carilion Roanoke Memorial Hospital Palliative Care Service and Associate Medical Director for Good Samaritan Hospice. She earned her bachelor's degree in biology from Carnegie Mellon University. She completed her medical degree at University of Pittsburgh School of Medicine and subsequent Family Medicine training at Lancaster General Hospital. After nearly 10 years of private practice she transitioned her focus to palliative and hospice medicine, completing a fellowship at Carilion Clinic. She is board certified in Family Medicine and Hospice and Palliative Medicine.

Kye Y. Kim, MD

Dr. Kim is a geriatric psychiatrist at the Carilion Clinic Center for Healthy Aging and Professor at the Virginia Tech Carilion School of Medicine's Department of Psychiatry and Behavioral Medicine. He earned his medical degree at Yonsei University, Seoul, South Korea and completed his psychiatry residency at State University of New York at Buffalo. Dr. Kim subsequently finished his geriatric psychiatry fellowship training at University of South Florida. He is board certified in Adult Psychiatry and Geriatric Psychiatry.

In: Palliative Care
Editor: Michael Silbermann

ISBN: 978-1-53616-199-1
© 2019 Nova Science Publishers, Inc.

Chapter 2

BEYOND QUALITY OF LIFE: AN APPROACH TO COMPLEXITY

Lodovico Balducci[*], *MD*
Moffitt Cancer Center, Tampa, FL, US

ABSTRACT

The influence of medical interventions on the patient's quality of life (QOL) represents a critical information to be able to formulate personalized treatment. Current methods of assessing QOL are quantitative and maybe misleading as it is shown with the description of two clinical cases. A more complete and more reliable estimate of QOL may be obtained with qualitative research and in particular with the use of narrative that allows patients to describe their own history with their own words and without the constrictions of a questionnaire.

The examination of two clinical cases through patient narratives has revealed the importance of sacramentality in fostering and supporting a patient's QOL. A sacrament is an object or an event whose importance resides in its meaning, not in its economic value. Mrs. Jones was a lady with terminal breast cancer who kept working as a licensed professional nurse until few days prior to her death to buy Christmas presents for her children's last Christmas together. Her QOL hinged around thos presents that did represent a sacrament.

Keywords: quality of life, cancer, narrative, qualitative research, sacraments, spirituality

INTRODUCTION

In a conference held at the Millsaps College in Jackson, Mississippi in 1984, Walker Percy, a renown American novelist, proclaimed: "the role of the literature is to find a response to questions like this one: why the only happy day in my uncle's life was the day the Japanese attacked Pearl Harbor?" In other words Percy recognized a discrepancy between our

---

[*] Corresponding Author's E-mail: Lodovico.balducci@moffitt.org.

feelings and the nature of the events that elicit those feelings. For his uncle a national tragedy provided an occasion of rejoicing rather than of distress or horror. This reaction is far from paradoxical. The recent suicides of a successful fashionist and a successful journalist, dismissed as manifestations of "depression," highlight the discrepancy between health, success, wealth, on one side and personal satisfaction with one's life on the other. It is dangerous to assume that this discrepancy derives exclusively from an imbalance of catecholamines in the human brain and it is still unproven that the pharmacological manipulation of this imbalance might prevent these tragedies. In any case this discrepancy may represent the main limitation to the evaluation of quality of life (QOL) in medicine [1].

The assessment of QOL that has become mandatory in most clinical trials, has represented a medical milestone, as it has highlighted the centrality of personal autonomy in the practice of medicine [2]. It implies that the value of health and survival are far from absolute and are subjected to individual procession and judgement. Only the individual patient has the right to decide whether the personal cost associated to a medical intervention is worth his/her while. This is even more true today when the aging of the population has been associated with increased prevalence of chronic diseases, whose treatment may cause serious discomfort and economic distress in exchange of negligible medical benefits. And it is especially true when a person's survival may be guaranteed only by the ongoing invasion of his/her body with endotracheal or feeding tubes and with intravenous lines, that recent technological advances have made possible.

In the early studies of QOL it has become soon clear that disease and medical treatment are only a component, and sometimes not the most important one, of this domain. To avoid the confusion deriving from non-medical parameters successive studies have focused on "Health Related Quality of Life" (HRQOL). HRQOL is assessed as the influence of disease and treatment on the physical, emotional, social and spiritual welfare of each individual [2]. This approach has produced important, novel, and sometimes unexpected results. It has revealed that partial mastectomy did not improve the HRQOL of women with breast cancer, as the major concern of these women was recurrence of the cancer rather than the loss of their breast [3]. The effects of breast preservation on HRQOL have emerged only after a number of clinical trials assured the patient that mastectomy and breast preservation were associated with comparable survival and risk of recurrence, but even then it has appeared to be marginal [4]. Another unexpected and practice changing result concerned the preference of patients who have been treated in Intensive Care Units [5]. The majority of these subjects were willing to repeat that experience if there was a chance to save again their lives. This finding surprised many medical caregivers convinced that the vast majority of patients considered intensive care an unbearable threat to their QOL.

At the meantime a main limitation of HRQOL emerged [1-2]. It fails to account for the complexity of the construct it is supposed to assess. QOL results from the interaction rather than from the sum of the different domains assessed. The word complexity derives from the Latin *cum Plexere* that means "to weave together". In other words QOL is best expressed by the design of a carpet than by the sums of the threads forming the carpet [6-7]. This complexity is revealed by a humorous assessment of a clinical trial in which a drug that cost approximately $10000.00 monthly produced an improvement in QOL. Somebody commented that the only meaningful study would have compared the QOL of patients receiving the drug and that of patients receiving $10000.00 each month free of taxes.

In this chapter we examine alternative ways to evaluate QOL and the influence of a spiritual perspective on QOL, after describing two clinical cases.

CLINICAL CASES

Mrs. Jones was a 47 year old licensed professional nurse with inflammatory breast cancer that presented to us for treatment. Despite her disease she was still working for a homecare agency, because she was the only breadwinner for her family. Her husband was permanently disabled from terminal colon cancer metastatic to the liver and she had two teen ager children attending high school. Her husband medical insurance had been cancelled after he lost his job, and her employment did not provide insurance benefits. She received free care at our institution. After an initial response to treatment with cyclophosphamide, doxorubicin, and paclitaxel, her cancer worsened and she developed liver metastases. Also, her pain in the edematous left arm worsened, but she was reluctant to take pain medications because she wanted to be able to work and to save money for her children's Christmas presents. She died at the beginning of the following year from liver failure.

The most remarkable aspect was this lady's attitude. Even prey of severe pain she was always smiling as a sign of gratitude for the health professionals who were trying to help her free of charge and she never expressed resentment or bitterness toward her disease, well aware that these sentiments would have not improved in any way her condition but would have only generated more angst and desperation. Though we did not have any specific discussion of religion, we learned that she belonged to an evangelical church that provided support for her and her family. The pastor and the church council helped her to find appropriate arrangements for her children prior to her death.

Mrs. Smith was a 47 year old woman with stage three C breast cancer that had undergone complete remission followed neo-adjuvant chemotherapy with carboplatin, docetaxel, trastuzumab and pertuzumab. She had received a mastectomy, breast reconstruction, one year adjuvant treatment with trastuzumab and after five years from the diagnosis was disease free. She was a professor of nursing at a major college and she and her husband of ten years had decided not to have children much before the development of cancer. After breast reconstruction she decided to divorce her spouse because she felt he had not been supportive of her and her needs and established a number of temporary romantic relations before settling down with a wealthy widower business owner fifteen years her senior. At that point she retired from her job and started traveling around the world. For the five years I took care of her I never saw Mrs. Smith smiling even once. Somehow I dreaded her visit because each time I had to listen to complains over which I had no control such as the concerns that trastuzumab might damage her heart, that chemotherapy had induced her menopause, that her spouse was an insensitive brute, that her cancer might have come back and we had already utilized all weapons available to take care of it. In her mind if her cancer where she attended with her husband two operas at the Metropolitan and several Broadway performances. When I asked her how much she had enjoyed her visit she started complaining that the rooms of the Astoria Hotel were too small to be comfortable, the heating inadequate and she had to wait for the hot water to shower. Not a world about the performances she had attended. According to our record Mrs. Smith was a member of one of the most prominent episcopal church in town and she was an active member of the church council. She never mentioned her faith or her church involvement.

Neither of these patients underwent a formal QOL assessment, but it is clear that such assessment might have been deceiving. From a health perspective the HRQOL of Mrs. Jones could have not been worse, yet she managed to cope with her disease in a very satisfactory and uplifting way. Mrs. Smith obtained a complete remission and likely a cure of her disease, but her successful treatment did not relieve her bitterness and her anger. In both cases the HRQOL was irrelevant to their outcome.

As health care professionals we can't help asking ourselves whether we should try to help these patients or whether their QOLs are outside the scope of medical practice. In this chapter it is assumed that we cannot witness suffering without taking care of it: if Mrs. Smith had disabling chronic arthritis instead of disabling chronic anger it would have behooved us to prescribe pain medications and to address her to the care of a proper specialist even if the arthritis was unrelated to the cancer we had been asked to manage. The decision to approach these problems begs three questions: how can we properly assess the QOL life of these individuals? What interventions are available? What can we learn from these cases to help other patients?

ASSESSMENT OF QOL

It is self-evident that any questionnaire to assess HRQOL would have fallen short in both cases and misinterpretation of the results might have worsened the QOL at least in the case of Mrs. Jones. For example, if we had concentrated on poor pain control we might have tried to prescribe stronger and more expensive medications that would have interfered with her main life goals: to continue to work to support her family and to save money for her children's Christmas present. Or we might have favored the divorce of Mrs. Smith assuming that the discord with her husband was an immediate consequence of the treatment, while most likely the disease did only allow pre-existing conflicts to surface. Another way to look at the issue is that one cannot tease out the health-related aspects of quality of life from the patient's personal history, and this attempt may lead to inappropriate clinical decisions, beside providing an information that is biased, at the very least.

A semi-structured interview involving a number of open end questions might have been more revealing, even if it would not have allowed the investigators to quantify the HRQOL of these patients [6-8].

It would have taught us that once her cancer had progressed and had become incurable the main goals of Mrs. Jones included to keep working until the end, to have enough money to pay for her husband funeral and for allowing her and her children a last Christmas feast, and to make sure that her children were properly cared for after her demise. Symptom control was a secondary goal and it was important only to the extent in which symptoms might have interfered with the achievement of her primary aims. We might also have recognized the source of her inner strength and become able to exploit it to reinforce and support her QOL. It would have been essential to know for example that she belonged to a church able to help in the management of her children and that faith in a benign deity underlie her peace of mind in face of her many challenges. Even fear of death was secondary as she had plenty to live for during her short life expectancy. She simply did not have the opportunity to think about her death, or maybe the same faith that made her persistent in her goals convinced her to be trusted to the hands of a benign deity that would have taken care of her even if she could not figure out how.

From Mrs. Smith we might have learned that she was unprepared to face the challenges of survivorship that in her case included medical menopause [9] and associated sexual difficulty such as reduced libido swinging moods and vaginal dryness, loss of interest in her profession as she identified a gap between her medical knowledge and her personal experience, and consequently she found the profession to which she had dedicated her life uninteresting. Also, concerns about how the treatment would have affected her attractiveness impinged negatively on her QOL. In her case even more than in the case of Mrs. Jones it would have been important to know her previous history. It looked like that her cancer had unleashed a number of inner conflicts that she had never felt the need to face prior to her disease. Why did she not want to have children? Was that because of an abusive childhood and adolescence during which she felt victimized? Did she experience a serious disease or emotional trauma in her youth during which she felt abandoned by her family and she had the impression to live again the same experience with her husband? Were her academic pursuits to which she had sacrificed her family life a way to escape the pain of being unable to establish close intimate relations? These were just a few of the questions that might have provided a clue to her distraught life and possibly a treatment of her distress.

What I am trying to say is that the best way to relate to a human experience is to elicit a narrative from the person trusted to our care [6-8]. A narrative is a favorite instrument of qualitative scientists interested in recognizing the way through which each design in each carpet of human life is obtained and to understand why the same amount of threads may produce completely different designs [8, 10-11].

The advantages of a narrative are self evident: by its nature the human experience Is loaded with ambivalences that are all but masked in a questionnaire with fixed answers. The unconstrained description of one's experience may reveal that the love for one's spouse and children may very well be present together with aversion and hostility, or that a provider acts particularly hostile to patients toward whom he/she proves the deepest compassion [12]. The acknowledgment and acceptance of this ambivalence may represent indeed the essential step for establishing meaningful human relationship; it is nothing less than the acceptance of our own humanity.

In John's Gospel Jesus refuses to answer Pilate's question "what is the truth?" [13] It is tantalizing to interpret this episode as a vindication of qualitative research. By refusing to answer Jesus was saying: "Nobody can coerce the truth within the boundaries of a concept: the truth is the complex human experience that every person needs to live on his/her own.

The discussion of the Techniques of Narrative based research is beyond the scope of this chapter [1, 8, 11-12]. It may be worthwhile to mention that these include observation of non verbal messages, repetitiveness of ideas and concepts, and analysis of the language.

In the case of Mrs. Jones her main messages came from her consistent smiles, that in addition to gratitude expressed satisfaction with her own life and peace of mind. Virtually at every encounter she talked about her children whereas she skirted questions related to her pain and she did not volunteer information about her husband, though she answered politely questions related to his health. From time to time she shared with us spontaneously information related to her patients that revealed her empathy for old and disabled people that she was proud to help in their activities of daily living. Unfortunately we failed to record these conversations, but from this brief summary one may infer that:

- Despite the proximity of death she felt still alive as long as she could take care of her children and of her patients. Clearly her maternity and her profession were the two poles that energized her life.
- She was happy to have a function in life and was grateful to her employer and her health care professionals that enabled her to perform her function to the very end.
- Even if she never put it in so many words, I believe it is safe to conclude that she was a person of faith. The content of her faith was clear: a benign deity, identified in her case with the Christian God, took care of each person of faith: we have the choice to trust this deity or to abandon ourselves to desperation, which in her worldview would have been unacceptable. She seemed to ask "why to make our last days more miserable when we have the option to believe that we will be taken well care of?" Unfortunately we have no way to establish the origin of her faith, whether a living tradition of her family or an act of faith in persons who had witnessed in front of her their Christian faith.
- Sacraments were an essential part of her faith. In the Jewish Christian tradition a sacrament is a material sign of a relation with the deity. In the Jewish tradition the two official sacraments are circumcision and the Pass-over supper; in the Christian one the baptism and the Lord supper. In addition to these however every human experience may become a sacrament. The main value of the poor presents that Mrs. Jones would have been able to buy to her children for Christmas was mainly sacramental, like the small mementos she received from her grateful patients or the small Christmas tree ornaments she had sown for the hospital staff. The value of these inexpensive objects consisted in what they represented, in the message they conveyed. I insist on this sacramental aspect of spirituality because I believe it is accessible to everybody, as the new age spirituality has taught us.
- The relation of Mrs. Jones with her dying spouse remains a puzzle and it is not worthwhile to speculate on it. Whatever the nature of this relation it did not interfere with her peace of mind.

Though Mrs. Smith spent many more years and many more words in our clinics one may almost conclude that unlike Mrs. Jones' her words were aimed to conceal rather than to expose her person. Her narrative may be rather obtained from what she did not express than from what she said. With her lack of pleasantness and her repeated complains she wanted definitely to let you know that she was unhappy . Some comparisons with Mrs. Jones are unavoidable: Mrs. Jones let us know she had been happy to clean the incontinence of a paralyzed wheel chair bound old lady, while Mrs. Smith expressed her disappointment with one of the most expensive hotels of New York City. Mrs. Jones' QOL was enhanced by a menial endeavor that many people would have found disgusting, while Mrs. Smith's was deteriorated by a luxury residence. If one is asked to identify the main difference between the two patients, one is tempted to say that Mrs. Jones' life was made meaningful by the sacraments she had discovered, while Mrs. Smith's appeared meaningless because of the absence of sacraments. This despite that both patients were active member of a Christian church and presumably professed some type of Christian faith.

Despite her loquacity Mrs. Smith did not convey any useful information about herself, her husband, her family, her friends, her beliefs. Her words were used to build a barrier to prevent other people from getting close to her rather than to provide a door to access her intimacy. We never could figure out to our dismay whether her complains represented a call for help, if she would have liked for somebody to destroy her barrier. Should I have the opportunity to take care of her again I may ask help to obtain her history. Her cancer might have represented the opportunity for her to obtain the help she had needed in her life, and I regret to think we have dropped the ball.

SPIRITUALITY AS A SOURCE OF RELIEF IN THE PRESENCE OF DISEASE AND DEATH

The history of Mrs. Jones contains important insights on the effects of religion on coping with overwhelming physical and emotional challenges and near death. Once again narrative might identify the elements of her spirituality that promise to be helpful to other individuals we meet in our practices.

Clearly, her Christian faith was the source of her inner strength. The beneficial effects of religion on quality of life have been well described [14-18]. Religiosity may foster peace of mind as well as emotional resilience through faith in a benign deity, through a number of practices that include prayer, meditation, and worship, through enhancement of positive character traits such as optimism, forgiveness, gratefulness, kindness and compassion that facilitates the communication with providers, caregivers and friends [13-15]. As the case of Mrs. Jones showed the benefits of religion may extend to practical aspects of cancer management such as finding a community available to support the patient and the patient's family.

The most common complication of religiosity is spiritual distress, generally related to feeling of guilt or abandonment by god [19]. Spiritual distress and spiritual pain may represent a severe cause of discomfort and are best managed by a chaplain who underwent clinical pastoral training. Every provider should be trained to recognize spiritual distress and spiritual pain, as these conditions may jeopardize a patient's quality of life as well as the treatment outcome [19].

As religion may be a major resource to the well being of the patient and the family, may provide social support, in addition to the moral one, and religious beliefs may occasionally be a source of distress and discomfort, it behooves the practitioner to investigate a patient's religious dimension. A simple screening test for this purpose is called FICA (acronym for Faith, Importance, Community and Assessment) that allows the practitioner to establish whether religion may represent an emotional, a spiritual and a social resource in a particular case [19].

Religious faith cannot be imposed. The patient history may inform us on which elements of religiosity are particularly relevant to QOL and whether some of these elements may be utilized in the management of individuals that do not profess any special religious belief. This is an urgent endeavor, as younger generations in the Western world are becoming more and more secularized and are less and less likely to belong to an organized form of religion or a specific church.

In describing the case of Mrs. Jones the sacramentality of her experience was highlighted. It was emphasized that the presents she was going to buy for her children's last family Christmas, the mementos she was proud to receive from her patients as a recognition of her assistance, the small Christmas tree ornaments she was sewing for thanking her nurses and her doctors had a sacramental value, that overwhelmed the scarce economic value.

In the Judeo-Christian tradition a sacrament is a physical sign of the presence of God in everyday life. The economic value of a wafer or of a sip of wine is a few cents, but the sacramental value is inestimable for the faithful for whom they represent the body and the blood of Christ and are the through of an intercourse with Christ.

Interestingly sacraments are a fundament of the mind, body and spirit integration movement, previously known as a New Age movement [20], a form of spirituality that has flourished in the Western World in the past two centuries. Without promoting the belief in a specific deity this movement holds that objects have a sacramental value, represent a conduit of spiritual union and participation.

The word Sacrament derives from the Latin *sacrum* that means reserved for a special use. The cheap sport Jackets that Mrs. Jones bought for her adolescent children in addition to being a piece of garments carried the love of a mother that had only few months to live and that wished to remain somehow in contact with her children. That value could only be carried by the jacket she chose, and no other jackets of the same fabric the same brand and the same measures. Only the jackets she had chosen had become sacred, a sacrament.

In every family, in every partnership, in every relationship there may be events that represent a sacrament, that create a human bondage that may last beyond one's death, like an essence of Bulgarian roses, one drop of which contains the extract of thousand petals withered centuries ago. In my experience the memory of these events represents a sacrament that comforts a person closed to die and provide a sense of eternity even for those who are unable to believe in a deity.

When we compare the histories of the two patients we recognize that religious faith needed to be translated into sacraments to affect a person's quality of life. Divorced from these practical consequences religiosity did not have much effect on QOL. A very important question to an increasingly secular society is whether sacraments may subsist even in the absence of a specific credence or even in the presence of professed atheism and agnosticism.

This is another important function of qualitative scientist, to help dying people to build a personal narrative out of valuable experiences buried under mountains of rubbish. Sacramentality appears as the hinge of spiritual health.

Conclusion

A French priest, Father Jacques Philippe stated: "a problem needs an artistic formulation more than a solution" and "human freedom is not so much the power to transform as a capacity to welcome novelty." I found these statements very germane to the chapter I finished to write.

The concern for QOL cannot be overstated: it has represented the first effective attempt to humanize a medicine that technology and science had divorced from human needs. The efforts to produce quantitative results might have jeopardized the value of HRQOL studied in clinical trials however. The two cases presented indicate how the determination of HRQOL might have been deceptive and potentially dangerous. Qualitative research, through narrative, promises to provide amore complete assessment of quality of life, of the importance of the spiritual dimension of QOL and of the discovery of personal sacraments in each individual story.

Purposefully, this chapter does not address the practical aspect of this endeavor, but it is not unreasonable to train all providers in basic narrative research technique and to complement these providers with the assistance of qualitative scientist.

REFERENCES

[1] Antaki C, Rapley M: "Quality of Life talk": the liberal paradox of psychology testing. *Discourse and society,* 1996, 7, 293-316.

[2] van Roij J, Fransen H, van de Poll-Franse L, et al: Measuring health-related quality of life in patients with advanced cancer: a systematic review of self-administered measurement instruments. *Qual Life Res* 2018, doi: 10.1007/s11136-018-1809-4.

[3] Kiebert GM, de Haes JC, van der Velde CJ: The impact of breast conserving treatment and mastectomy on the quality of life of early stage breast cancer patients: a review. *J Clin Oncol,* 1991, 9, 1059-1070.

[4] Hartman-johensen OJ, Kārensen R, Schlichting R et al: Survival is better after breast conserving surgery than mastectomy for early breast cancer. A registry-based follow-up study of Norwegian women primarily operated between 1998 and 2008. *Ann Surg Oncol,* 2015, 22, 3836-3845.

[5] Langerud AK, Rustøen T, Småstuen MC, et al.: Health-related quality of life in intensive care survivors: Associations with social support, comorbidity, and pain interference. *PLoS One* 2018 Jun 25;13(6):e0199656. doi: 10.1371/journal.pone.0199656.

[6] Overcash JA: Using narrative research to understand the Quality fo Life of Older Women with breast cancer. *Oncol Nurs Forum,* 2004, 31, 1153-1159.

[7] Hartog I; scherer.-Rath M; Kruizinga R et al: Narrative meaning making and integration: Toward a better understanding of the way falling ill influences quality of life. *J Health Psychol,* 2017 Sep 1:1359105317731823. doi: 10.1177/1359105317731823.

[8] Bochner, A. & Ellis, C. (2016) *Evocative Autoethnography: Writing Lives and Telling Stories.* New York: Routledge.

[9] Dohou J, Mouret-Reynier MA, Kwiatkowski F, et al: A Retrospective Study on the Onset of Menopause after Chemotherapy: Analysis of Data Extracted from the Jean Perrin Comprehensive Cancer Center Database Concerning 345 Young Breast Cancer Patients Diagnosed between 1994 and 2012. *Oncology,* 2017, 92, 255-263.

[10] Mishler EG (1991). *Research Interviewing: context and narrative.* Harvard University Press 1991.

[11] Morgan MS, Wise MN: Narrative Science and Narrative knowing: Introduction to special issue on Narrative science. *Stud Hist Philos Sci* 2017, 62, 1-5.
[12] Balducci L: The hateful patient, *J Med Person,* 2013, 11, 113-117.
[13] *The Gospel of John,* 18, 386.
[14] Balducci L: Geriatric Oncology, spirituality and palliative care. *J pain Symptom Manag* 2018, 2018 Jun 13. pii: S0885-3924(18)30254-9. doi: 10.1016/j.jpainsymman.2018.05.009.
[15] Bai M; Lazemby M: A systematic review of associations between spiritual well-being and quality of life at the scale and factor levels in studies among patients with cancer. *J pall Med,* 2015, 18, 286-298.
[16] Panzini RG; Mosqueiro BP; Zimpel RR et al.: Qualiy of life and spirituality. *Int Rev Psychiatry,* 2017, 29, 263-282.
[17] Koenig HG: religion, Spirituality, and Health: a review and update. *Adv Mind Body Med,* 2015, 29, 19-26.
[18] *PDQ Supportive and palliative care editorial board: Spirituality in Cancer care,* published online, 2016.
[19] Puchalski CP; king SDW; Ferrell BR: Spiritual Considerations. *Hematol Oncol Clin N. America* 2018, 32, 505-517.
[20] Anonymous: *New Age,* Wikipedia.

BIOGRAPHICAL SKETCH

Lodovico Balducci, MD

Lodovico Balducci MD is Senior Member Emeritus of the Moffitt Cancer center and Professor Emeritus of the University of South Florida College of Medicine in Tampa, FL.

In the Supplement of the ASCO evening Time in March 2015 Balducci was called "the Father of Geriatric Oncology" and was indicated as one of the ten most influential oncology in our time. Since 1993 until 2017 he has directed at the Moffitt Cancer Center the first program in the world in Geriatric Oncology and his program became a model for the whole world. Balducci published 7 textbooks of Geriatric Oncology and Hematology and approximately four hundred articles dedicated to the topic. For his innovative research he has received numerous international award that include:

2002: Sigismondo d'oro at his hometown of Rimini recognizing him as citizen of the year.
2003: First Paul Calabresi award of the International Society of Geriatric Oncology (SIOG) in Rome Itali.
2007: First BJ Kennedy award for excellent research in geriatric Oncology by the American Society of Clinical Oncology (ASCO) in Chicago.
2009: Claude Jacquillat award of the International Society of Anticancer Research in Paris.
2009: Mehdi Tavassoli award of the University of Mississippi School of Medicine, in Jackson, MS.
2009: Nimmo professorship from the University fo Southern Australia in Adelaide, Australia.

2015: Enzo Piccinini award of the University of Modena in Modena, Italy.
2017: Lifetime achievement award from the SIOG in Warsaw.

A second vocation for Balducci has been the literature. He has published a memoir entitled "Megalies" in 2014 by the publisher "Resources" of Eugene Oregon and two collections of poems in 2018.

In 2017 he won the Artemisia award in Bari Itali for his monologue entitled "Job" where the biblical character of Job is a young woman dying of breast cancer. His work will be produced in Bari in October 2017 by the director Antonio Minelli.

In: Palliative Care
Editor: Michael Silbermann

ISBN: 978-1-53616-199-1
© 2019 Nova Science Publishers, Inc.

Chapter 3

USING EVIDENCE TO IMPROVE PALLIATIVE CARE PRACTICE

Regina M. Fink[1],, PhD and Jeannine M. Brant[2],†, PhD*

[1]Interprofessional Master of Science in Palliative Care Program,
University of Colorado Anschutz Medical Campus,
School of Medicine and College of Nursing, Aurora, CO, US
[2]Billings Clinic, Billings, MT, US

ABSTRACT

Healthcare providers aim to incorporate best evidence into practice to provide quality patient care and improve patient outcomes. Evidence-based practice provides a framework for examining clinical questions related to palliative care, searching for and critically appraising the literature, translating evidence into practice to make the best patient care decision, and evaluating the outcomes of the practice change. This chapter describes the five-step evidence-based practice process and explores strategies to create a culture that questions practice and is empowered to explore and implement evidence.

Keywords: palliative care, evidence-based practice, levels of evidence, critique, journal club, translating research into practice

INTRODUCTION

Health care professionals around the world strive to incorporate the best evidence into practice to provide quality patient care and improve patient outcomes. The Institute of Medicine aims that by 2020, at least 90% of clinical decisions be evidence-based [1]. Palliative care professionals are equally charged with this task as providing evidence-based care will lessen physical symptoms, psychological distress, and alleviate social and spiritual

---

* Corresponding Author's E-mail: regina.fink@ucdenver.edu.
† Corresponding Author's E-mail: jbrant@billingsclinic.org.

suffering to optimize quality of life. Evidence-based practice (EBP) is "the conscientious, explicit and judicious use of current best evidence in making decisions about the care of the individual patient [2]." At the core of EBP is the integration of patient values and preferences [3]. This philosophy of patient-centered care closely aligns with the palliative care philosophy and practice.

The goal to consistently incorporate evidence into palliative care practice may seem insurmountable. Searching for and accessing the most recent evidence, reviewing current literature, critiquing and synthesizing studies, and then deciding which evidence to implement may be time consuming and requires effort beyond available resources. Most important is to focus on one area of practice, such as palliative care, and then identify a question within that scope, such as a physical symptom. Next, the five steps of EBP can be addressed and include: 1) asking the question, 2) finding the evidence, 3) critically appraising the literature, 4) integrating or translating evidence into practice to make the best patient care decision, and 5) evaluating the outcomes of the practice change. This chapter will apply this process using mucositis as an example and illustrate how a palliative care team can navigate the five EBP steps and tackle topics, one-by-one, to progressively implement current evidence into practice and improve patient outcomes. This process can foster an environment that continuously follows these processes to create a culture of evidence-based palliative care [4].

ASKING THE QUESTION

A mock case scenario will be used to illustrate the EBP process: A palliative care team met with a patient and their family earlier in the day, and the patient was to undergo a combined regimen of radiation and chemotherapy for a new diagnosis of head and neck cancer. The team's goal was to discuss possible complications with the disease and related treatment and to discuss strategies to minimize symptoms during treatment. The organization has a protocol for prevention of mucositis for this population that consists of chlorhexidine mouth rinses after meals and at bedtime. However, a nurse on the team mentions that she recently read an article that suggested a different set of interventions for mucositis prophylaxis. Because the team desires to practice according to the most up-to-date evidence, they develop a question as the first step of the EBP process. They ask, "What is the best intervention(s) for preventing mucositis in patients undergoing combined chemotherapy and radiation therapy for head and neck cancer?

Table 1. PICOT format for evidence-based questions

Acronym	Definition	Example
P	Population – the patient population	Patients with head and neck cancer Undergoing combined radiation therapy and chemotherapy
I	Intervention – the therapies or treatments given to the patient	Best treatment for mucositis prophylaxis
C	Control – this could be the comparison or the alternative therapy for the patient	Chlorhexidine mouth rinses
O	Outcome – the outcome that is sought, e.g., improvement of symptoms, mortality, etc.	Prevention of mucositis
T	Time – the time frame, which is optional	Could be four times per day mouth rinses Prophylactic or prevention are other time-related terms

Asking the right question in the right format is important to clearly identify the problem and to find the right evidence to answer the question [5]. PICOT provides one method to formulate a question with consideration to specific criteria [6, 7]. The PICOT format allows the question to have direct application to the problem presented to clinicians. Table 1 includes the PICOT components along with an extrapolation of the mucositis example.

FINDING THE EVIDENCE

The second step in EBP is finding adequate evidence to answer the question [8-10]. In addition to formulating the question, PICOT is used to facilitate the search of evidence. For example, when searching PubMed, the term "mucositis" yields 8,894 results. Adding the terms "prevention," "chemotherapy," and "radiation therapy" condenses the yield to 334 citations; results are further scaled down to 261 with the addition of "head and neck cancer." A potential exists for a search to become too narrow; therefore, the exact patient population may need to be eliminated. For example, rather than using a specific type of cancer in the search, simply using the word "cancer" may increase results in some cases.

Table 2. Levels of evidence

Level of Evidence	Description	Mucositis Example
Level 1	Systematic reviews or meta-analyses of randomized controlled trials (RCTs)	Cardona, A., Balouch, A., Abdul, M. M., Sedghizadeh, P. P., & Enciso, R. (2017). Efficacy of chlorhexidine for the prevention and treatment of oral mucositis in cancer patients: a systematic review with meta-analyses. *J Oral Pathol Med*, 46(9), 680-688. doi:10.1111/jop.1254915
Level 2	RCTs	Demir Dogan, M., Can, G., & Meral, R. (2017). Effectiveness of Black Mulberry Molasses in Prevention of Radiotherapy-Induced Oral Mucositis: A Randomized Controlled Study in Head and Neck Cancer Patients. *J Altern Complement Med*, 23(12), 971-979. doi:10.1089/acm.2016.042516
Level 3	Quasi-experimental studies without randomization	Meca, L. B., Souza, F. R., Tanimoto, H. M., Castro, A. L., & Gaetti-Jardim Junior, E. (2009). Influence of preventive dental treatment on mutans streptococci counts in patients undergoing head and neck radiotherapy. *J Appl Oral Sci*, 17 Suppl, 5-12.17
Level 4	Case control or cohort studies	Miah, A. B., Schick, U., Bhide, S. A., Guerrero-Urbano, M. T., Clark, C. H., Bidmead, A. M., . . . Nutting, C. M. (2015). A phase II trial of induction chemotherapy and chemo-IMRT for head and neck squamous cell cancers at risk of bilateral nodal spread: the application of a bilateral superficial lobe parotid-sparing IMRT technique and treatment outcomes. *Br J Cancer*, 112(1), 32-38. doi:10.1038/bjc.2014.55318
Level 5	Systematic reviews of descriptive or qualitative studies	McGuire, D. B., Fulton, J. S., Park, J., Brown, C. G., Correa, M. E., Eilers, J., . . . Lalla, R. V. (2013). Systematic review of basic oral care for the management of oral mucositis in cancer patients. *Support Care Cancer*, 21(11), 3165-3177. doi:10.1007/s00520-013-1942-019
Level 6	Descriptive and qualitative studies	Kroner, A., Aerts, E., Schanz, U., & Spirig, R. (2016). [Mouthrinse in oral mucositis in the context of allogeneic stem cell transplantation: a qualitative study]. *Pflege*, 29(1), 21-31. doi:10.1024/1012-5302/a00046520
Level 7	Expert opinions, anecdotal cases and reports, clinical guidelines	AAOM Clinical Practice Statement: Subject: Dental Evaluation Before Head and Neck Radiotherapy. (2016). *Oral Surg Oral Med Oral Pathol Oral Radiol*, 122(5), 564-565. doi:10.1016/j.oooo.2016.05.01921

The next step in the search process is to narrow results by looking at the Levels of Evidence. An understanding of how various levels of evidence are reported and how this literature is organized will help the researcher retrieve the highest levels of evidence for a particular clinical question. The level of evidence approach is an explicit way of ranking evidence. For example, the strongest evidence for therapeutic interventions is provided by meta-analysis or systematic review of randomized, double-blind, placebo-controlled trials involving a homogeneous patient population and condition, especially those that have sufficient statistical power to support negative findings. In contrast, patient testimonials, case reports, and even expert opinion have little value as sound evidence due to biases inherent in observation and reporting of cases, difficulties in ascertaining who is an expert, and more.

If a team decided to conduct a research study to test an intervention for mucositis, it would be important to look at all evidence that exists. But when looking for evidence to change practice, clinicians should seek the strongest level of evidence available to answer the question. Levels range from 1 to 7 with 1 being the strongest evidence. Level 1 evidence is especially notable for busy clinicians. This level includes systematic reviews and meta-analyses of studies, which means that researchers have already compiled available research studies and other evidence to date for a particular topic. Filters within the search engine can tailor the search to include these. When applying that filter to this search example, 26 systematic reviews or meta-analyses arose for review. Reading and reviewing the abstracts of the 26 citations will help to further narrow down the search. For example, included in this list were studies about the management of mucositis pain, which are not relevant to the palliative care team's current question. A description of the 7 levels of evidence are included in Table 2.

CRITICALLY APPRAISING THE LITERATURE

Critiquing research articles is a crucial step in determining whether the available evidence can be applied to one's current practice. The team should ask the following questions:

- Does the recent literature support my current practice?
- Is the literature strong enough to propose a practice change?
- Would it be valuable to replicate the reviewed research in my setting or population?

Table 3. Critical appraisal of a research article

	Quantitative Study	Qualitative Study
Research Problem and Purpose	What is the purpose of the study? Is it clearly identified? What are the research question(s) and/or hypotheses?	What is the purpose of the study? Is it clearly identified? Identify why the phenomenon requires a qualitative format? Is the research question one that tries to explore, describe, or expand knowledge about how reality is experienced?
Review of Literature/ Background	<ul><li>Do the authors specify a theoretical/conceptual framework guiding the study? If so, please specify.</li><li>Is the literature review relevant to the study purpose?</li><li>Is the literature review logically and clearly organized?</li><li>Does the review primarily use current literature? (published within the last 5 years; unless a "classic")</li></ul>	

	Quantitative Study	**Qualitative Study**
Research Design	What type of design was used? • Systematic Review, Meta-analysis, Experimental, Quasi-experimental, Correlational, Case control, Cohort, Exploratory, Descriptive, Survey, Other_____ • None specified	What type of design was used? • Qualitative Descriptive, Ethnography, Phenomenology, Hermeneutics, Grounded Theory, Historical, Case Study, Other_____ • None specified

Research Methods	• Institutional review board approval?
	• Does the research methodology make sense in light of the research question?
	• Population
	• Sample (size, selection, adequate and appropriate)?
	• Type of sampling method was used?
	• probability (randomization), non-probability (convenience), or purposive
	• Inclusion and exclusion criteria
	• Setting
	• Key variables, if applicable:
	  o Independent: (causes the effect that is being studied)
	  o Dependent: (the outcome or effect thought to result from the independent variable)
	  o Research or Study: (characteristics or qualities being measured or described)	

Data Collection, Measurement, and Analysis	• Describe data collection methods • List instruments/tools used with reliability and validity • Describe data analysis procedures • List statistics used to analyze data. Are they appropriated for the questions/hypotheses and levels of measurement?	• Describe data collection methods and analysis • Is data saturation described • Credibility: Does the researcher describe going back to the participants to validate the findings? • Auditability: Are enough examples given that the reader can follow the **researcher**'s reasoning process throughout the study? Is the research process described step-by-step? • Fittingness: Are the findings described in enough detail to be useful to practice, research, and/or theory? Are the results useful for guiding your practice?
Findings/Results	• Tables and figures clear and relevant? • Results organized logically and presented clearly? • Briefly describe results and the conclusions drawn from them. Are the conclusions consistent with the results? • Are the conclusions discussed in relation to the theoretical/conceptual framework? • Does the researcher place the report in the context of what is already known about the focus of the study or phenomenon?	
Conclusions	• Are there answers to the all research question(s)/ hypotheses asked in this study? If not, which one(s) were left unanswered?	• Do the themes/theory/process presented make sense in light of the data provided?
Limitations and Bias	List the strengths, limitations, and biases. Are the limitations/biases concerning enough to cause you to question the validity of the results?	
Significance, Implications, Future Research	Is this study significant to my practice? If so, how is it significant? Are the implications for practice clearly stated? Are suggestions for future research included? If so, what are they?	
Level of Evidence	What is the level of evidence for this study?	

Adapted from University of Colorado Hospital/Health System, Aurora, CO, Professional Resources Research Critique Forms, 2014.

A structured critique form, used to guide the critical appraisal of the research, provides an unbiased systematic method to research evaluation. Critique forms help to promote discussion and improve the educational value. Critique forms should also reflect the quantitative or qualitative research methods of the article. Table 3 provides examples of key questions to use when critiquing a research article. Creating user-friendly critique forms or checklists demonstrate how to critically analyze a research article and provide a framework for dialogue.

JOURNAL CLUB

A journal club is an educational forum to bring together participants from similar or different disciplines to critically appraise a research article relevant to a shared area of expertise or clinical practice. Journal clubs may be unit-based, service-based, or system-based (i.e., hospital- or agency-wide). Journal clubs can also be held in an academic setting (School of Medicine, College of Nursing, etc.). Journal clubs are used to narrow the research-practice gap by providing a welcoming environment to discuss scientific merit of relevant research. Journal clubs can make a difference in health care team attitudes towards research, including reducing perceived barriers to translating research into practice. Through journal club discussion, participants can determine if research findings should be implemented into clinical or professional practice, to promote improved patient care and positive outcomes. Journal clubs have added benefits such as refining of professional reading habits, emboldening research awareness, enhancing critical thinking skills, and facilitating the use of best evidence into practice [11]. Additionally, journal clubs create an environment of life-long learners, nurturing collegiality and interprofessional collaboration.

For the given example, to examine evidence-based protocols for mucositis prophylaxis, the palliative care team decides to hold a journal club to discuss the current evidence. They use a systematic review, which summarized several studies on the topic. Various mucositis strategies are discussed, including the fact that chlorhexidine is no longer a suggested management strategy. The journal club format allowed all team members to discuss this change in practice without specific reference to a participant's *personal* practice, encouraging a "safe" place for participants to learn and explore their personal practice and encouraging adoption of best evidence into practice.

To maximize a journal club's success, it is wise to have a leader who is skilled in research critique. The leader's role is to orchestrate and guide the journal club process. This individual provides mentorship, directs the discussion, and encourages participants to critique the research article and develop skills in interpretation of research findings. It is helpful if the leader provides a formal written critique of the research article at the conclusion of the journal club, allowing participants to compare their critique. New knowledge and re-examination of practice is ongoing. While journal clubs provide an exceptional venue for actively exploring current evidence and practice through dialogue, engaging participants can be challenging. Successful journal club strategies are included in Table 4.

Online journal clubs provide an alternative to an in-person meeting. Participants can critique and comment on the article using an electronic platform. Some healthcare professional organizations and journals offer online journal clubs so that the participant can access the online article, respond to the article, read others' responses, or e-mail a critique to a colleague. When participating in online journal club blogs, the purpose is to post brief comments and ideas about the article so that others can read and respond. Online journal club benefits include: networking with colleagues from all over the world; gathering new insights; and sharing stories, successes, and lessons learned from the journal article. Providing a discussion of the science and evidence behind practice change is more likely to result in adoption of evidence rather than simply publicizing new practice guidelines. Dialogue facilitates understanding; journal clubs are a medium fostering this process.

Table 4. Journal club guidelines

Activity	Instructions
Schedule	Explore the best day/time for the healthcare team. Be consistent to help establish a "routine."
Invite	Participants can include all healthcare providers interested in the topic or more focused dependent on the article for review
Publicize	Post flyers and send electronic communication about journal club logistics (time, place, article citation, and how the participant can access the critique form)
Choose article	The article topic may be driven by a patient problem, changes in practice that have not been well implemented in the practice area or burning clinical question. Journal clubs are most effective when the topic for discussion can be immediately relayed back into clinical practice or raises questions about the status quo in practice.
Access article	Explore ways to share the article before journal club. Discussions are most rich when the participants have read the article prior to attending journal club. Be aware of copyright laws; do not mass produce the article. Post instructions on how to access the article through the health sciences library or online literature resources such as PubMed or Google Scholar (http://scholar.google.com). A small fee may be required to download the full text article in some settings.
Critique	Critiquing the literature is most effective when participants can follow a form that guides the reader in the critical analysis process of the research article.
Host journal club	Open with a question, "Who read the article and what are your initial impressions?" After a general discussion, proceed through the critique form engaging participant dialogue in the review process.
Summarize	Post a copy of your highlighted article and critique form for staff unable to attend. A summary of the journal club dialogue can be an effective means to increase peers' awareness or generating interest for future journal club forums.

TRANSLATING RESEARCH INTO PRACTICE

While critiquing the literature is a critical step, it is not the final step. It should be followed with careful assessment of one's clinical practice and patient population based on the evidence, to determine if the change can be successfully translated into practice. The following steps should be considered when assessing the need and success of a practice change based on critique results:

1. Disseminate knowledge learned from your evidence-based literature review to appropriate staff and stakeholders.
2. Determine if the proposed change in practice is applicable to your clinical setting. OR Is it necessary to replicate the research in your practice setting and population?
3. Assess staff readiness to support a potential practice change.
4. Analyze whether the practice change will result in better patient outcomes.
5. Develop a plan to educate staff on the proposed practice change.
6. Discuss potential barriers to the proposed practice change.
7. Consider the financial implications related to the practice change and resources needed.

Table 5. Palliative care evidence-based practice resources

Organization	Website
Center to Advance Palliative Care (CAPC)	https://www.capc.org/about/capc/
	https://getpalliativecare.org/resources/
End of Life/Palliative Education Resource Center (EPERC) - CAPC- Fast Facts	https://www.capc.org/fast-facts/
National Palliative Care Research Center	http://www.npcrc.org/
National Hospice and Palliative Care Organization	http://www.nhpco.org/
Hospice and Palliative Nurses Association (HPNA)	http://hpna.advancingexpertcare.org/
End of Life Nursing Education Consortium (ELNEC)	http://www.aacn.nche.edu/elnec
Education in Palliative and End-of-Life Care	http://www.epec.net/
American Association of Hospice and Palliative Medicine (AAHPM)	http://aahpm.org/
World Health Organization	http://www.who.int/cancer/palliative/en/
Global Atlas of PC at EOL	http://www.who.int/nmh/Global_Atlas_of_Palliative_Care.pdf
International Palliative Care Resource Center	http://www.ipcrc.net/
The International Program of the Harvard Medical School Center for Palliative Care (MGH)	http://www.massgeneral.org/palliativecare/education/international_program.aspx

The nature and scope of any recommended practice change will determine what avenues should be taken next to begin the change process. If a study is to be replicated, then protocols for conducting research in your setting must be followed. Is the potential practice change limited to your care area or can and should it be implemented throughout your organization or system? Knowledge gained through careful critique of current literature can validate your current practice or support the need to change practice using innovative and efficient new strategies.

Multiple resources exist for implementing EBP change into palliative care practice (Table 5). National and international resources should be also explored for implementing EBP change. For example, implementation frameworks can assist clinicians in translating evidence into practice. The Iowa Model is one framework that can provide teams with a multi-step process for EBP success [12]. Another valuable resource is the Oncology Nursing Society (ONS) *Putting Evidence Into Practice* (PEP)™ framework, which provides EBP recommendations for exemplary oncology clinical practice (www.ons.org). EBP teams, comprised of ONS members are led by a research nurse scientist to coordinate the critique and synthesis effort. Clinical practice issues are addressed; evidence is searched for, critiqued, and synthesized. Dissemination occurs through the online PEP website and through published systematic reviews. For example, the most recent mucositis systematic review was published in 2014 [13]. A unique feature of the PEP card is the use of the three-colored stop light (green, yellow, red) system. Green supports the evidence is strong enough that it should be used in practice; yellow suggests caution in using the evidence; and red indicates the evidence shows the evidence ineffective and not recommended for practice.

EVALUATING THE CHANGE

The final step in the EBP process is to evaluate the change to determine the success of the implementation. Too often, EBP changes are made, but may not be followed consistently. Additionally, implementation barriers arise in real world settings, and the team may need to evaluate barriers. Evaluation also includes celebrating successes, and baseline and follow-up data can be used to document positive impacts on patient care and clinical practice [14].

CONCLUSION

Practicing according to the best evidence requires a team of healthcare professionals and an organizational culture that values change, based on research and other forms of evidence to optimize patient outcomes. Mentoring and engaging others and creating a culture that questions practice and is empowered to explore and implement new evidence to maximize patient care are essential ingredients to effective dissemination and implementation of EBP. Palliative care teams can use these processes to tackle individual patient symptoms and clinical problems, one at a time, to provide patients with consistent EBP approaches to care to alleviate suffering and improve quality of life.

DISCLOSURE STATEMENT

Regina Fink reports no commercial or financial conflicts of interest. Jeannine Brant is on speaker's bureaus for Insys and Genentech. The authors alone are responsible for the content and writing of this manuscript.

REFERENCES

[1] Institute of Medicine. *The Future of Nursing: Leading Change, Advancing Health*. 2010. Accessed March 3, 2015, 2015.

[2] Sackett D. L., Strauss SE, Richardson WS, Rosenberg W, Hayes RB. *Evidence-based medicine: How to practice and teach EBM, 2nd ed.* New York: Churchill Livingstone; 2000.

[3] Goode CJ, Fink RM, Krugman M, Oman KS, Traditi LK. The Colorado Patient-Centered Interprofessional Evidence-Based Practice Model: a framework for transformation. *Worldviews Evid Based Nurs.* 2011;8(2):96-105.

[4] Melnyk BM. Building cultures and environments that facilitate clinician behavior change to evidence-based practice: what works? *Worldviews Evid Based Nurs.* 2014;11(2):79-80.

[5] Stillwell SB, Fineout-Overholt E, Melnyk BM, Williamson KM. Evidence-based practice, step by step: asking the clinical question: a key step in evidence-based practice. *Am J Nurs.* 2010;110(3):58-61.

[6] Stern C, Jordan Z, McArthur A. Developing the review question and inclusion criteria. *Am J Nurs.* 2014;114(4):53-56.
[7] Riva JJ, Malik KM, Burnie SJ, Endicott AR, Busse JW. What is your research question? An introduction to the PICOT format for clinicians. *J Can Chiropr Assoc.* 2012;56(3):167-171.
[8] Fineout-Overholt E, Melnyk BM, Stillwell SB, Williamson KM. Evidence-based practice step by step: Critical appraisal of the evidence: part I. *Am J Nurs.* 2010;110(7):47-52.
[9] Fineout-Overholt E, Melnyk BM, Stillwell SB, Williamson KM. Evidence-based practice, step by step: critical appraisal of the evidence: part II: digging deeper--examining the "keeper" studies. *Am J Nurs.* 2010;110(9):41-48.
[10] Fineout-Overholt E, Melnyk BM, Stillwell SB, Williamson KM. Evidence-based practice, step by step: Critical appraisal of the evidence: part III. *Am J Nurs.* 2010;110(11):43-51.
[11] Melnyk BM, Fineout-Overholt E. *Evidence-based practice in nursing and healthcare: A guide to best practice.* 2nd Ed. Philadelphia Lippincott, Williams & Wilkins; 2011.
[12] Iowa Model C, Buckwalter KC, Cullen L, et al. Iowa Model of Evidence-Based Practice: Revisions and Validation. *Worldviews Evid Based Nurs.* 2017;14(3):175-182.
[13] Eilers J, Harris D, Henry K, Johnson LA. Evidence-based interventions for cancer treatment-related mucositis: putting evidence into practice. *Clin J Oncol Nurs.* 2014;18 Suppl:80-96.
[14] Fineout-Overholt E, Williamson KM, Gallagher-Ford L, Melnyk BM, Stillwell SB. Following the evidence: planning for sustainable change. *Am J Nurs.* 2011;111(1):54-60.
[15] Cardona A, Balouch A, Abdul MM, Sedghizadeh PP, Enciso R. Efficacy of chlorhexidine for the prevention and treatment of oral mucositis in cancer patients: a systematic review with meta-analyses. *J Oral Pathol Med.* 2017;46(9):680-688.
[16] Demir Dogan M, Can G, Meral R. Effectiveness of Black Mulberry Molasses in Prevention of Radiotherapy-Induced Oral Mucositis: A Randomized Controlled Study in Head and Neck Cancer Patients. *J Altern Complement Med.* 2017;23(12):971-979.
[17] Meca LB, Souza FR, Tanimoto HM, Castro AL, Gaetti-Jardim Junior E. Influence of preventive dental treatment on mutans streptococci counts in patients undergoing head and neck radiotherapy. *Journal of Applied Oral Science : Revista FOB.* 2009;17 Suppl:5-12.
[18] Miah AB, Schick U, Bhide SA, et al. A phase II trial of induction chemotherapy and chemo-IMRT for head and neck squamous cell cancers at risk of bilateral nodal spread: the application of a bilateral superficial lobe parotid-sparing IMRT technique and treatment outcomes. *Br J Cancer.* 2015;112(1):32-38.
[19] McGuire DB, Fulton JS, Park J, et al. Systematic review of basic oral care for the management of oral mucositis in cancer patients. *Support Care Cancer.* 2013;21(11):3165-3177.
[20] Kroner A, Aerts E, Schanz U, Spirig R. [Mouthrinse in oral mucositis in the context of allogeneic stem cell transplantation: a qualitative study]. *Pflege.* 2016;29(1):21-31.
[21] AAOM Clinical Practice Statement: Subject: Dental Evaluation Before Head and Neck Radiotherapy. *Oral Surgery, Oral Medicine, Oral Pathology and Oral Radiology.* 2016;122(5):564-565.

BIOGRAPHICAL SKETCHES

Regina M. Fink, PhD, APRN, FAAN

Position Title: Full Professor, School of Medicine and College of Nursing

Education/Training:

Villanova University, Villanova, PA	BSN	05/1977	Nursing
University of Colorado, Aurora, CO	MS	08/1979	Nursing
University of Colorado, Aurora, CO	PhD	05/1999	Nursing

Personal Statement: Throughout my career, I have held many positions, clinical nurse specialist, educator, research nurse scientist, and co-investigator. I am co-director of and teach in the Interprofessional Master of Science in Palliative Care (MSPC) and Graduate Palliative Care Certificate programs at the University of Colorado at the Anschutz Medical Campus. As a Nurse Scientist and Associate Professor, I consult with nurses and other healthcare professionals on research, quality improvement, and evidence-based practice (EBP) projects and mentor students in the conduct of their Capstone, DNP, and PhD research projects. A national and international lecturer on pain, palliative care, and EBP with multiple publications (60+ peer reviewed articles, chapters, and 5 books), I have focused my 40 year nursing career on caring for persons with cancer, pain, and symptoms, focusing on improving quality of life and have been a co-Investigator on university-funded, NINR, AHRQ, and other grants. I have successfully co-conducted a fully powered RCT of a patient navigator intervention for Latinos with advanced cancer funded by the American Cancer Society and am currently a co-investigator on a RO1 that is testing the effect of a patient navigator intervention for Latinos with non-cancer advanced illness. I am also involved with advance care planning outreach to Colorado rural and underserved communities. I have specific expertise in key research areas including quantitative and qualitative analysis, instrument development, survey research, focus groups, and secondary data analysis. I have administered research projects and collaborated with other researchers. I realize the importance of frequent communication among team members and a realistic research plan, budget, and timeline. I am adept at establishing relationships and networking with healthcare professionals at multiple research community sites.

Positions and Honors

Positions and Employment

1977-1978	Clinical RN, Investigational Chemotherapy, Memorial Sloan-Kettering Cancer Center, NY, NY
1978-1979	Clinical RN, 8W CRC, University of Colorado Health Sciences Center, Denver, CO
1979-1981	Assistant Head Nurse, Oncology Unit, Rose Medical Center, Denver, CO
1981-1986	Oncology Clinical Nurse Specialist/Program Manager, P/SL Medical Center, Denver, CO

1986-1989	Oncology Clinical Nurse Specialist, Hematology/Oncology Associates, Denver, CO
1990-1995	Oncology Clinical Nurse Specialist, University of Colorado Hospital
1990-1998	Clinical Faculty, University of Colorado College of Nursing, Denver, CO
1995-1998	Acute Pain Clinical Nurse Specialist, University of Colorado Hospital, Denver, CO
1998-2015	Research Nurse Scientist, University of Colorado Hospital, Aurora, CO
10/98-present	Associate Professor and Co-Director MSPC, University of Colorado Anschutz Medical Campus, School of Medicine and College of Nursing, Aurora, CO

Selected Awards, Certifications, and Professional Memberships

1978-present	State of Colorado, Nursing and Advanced Practice Nurse Licenses
1981-present	Member, American Pain Society
1981-present	Member, Oncology Nursing Society and Metro Denver Oncology Nursing Society
1995-present	Member, American Society of Pain Management Nurses
1995-present	Member, Sigma Theta Tau, Member at Large, Alpha Kappa Chapter
1996-present	Advanced Oncology Certified Nurse (AOCN)®, Oncology Nursing Society
2000-present	Member, American Nurses' Association, Colorado Nurses' Association,
2001-present	Fellow, American Academy of Nursing
2010-2013	Senior Research Advisor, Hartford Institute for Geriatric Nursing, NYU, New York
2014-present	Member, Hospice and Palliative Nurse's Association (HPNA)
2015-present	Certified Hospice and Palliative Care Nurse (CHPN), HPNA

Honors

1993	International Oncology Nursing Fellowship Award
1994	Medallion for Leadership in Nursing Practice & Health Care Delivery, Villanova University College of Nursing, Villanova, PA
1995	Florence Nightingale Award Recipient, State of Colorado
2001	Fellow in the American Academy of Nursing
2008	AJN Book of the Year (Gates RA, Fink RM. Oncology Nursing Secrets, 3rd edition, 2009)
2012	Magnet Nurse of the Year, University of Colorado Hospital
2013	Karen Smith Lastreto Mentor Award, Sigma Theta Tau
2013-2017	Invited Presenter, International Middle East Cancer Consortium and Oman Cancer Association

Contributions to Science

1. My early research endeavors include the development and testing of an instrument (the Casey-Fink Graduate Nurse Experience) to measure the graduate nurse transition into clinical practice which is used by the University Health System Consortium and the American Association of Colleges of Nursing in their extensive research and development of a national nurse residency program. In collaboration with Kathy Casey,

RN, MSN, I also developed reliable and valid instruments to measure readiness for practice (Casey-Fink Readiness for Practice Survey) and nurse retention (Revised Casey-Fink Nurse Retention Survey). These instruments are available for use nationally and internationally by researchers. https://www.uchealth.org/professionals/Pages/Casey-Fink-Survey-Instruments.aspx.
   a. Casey K, Fink RM, Krugman M, Propst J. The graduate nurse experience. *Journal of Nursing Administration* 2004;34(6):303-311.
   b. Fink RM, Krugman ME, Casey K, Goode CM. The graduate nurse experience: Qualitative residency program outcomes. *Journal of Nursing Administration* 2008;38(7/8):341-348.
   c. Casey K, Fink RM, Jaynes C, Campbell L, Cook P, Wilson V. Readiness for practice: The senior practicum experience. *Journal of Nursing Education* 2011;50(11):646-652.
   d. Buffington A, Zwink J, Fink RM, DeVine D, Sanders C. Factors affecting nurse retention at an academic magnet hospital. *Journal of Nursing Administration* 2012;42(5):273-281.

2. Previous pain research includes being a co-investigator on an AHRQ grant, *Improving Pain Management in Nursing Homes,* where I was responsible for developing and implementing educational and behavioral interventions in 12 Colorado nursing homes, coordinating the internal pain teams, conducting pain rounds, and consultations. Additionally, I analyzed medication orders and pain medication administration in nursing home residents. I developed and disseminated a nursing home toolkit to improve pain management in nursing homes. The MDS 3.0 includes pain assessment documentation based on our work. Other pain research included measuring pain perceptions and medication taking in palliative care patients. Clinical innovations have included the development of a nationally distributed pain assessment guide (WILDA) that has been translated into multiple languages, analgesic reference guide, and pain assessment video to hospitals, hospices, and home care agency staff.
   a. Jones KR, Fink RM, Hutt E, Vojir C, Pepper G, Clark L, Scott J, Martinez R, Vincent D, Mellis B. Translation research in long-term care: Improving pain management in nursing homes. *Worldviews on Evidence-Based Nursing* 2004;1(S1):S13-S20.
   b. Jones KR, Fink RM, Pepper G, Hutt E, Vojir CP, Scott J, Clark L, Mellis BK. Measuring pain intensity in nursing home residents. *Journal of Pain and Symptom Management* 2005;30(6):519-527.
   c. Hutt E, Pepper G, Fink RM, Vojir C, Jones, KR. Assessing the appropriateness of pain medication prescribing practices in nursing homes. *Journal of the American Geriatric Society* 2006;54:231-239.
   d. Hutt E, Fink RM, Nelson-Marten P, Jones J, Kutner JS. Measuring pain perceptions and medication taking behavior at the end of life: A pilot study. *American Journal of Hospice and Palliative Medicine* 2013;23 epub ahead of print.

3. My palliative care research includes being a co-investigator on an NIH grant on Palliative Care, where I integrated palliative care and pain management content into the curricula of nursing and medical schools. I developed and conducted a palliative care

needs assessment in rural Rocky Mountain hospitals and I collaborated with health care professionals in 15 Middle Eastern countries through the Middle Eastern Cancer Consortium (MECC) to replicate this work. I presented these findings in Ankara Turkey at the 2014 MECC Palliative Care meeting and have traveled extensively to Muscat Oman to conduct a needs assessment and teach Middle Eastern healthcare providers. I was a co-investigator on an ACS Funded grant, "Apoyo con Carino: Patient Navigation to Improve Palliative Care for Latinos with Advanced Cancer." I collaborated with an interdisciplinary team of palliative care health care professionals to conduct a systematic review of rural palliative care research. I am a co-investigator on an NINR funded grant, "Apoyo con Cariño: Patient Navigation to Improve Palliative Care for Seriously Ill Latinos."

    a. Fink RM, Oman KS, Youngwerth J, Bryant L. A palliative care needs assessment in rural hospitals, *Journal of Palliative Medicine* 2013;16(6):638-644.

    b. Silbermann M, Fink RM, Min SJ, Mancuso MP, Brant J, et al. Evaluating palliative care needs in Middle Eastern countries. *Journal of Palliative Medicine*; 2015;18(1):18-25.

    c. Fischer SM, Cervantes L, Fink RM, Kutner JS. Apoyo con Carino: A pilot RCT of a patient navigator intervention to improve palliative care outcomes for Latinos with serious illness. *Journal of Pain and Symptom Management* 2015;49(4):657-65.

    d. Bakitas MA, Elk R, Astin M, Ceronsky L, Clifford KN, Dionne-Odom JN, Emanuel LL, Fink RM, Kvale E, Levkoff S, Ritchie C, Smith T. A systematic review of rural palliative care research: A new frontier. *Cancer Control* 2015;22(4):450-64.

    e. Fischer SM, Kline DM, Min SJ, Okuyama S, Fink RM. Apoyo con Cariño: Strategies to Promote Recruiting, Enrolling, and Retaining Latinos in a Cancer Clinical Trial. *Journal of the National Comprehensive Cancer Network.* 2017;15(11):1392-9.

4. In addition to the contributions described above, I have collaborated with an interdisciplinary team of health care professionals to conduct research and quality improvement to improve catheter associated urinary tract infections (CA-UTI) both locally and nationally.

    a. Fink RM, Gilmartin H, Richard A, Capezuti E, Boltz M, Wald H. Indwelling urinary catheter management (IUC) and CAUTI prevention practices in Nurses Improving Care for HealthSystem Elders Hospitals. *American Journal of Infection Control* 2012;40(8):715-720.

    b. Oman KS, Makic MBF, Fink RM, Schraeder N, Hulett T, Keech T, Wald H. Nurse-directed interventions to reduce catheter-associated urinary tract infections. *American Journal of Infection Control* 2012;40(6):548-553.

    c. Scott R, Oman KS, Makic MB, Fink RM, Braaten J, Severyn F, Wald H. Reducing indwelling urinary catheter use in the Emergency Department: A successful quality improvement initiative. *Journal of Emergency Nursing* 2014; 40(3):237-244.

    d. Wald H, Richard A, Bandle B, Fink RM, Boltz M, Capezuti E. Building capacity in HAI prevention research: NICHE and the STOP CAUTI workgroup. *Advances in the Prevention and Control of HAI Infections:* 2014 AHRQ Publication.

Additional Information: Research Support and/or Scholastic Performance

Ongoing Research Support
    NINR   (Fischer, PI)   1R01NR016467-01   9/26/2016-7/31/2020
"Apoyo Con Carino: Patient Navigation to Improve Palliative Care for Seriously Ill Latinos"
A multi-site randomized controlled trial of the patient navigator intervention to evaluate the efficacy of the intervention to increase advance care planning, improve pain management, and increase hospice utilization for Latinos with advanced medical illness in Colorado.
    Role: Co-Investigator (0.25 FTE)

    Colorado Health Foundation (Handel, PI)   6/01/16-11/01/18
    Conversations about Advance Care Planning in Underserved Populations
    Role: Co-investigator (0.05 FTE)

Jeannine M. Brant, PhD

Position Title: Oncology Clinical Nurse Specialist and Nurse Scientist

Contact Information: Email: jbrant@billingsclinic.org

Education/Training:

Montana State University, Bozeman, MT	BSN	1984	Nursing
University of California, San Francisco, CA	MS	1990	Oncology Nursing
University of Utah, Salt Lake City, UT	PhD	2008	Nursing Research

Personal Statement: I have been an oncology nurse for almost 35 years with 30 years of research experience. I began my research career as a research assistant in graduate school and have also served as a co-investigator, principal investigator, and research mentor for other nurses and health care professionals conducting research. I have participated in all aspects of the research process including study design, implementation and data collection, data analysis, and dissemination. Retrospective and prospective designs, mixed methods using qualitative and quantitative methods, cross-sectional and longitudinal studies are all within my repertoire. I also had the privilege of serving on the Clinical Trials Blue Ribbon Panel for the Moonshot initiative. In addition, I have worked extensively with global, rural and American Indian populations, and my goal is always to encourage these populations to participate in research so that interventions may be more generalizable to diverse populations.

Positions and Honors:

Professional Positions and Research-Related Activity
1984-1986   Oncology Staff Nurse/Charge Nurse, Deaconess Medical Center, Billings, MT

1985-present	Member, Oncology Nursing Society (ONS) and American Pain Society (APS)
1986-1987	Intensive Care Unit Staff Nurse, Deaconess Medical Center, Billings, MT
1987	Outpatient Chemotherapy Nurse, Billings Clinic, Billings, MT
1988-1990	Oncology Charge Nurse, Redding Medical Center, Redding, CA
1990	Research Assistant, Pediatric Pain Study, University of California, San Francisco
1990-2008	Oncology Clinical Nurse Specialist & Pain Consultant, Cancer Support Group Facilitator, St. Vincent Healthcare, Billings, MT
1991-2004	Director, Women Reaching for Wellness; a cancer education and research collaborative to address health care disparities in American Indian women ($800,000 funding history)
1992-present	Reviewer Positions: ONS national publications: Recycling Our Ideas, ONS Biotherapy Guidelines, Psychosocial Module in Oncology Nursing, Bone Marrow Transplant Module, Clinical Manual for the Oncology Advanced Practice Nurse, Case Management Module, Congress abstracts; Journal/Publication Reviewer: American Nurses' Association Standards of Nursing Practice, Clinical Journal of Oncology Nursing, Oncology Nursing Forum, American Journal of Nursing, Journal of Pain and Symptom Management, Oncology Nursing Forum, European Journal of Oncology Nursing, Journal of Clinical Oncology, Cancer Practice; Reviewer of National Cancer Institute publications: Eating Hints, Chemotherapy and You
1994-present	Editorial Positions: ONS Scan in Oncology Nursing (1997-1998); Standards of Oncology Nursing Practice (2003, 2011), Clinical Journal of Oncology Nursing (2002-2005), Journal of Advanced Practitioners in Oncology (2009-present)
1991-present	Affiliate Assistant Professor, Montana State University, Bozeman, MT
2002-present	Affiliate Faculty Member, University of Southern Indiana pain certification program
2004-present	Affiliate Faculty Member, University of MT Geriatric Education; pain and palliative care
2009-present	Nurse Scientist and Oncology Clinical Nurse Specialist, Billings Clinic, Billings, MT
2009-present	Associate Editor, Journal of Advanced Practitioners in Oncology
2009-present	Team Member, Putting Evidence into Practice Pain Guideline Team
2012-present	Team Member, Oncology Nursing Society Grants Review Team
2013-2014	Auditor, American Society of Clinical Oncology (ASCO) Quality Oncology Practice Initiative (QOPI)
2013-present	Planning Committee, ASCO Palliative Care Symposium
2013-present	Executive Committee, National Cancer Institute, Palliative Care in the Middle East
2014-present	Principal Investigator, Montana Cancer Consortium Cancer Control Delivery Research
2014-present	Committee Member, Alliance Research Base Symptom Management Committee
2015-present	International Liaison, Palliative Care in the Middle East ONS Liaison

2016   National Palliative Care Steering Committee, American Nurses Association
2017   Joe Biden Blue Ribbon Panel, National Cancer Institute

Honors/Awards:

American Cancer Society Master's Scholarship, 1988-1990; Golden Eagle Award given by CINE for "New Horizons: Management of Chemotherapy-Induced Emesis" educational video (national award), 1992; Gold Spirit Award for Communications given by the Catholic Health Association of the United States for "Standing Strong Against the Cancer Enemy" cancer prevention video for American Indians (national award), 1994; Innovative Health Care Award given by the Montana Hospital Association for "Standing Strong Against the Cancer Enemy" cancer prevention video (statewide award), 1994; Who's Who in American Nursing (national award), 1994; "International Health and Medical Film Festival Finalist" for the film "Standing Strong Against the Cancer Enemy" (national award), 1995; "Profiles in Progress" Award given by Zeneca Pharmaceuticals for the "Indian Women Reaching For Wellness Program" (national award), 1995; ONS/AMGEN Award for Excellence in Patient/Public Education (national award) 1997; ONS/Schering Oncology/Biotech Clinical Lectureship (national award), 1998; Montana Public Health Association President's Award – "Women Reaching for Wellness Program" (statewide award), 2000; Marsha Liebman New Writer Award – Coauthor and Mentor of nurse who received the award, "When a Parent Dies of Cancer" (national award), 2002; Oncology Nursing Society/Purdue Pharma Excellence in Pain Management Award (national award), 2004; Oncology Nursing Society Doctoral Scholarship, 2005 (national); American Cancer Society Doctoral Scholarship (national), 2005-2008; Nurse educator, researcher, and pain consultant for the Middle Eastern Cancer Consortium (international), 2010-2012; Montana State University Nursing Distinguished Alumni Award (state), 2013; Fellow American Academy of Nursing 2014; Best Poster World Congress of Psycho-Oncology 2015; Yellowstone Valley Women's Magazine Cover Photo and Story 2015, Oncology News Cover Photo and Story 2017; Mary Padzur Advanced Practice Award, 2018.

Contribution to Science:

1. Global Palliative Care: I have made significant contributions to palliative care science around the globe, particularly in collaboration with the Middle Eastern Cancer Consortium (MECC). I currently serve as the Oncology Nursing Society US liaison to the program. Through this National Cancer Institute funded initiative, our team has trained over 1000 nurses throughout the Middle East in palliative care. We have conducted multi country research, evaluating palliative care needs in Middle Eastern countries, and I have personally mentored scientists from throughout the Middle East in palliative care study design and dissemination of findings. Most recently, my Israeli physician colleague and I published a two-part supplement on Palliative Care Nursing in Palliative Care and Medicine. Select contributions include:

   Kav, S., Brant, J. M., & Mushani, T. (2018). Perspectives in International Palliative Care. *Semin Oncol Nurs*. doi:10.1016/j.soncn.2018.06.009
   Brant, J. M., Newton, S., & Maurer, M. A. (2017). Pain Management in the Middle East: Building Capacity with Global Partners. *Oncol Nurs Forum*, 44(4), 403-405. doi:10.1188/17.onf.403-405

Brant, J. M. (2017). Holistic total pain management in palliative care: Cultural and global considerations. *Palliative Medicine and Hospice Care*, S32-S38. doi:10.17140/ PMHCOJSE-1-108

Brant, J.M., Kav, S. (2016). Leading the global transformation of healthcare. In M. Gullatte (Ed). *21st Century Nursing Leadership*. Pittsburgh: ONS Press.

Kennedy Sheldon, L., Brant, J., Shaughnessy Hankle, K., Bialous, S., Lubejko, B. (2016). Promoting cancer nursing education, training, and research in countries in transition. In M. Silbermann (Ed) *Cancer Care in Countries and Societies in Transition*. Switzerland: Springer, pp. 473-493.

Brant, J.M. (2015). Palliative care nursing: Looking back, looking forward. *J Palliat Care Med*, S5:1 Supplement found at: http://www.omicsgroup.org/journals/ArchiveJPCM/specialissue-palliative-care-and-nursing-S5.php

Silbermann, M., Fink, R.M., Min, S.J., Mancuso, M.P., Brant, J. …. Strode, D. (2015). Evaluating Palliative Care Needs in Middle Eastern Countries. *J Palliat Med*, 18(1), 1-8. DOI: 10.1089/jpm.2014.0194

2. Pain Care Quality: Pain care quality is lacking in US hospitals. Through an iterative process, our research developed the Pain Care Quality Surveys (PanCQ), which measured the quality of care related to the assessment and management of pain. In a subsequent study, we disseminated the surveys as quality indicators through The National Database of Nursing Quality Indicators (NDNQI). We were able to secure 326 hospitals as research sites, facilitated 326 IRB approvals, and gathered pain care quality data on over 20,000 patients at baseline and another 20,000 patients for the follow-up visit. Hospitals scoring the lowest were randomized to Communities of Practice (COP), where they met via phone conference to discuss quality improvement plans plus a Pain Care Quality Toolkit which we developed through the study, a COP alone, or to a Control group. Hospitals showed improved pain scores in all groups. I served as a co-investigator on the study, and as a pain expert was also accountable for the development of the online toolkit. Additionally, I facilitated three Communities of Practice. This was the first attempt nationwide to measure nursing pain care quality in US hospitals. Hospitals were able to benchmark scores with one another and improve pain care over time. Organizations across the country continue to use the surveys for quality and research purposes. Some of the papers are included below:

Brant, J. M., Keller, L., McLeod, K., Yeh, C., & Eaton, L. H. (2017). Chronic and Refractory Pain: A Systematic Review of Pharmacologic Management in Oncology. *Clin J Oncol Nurs*, 21(3), 31-59. doi:10.1188/17.CJON.S3.31-53

Brant, J. M., Rodgers, B. B., Gallagher, E., & Sundaramurthi, T. (2017). Breakthrough Cancer Pain: A Systematic Review of Pharmacologic Management. *Clin J Oncol Nurs*, 21(3), 71-80. doi:10.1188/17.CJON.S3.71-80

Tavernier, S. S., Guo, J. W., Eaton, J., Brant, J. M., Berry, P., & Beck, S. L. (2018). Context Matters for Nurses Leading Pain Improvement in U.S. Hospitals. *Pain Manag Nurs*. doi:10.1016/j.pmn.2018.05.003

Beck, SM, Brant, JM, Donahue, R, Smith, EL, Towsley, GL, Berry, PH, Guo, JW, Al-Qaaydeh, S, Pett, MA, Donaldson, G. (2015). Oncology nursing certification and relationships to nurses' pain knowledge and attitudes, pain care quality, and pain outcomes. *Oncology Nursing Forum*, 43(1):67-76. doi: 10.1188/16.ONF.67-76

Pett, M. A., Beck, S. L., Guo, J. W., Towsley, G. L., Brant, J. M., Lavoie Smith, E. M., . . . Donaldson, G. W. (2012). Confirmatory Factor Analysis of the Pain Care Quality Surveys (PainCQ((c))). *Health Serv Res*. doi:10.1111/1475-6773.12014

Beck, S. L., Towsley, G. L., Pett, M. A., Berry, P. H., Smith, E. L., Brant, J. M., & Guo, J. W. (2010). Initial psychometric properties of the Pain Care Quality Survey (PainCQ). *J Pain*, 11(12), 1311-1319. doi:10.1016/j.jpain.2010.03.008

3. Cancer Screening and Cancer Services in American Indian (AI) Populations: My work with AIs began with a visit to two Montana (MT) Indian reservations in the 1990's. Seeing significant cancer disparities, I wrote an educational grant which led to development of AI Women Reaching for Wellness Program, which over 15 years spread from 2 reservations to 8, received $840,823 supporting 3 full-time employees, educated over 20,000 AI women, increased mammography in AI women from 5/year to over 200/year, and produced an award-winning film, Standing Strong Against the Cancer Enemy with over 200 copies nationally distributed. As Director and Principal Investigator of the AI Women Reaching for Wellness Program, our team successfully launched cancer education opportunities and screening services throughout AI reservations in Montana. At the time, women were being diagnosed with late stage disease; the five year breast cancer survival rate in AIs was less than 60% compared to 85% now.

Haozous, E. A., Knobf, M. T., & Brant, J. M. (2011). Understanding the cancer pain experience in American Indians of the Northern Plains. *Psychooncology,* 20(4), 404-410. doi:10.1002/pon.1741

Brant, J. M., Fallsdown, D., & Iverson, M. L. (1999). The evolution of a breast health program for Plains Indian women. *Oncol Nurs Forum*, 26(4), 731-739. Retrieved from http://www.ncbi.nlm.nih.gov/pubmed/10337651

Brant, J., Ishida, D., Itano, J., Kagawa-Singer, M., Palos, G., Phillips, J., Tejada-Reyes, I. (1999). *Oncology Nursing Society Multicultural Outcomes: Guidelines for Cultural Competence*. U.S.A.: Oncology Nursing Press. https://www.google.com/?gws_rd=ssl#q=ONS+multicultural+outcomes+Brant

Brant, J. (1996). Breast cancer challenges in American Indian women. In K. Hassey Dow (Ed.) *Contemporary Issues in Breast Cancer*. Boston: Jones and Bartlett.

4. Development of the Dynamic Symptom Model: During my PhD program, a conceptual model was lacking that would illustrate my research aims that examined symptom trajectories in patients with cancer. I began studying symptom models and developed a model that both guided my research and served as my theoretical framework. I continue to revise and use the model, have been a guest lecturer at PhD classes around the country to discuss the model; the model has been cited by over 25 research scientists who are using the model as their theoretical framework to guide research. Some of my studies and papers that include the model are listed below.

Brant, J. M., Blaseg, K., Oliver, D., & Aders, K. (2012). Quality of Life Trajectories of Breast Cancer and Lymphoma Survivors Enrolled in A Survivorship Program. *Oncology Nursing Forum*, 39, E540. doi:10.1188/12.ONF.E548-E590

Brant, J. M., Beck, S., & Miaskowski, C. (2010). Building dynamic models and theories to advance the science of symptom management research. *J Adv Nurs*, 66(1), 228-240. doi:10.1111/j.1365-2648.2009.05179.x

5. Organizational Nurse Scientist: I have worked as a nurse scientist in a fully integrated health care organization over the last 7 years. The role is not well defined, and outcomes are lacking. I have developed the nurse scientist role and have disseminated outcomes and role specifics. Under my leadership (since 2012), nurses have submitted over 60 abstracts to national meetings including Magnet, ONS, and the ANA Quality Conference and 25 have been accepted– prior to my presence, 2 had been presented at national meetings. Nurses are also actively engaged in research under my mentorship, investigating topics such as Predictors of Opioid-Induced Oversedation, Navigating the Transition of Cancer Survivorship, and Incorporating Palliative Care Into the Medical Home. Select publications:

Brant, J. M., & Mayer, D. K. (2017). Precision Medicine: Accelerating the Science to Revolutionize Cancer Care. *Clin J Oncol Nurs*, 21(6), 722-729. doi:10.1188/17.CJON.722-729

Brant, J.M., Stringer, L., Peterson, L., Herbert, S. Coombs, N. (2018). Predictors of Oversedation in Hospitalized Patients. *American Journal of Health System Pharmacists*.

Brant, J. M. (2015). Bridging the Research-to-Practice Gap: The Role of the Nurse Scientist. *Semin Oncol Nurs*, 31(4), 298-305. doi:10.1016/j.soncn.2015.08.00

Full publication list:
http://scholar.google.com/citations?user=ECfsQr0AAAAJ&hl=en

Research Support
HHSP233201500015I (Brant: PI)   11/01/2015 – 10/31/2020
Agency for Health Research and Quality
AHRQ Acceleration Change and Transformation in Organizations and Networks (ACTION) III

The goal of ACTION III is to promote and accelerate the development, implementation, dissemination and sustainability of evidence-based innovation in health care delivery to measurably improve the effectiveness, safety, quality and efficiency of health care in the U.S. In support of this goal, ACTION II will support practice-based research focused on achieving one or more of the following four objectives: Test or expand investigation of innovations that are new to the health care field, (proofs of concept); Implement, in additional settings, interventions or improvement approaches that have been demonstrated to have worked in a limited type or number of settings; Spread, or take to scale, one or more proven innovations or delivery system improvements.

1UG1CA189872 (CCDR PI: Brant)   8/1/2014 – 7/31/2019
NCI
Montana Cancer Consortium NCI Community Cancer Research Program (NCORP)

Through this research initiative, our team examines how social factors, financing systems, organizational structures and processes, health technologies, and healthcare provider and individual behaviors affect cancer outcomes, access to and quality of care, cancer care costs, and the health and well-being of cancer patients and survivors. I serve as PI for the Montana region which extends into northern Wyoming and northern Idaho.

Grant Number NA (PI: Brant)   3/1/2014 – 8/30/2018
Billings Clinic and Carevive
Addressing Quality Cancer and Survivorship Care: Pilot Testing the Carevive Care Planning System

Our team is exploring, from both patient and provider perspectives - the feasibility, usability of, and acceptability and satisfaction of a novel electronic platform, the Carevive Care Planning System. Secondary outcomes include patient's perceptions of quality and coordination of care, self-reported adherence to recommended tasks, self-reported goals and concerns at each visit, patient satisfaction with the care team, and health care utilization. The platform also includes a Cancer Survivorship Planning System, which we are testing as well. This mixed methods study, conducted at Billings Clinic and Moffitt Cancer Center includes mixed methods with qualitative interviews and quantitative analysis of common symptoms, recommended tasks generated by the provider, and patient goals, visit concerns, and satisfaction.

1 PAWOS000019-01-00 (PI: Brant)   9/1/2015 – 8/30/17
Office of the Assistant Secretary for Health (OASH)
Development of Systems for Trauma-Response Education and Supportive Solutions (DE-STRESS)

The purpose of this project is to engage our community in a coordinated response to adverse childhood experiences, through trauma-informed responses, in order to improve the physical and mental health status of our citizens. Using the OASH/HHS trauma-informed platform, this multi-pronged approach will inform and influence the continuum of care and develop pathways to create a trauma-informed community and trauma-responsive systems addressing the three R's: Realize, Recognize, and Respond as identified by the National Center for Trauma-Informed Care (NCTIC).

CCEWH111023 (PI: Neary)   9/01/2011 – 8/31/2016
DHHS Office of Women's Health,
Coalition for a Healthier Community Program

A Coalition of the County Health Department and two local hospitals will implement evidence-based health interventions through a public health systems approach that is gender-based, cost-effective, sustainable, and that addresses identified community health issues that adversely affect the health of Yellowstone County's women and girls. The Coalition seeks to accommodate and transform gender norms to increase physical activity and increase sense of self-worth for women in Yellowstone County. Interventions include community based organization groups, citizen groups, and a county-wide social marketing campaign. I serve as Lead Evaluator for the study.

Grant Number NA (PI: Blaseg) 9/01/2014 – 8/30/2017
Billings Clinic Foundation: Exploring Symptoms and Experiences Associated with Aromatase Inhibitor Therapy in Women from the Northern Rockies Region

Mixed methods are used to explore the symptom patterns, quality of life (QOL), and personal experiences of female breast cancer survivors taking aromatase inhibitors (AIs); to identify individual characteristics that predict temporal patterns of change. We follow these women longitudinally through Aromatase Inhibitor therapy; conduct qualitative interviews when women choose to discontinue therapy. I serve as Co-Investigator and Lead Evaluator.

In: Palliative Care
Editor: Michael Silbermann

ISBN: 978-1-53616-199-1
© 2019 Nova Science Publishers, Inc.

Chapter 4

RESEARCH TOOLS AND APPROACHES TO REDUCE THE SUFFERING OF CANCER PATIENTS IN DEVELOPING COUNTRIES

Lidia Schapira[1],*, MD and Karl Lorenz[2], MD
[1]Cancer Survivorship Program at the Stanford Comprehensive Cancer Institute;
Medicine at Stanford University, Stanford, CA, US
[2]VA Palo Alto-Stanford Palliative Care Program;
Medicine at Stanford University, Stanford, CA, US

ABSTRACT

Finding solutions to the global challenge of providing timely and comprehensive palliative care requires a multipronged approach and a receptive and collaborative learning community. Great strides have been made in providing relief of pain in low resource settings through partnerships involving healthcare professionals and local authorities, through the implementation of incremental and culturally attuned interventions. The demonstration of efficacy of palliative interventions through research led professional societies to call for early incorporation of palliative care for patients with cancer in more affluent settings, such as the United States. Barriers to widespread implementation include the limited numbers of palliative care specialists and resistance among all sectors of the population including patients, administrators and healthcare professionals. A generalist approach to palliative care that incorporates incremental steps combined with research and advocacy, holds more promise for resource constrained settings.

Keywords: suffering, palliative, global, pain, solutions, research

---

* Corresponding Author's E-mail: schapira@stanford.edu.

GLOBAL AIM TO REDUCE SUFFERING

A young woman lay quietly in her bed in the oncology ward of the city's main teaching hospital. A large disfiguring mass protruded from her right cheek extending to her face and neck. She was receiving treatments to mitigate her pain. The doctor sat at the side of her bed and asked about her concerns. She spoke frankly about how worried and sad she was at the thought of leaving her children, and of all the complex emotions she felt when she thought how her death would affect them.

Although this scene took place in Gabarone, Botswana, one could easily imagine a similar scenario in Boston or London. A mother of young children is hospitalized for pain management resulting from advanced cancer, and a palliative medicine clinician, acting as consultant to the medical team explores her understanding of illness and sources of distress and supports her coping needs. At its heart, palliative care is an approach and practice that engages concerns of the whole person, and many of the fundamental quality of life-related concerns it addresses transcend geography and culture.

Palliative care relieves and prevents the suffering associated with serious illness. The pervasive impact of illness requires every clinician to master essential skills in palliative care. Effective palliative practice employs multidisciplinary approaches that are applied to cancer and other serious conditions, and its benefits embrace both individual patients and families, encompassing both illness and bereavement. Recent models suggest palliative care can be delivered in a cost-effective manner; rather than burdening health systems, palliative care can assist in matching care intensity to appropriate treatment opportunities.

Despite this simple goal and relatively uncomplicated construct, the fact remains that a large number of patients die in pain, especially in the poorest regions of the world, while others in more affluent countries suffer the consequences of overly aggressive and highly technical interventions in the last years or months of their lives. In both contexts, commercially and technologically focused care is pursued at the expense of human solutions and community-focused support. Palliative care calls for an equipoise in healthcare investment focused on the wellbeing of patients, families, and communities.

In this chapter we examine the nature of several common barriers that have time and again hindered the implementation of palliative care in both well-resourced and under-resourced settings. We also describe inspiring examples of successful initiatives built with idealism and resolve, using strategies that addressed the needs of a community and came up with solutions that were adapted to best utilize local resources.

REALIZING THE GOAL

The goal of relieving pain is historically central to the mission of medicine. Elizabeth Kubler Ross, in one of the foundational texts of palliative practice, On Death and Dying wrote in 1969, "Our goal should not be to have specialists for dying patients, but to train our hospital personnel to be comfortable in facing such difficulties…" (Kubler Ross). While there has been much emphasis in oncology on specialty palliative practice, we are reminded that the goal of relieving suffering is a central task for all clinicians.

In sub-Saharan Africa, which accounts for 12% of the world's population and has the world's highest mortality rates from communicable and non-communicable diseases, there are barriers to the most basic health care services (Stulac). In the case of oncology, many cancers are diagnosed at an advanced stage, and few are curable, so palliative care is urgently needed. More than 1 million people are estimated to die in pain in Africa each year, so that improving access to analgesic drugs is a global priority (O'Brien).

Uganda emerged at the top of the list among African countries that provide pain relief after South Africa, and provides an inspiring case study from which we can learn many valuable lessons. Uganda's success is largely due to the vision of Anne Merriman, a British palliative care specialist who founded Hospice Africa in Uganda (HAU) in 1992, to initiate and support palliative care for all of Africa following a feasibility study in 4 countries (O'Brien) Hospice Africa was established as a culturally acceptable model for hospice services that could be adapted to other countries.

Hospice Africa Uganda which celebrates 25 years of service in 2018, provided a model for holistic care that included pain control with oral morphine. Dr. Merriman's introduction of affordable oral morphine suitable for use in the home revolutionized dying in Africa. Oral morphine is reconstituted locally with imported morphine powder, water and preservative and food dye to show the strength of the formulation. Listed as an essential medicine by the World Health Organization, morphine is not protected by patent and can cost as little as U.S. $0.01 per milligram (Foley).

The Ministry of Health in Uganda expressed its support for this ambitious goal by including the provision of palliative care for non-communicable diseases in its mission statement and its Health Sector Strategic and Investment plan (O'Brien). Although access remains challenging, since 2004 the Ugandan Government provides free morphine to anyone, as long as it is prescribed by a registered prescriber. Recognizing a physician shortage, nurses can obtain training in palliative care through a certificate program and this enables them to prescribe morphine. An institute of HAU has trained over 10,000 health care professionals from various countries.

Presently, Merriman heads Hospice Africa's International Programs, supporting new initiatives in Tanzania, Nigeria, Cameroon, Sierra Leone, Malawi, Ethiopia, Zambia, Sudan and Rwanda, and more recently training others from 11 Francophone countries to suit their different health service and needs. 12 African countries have adopted the morphine reconstitution formula and 17 have access to some type of oral morphine.

Dr. Merriman's simple goal can be summarized briefly and specifically: *to provide palliative care for all.* From her powerful example we learn that implementation of this goal required not only a transformative vision, but also determination to work through multiple steps: identifying partners and obtaining their trust, working collaboratively to change cultural practices about something as fundamental as the care of dying patients and building the professional capacity to deliver this care to those who needed it most.

AMPLIFYING THE MESSAGE THROUGH RESEARCH

As we explored in the prior section, Dr. Merriman's vision and strategic approach led to a radical change in the approach to dying patients and the care of the terminally ill. In addition to the training of professionals, Merriman and her colleagues have influenced practice through academic publications that addressed the need to control pain, the impact of serious illness on families and caregivers and the role of volunteers in delivery of basic palliative care.

In a study led by Dr. James Cleary, researchers examined data on availability and accessibility of opioids for managing cancer pain in 25 African countries. They found that many countries had restricted formularies of opioids and even when opioids were on formulary they were often unavailable, thus limiting access by over-regulation (Cleary). By publishing their findings in a high impact journal, Cleary and others have drawn the attention of world relief organizations and world health policy bodies to the dire needs of those dying from cancer in Africa and other low resource settings.

Another important topic for discussion and research is the implementation of palliative services. There is agreement that the best models for delivery of care need to be tailored to meet the needs of the population at a local and regional level, so it is imperative to collect at least some data about the population of interest. In resource constrained settings there is widespread agreement that palliative care needs should be addressed in the community and integrated into primary care (Osman). These needs may be best addressed by healthcare professionals working collaboratively with community health workers and even trained volunteers. Merriman's research team conducted a qualitative study of community volunteers in Uganda. Understanding that the expansion of palliative care depended in large measure on the availability of volunteers, they evaluated the motivation for becoming a volunteer and the personal impact of the role. Using semi-structured individual and group interviews they sampled 43 volunteers and found that the cultural wish to help people was a key driver as well as a sense of pride (Jack). Hospice workers, whether trained volunteers or professionals, need to understand the challenges faced by informal caregivers in the home. Collaborating with international social scientists, the HAU team published a study of 62 caregivers. The most frequent areas of need reported were financial – including the need for free medication for patients and opportunities for income generation for caregivers, as well as the need for specific caregiver training (Emmanuel). The investigators demonstrated that caregivers faced financial and personal hardship, and proposed that hospices could train and also provide opportunities for paid employment.

In the examples given in the preceding paragraphs we note that qualitative research provided important knowledge that informed the design of future interventions as well as policy. The findings helped define and refine models of care, staffing requirements, roles and training needs of team members and patients and families in need of services, and the need for the availability of opioid analgesics to relieve pain and suffering. HAU provides an ideal setting for additional research focused on the evaluation of established practices that could inform the adoption and revision of its successful model.

DECONSTRUCTING CHALLENGES

More than twenty million people worldwide need palliative care at the end of life and this number doubles if one considers early integration of palliative care for patients and families struggling with a life-altering illness such as cancer. This may seem daunting, given well described and recognized challenges in providing access and the limited availability of trained palliative medicine professionals.

Palliative care can begin early in the course of treatment for any serious illness that requires management of pain, or other distressing symptoms. In countries with a robust infrastructure for health care services, deaths from cancer are not usually sudden, but more often occur as a consequence of a prolonged illness that was managed over months or years, through many ups and downs. These long trajectories of illness afford patients and doctors many opportunities to establish deep connections and to discuss a person's wishes for end of life care through a process often referred to as advance care planning.

In more affluent settings, palliative medicine specialist clinicians can play an important role as mediators of communication, especially in situations that are medically complex, both in inpatient and outpatient settings. With specialized training in communication skills, palliative care physicians and advance practice nurses routinely explore a patient's understanding of illness and prognosis, clarifying the goals of treatment through an iterative process designed to help a patient come to terms with concepts that are emotionally complex. Discussions of 'goals of care' is currently interpreted as conversations about the dying process and the clarification and documentation of a patient's preferences for or against aggressive interventions required to sustain life in the setting of an incurable illness such as advanced cancer.

The role of palliative medicine in improving the experience of dying patients received considerable attention in the lay press in recent years and is now more openly debated in public forums. A 2014 report published by the Institute of Medicine in the United States called for government and private payers and providers to ensure comprehensive care for individuals with advanced serious illness who are nearing the end of life (IOM report). The report stated that improved communication between doctors and patients and more engagement of patients in advance care planning would result in broader acceptance of palliative care, noting this would eventually lead to avoidance of expensive hospitalizations and use of intensive care in the final weeks and months of life.

The American Society of Clinical Oncology (ASCO) issued a practice guideline in 2017 endorsing the integration of early palliative care for patients with advanced cancer (Ferrell).The guideline defined palliative care as a medical subspecialty comparable to oncology, and defined the population in need as patients with solid tumors with distant metastases, patients with a prognosis of 6 to 24 months, and those newly diagnosed with metastatic cancer. ASCO's guideline reviewed the tasks associated with provision of palliative care and these include: building rapport and relationships with the patient and family caregivers; managing symptoms including distress; exploring the patient's understanding of illness and prognosis; clarifying the goals of treatment, supporting the patient's coping needs and helping with medical decision making and coordination of care. It is worth noting that the panel convened for the purpose of issuing this guideline was influenced by available evidence gathered through rigorous research, including randomized clinical trials. These were reviewed and are quoted in the body of the guideline as justification for the panel's recommendations.

As we reflect on the common goal of providing relief from suffering, it is interesting to contrast models of specialized palliative care for inpatients and outpatients receiving treatment for cancer in the US with those of a generalist approach to palliation that is more deeply rooted in primary care and employs informal caregivers and volunteers that has emerged in resource constrained settings. Interestingly, current research in more affluent settings is exploring novel approaches to expanding the palliative care workforce through training volunteers to act as mediators in communication, demonstrating the potential for learning from successful experiments across the globe (Patel).

LEARNING FROM PATIENTS AND PHYSICIANS

Dr. Elizabeth Kubler Ross emphasized the importance of creating an organizational culture that is compassionate and respectful. Many years later, Kenneth Schwartz, a healthcare lawyer and non-smoker diagnosed with advanced lung cancer in his early 40's, echoed her perspective in an essay published in The Boston Globe (Schwartz).

Schwartz wrote he recognized that in a high-volume setting, the atmosphere tends to

"stifle a caregiver's inherent compassion and humanity. But the briefest pause in the frenetic pace can bring out the best in a caregiver and do much for a terrified patient. I cannot emphasize enough how meaningful it was to me when caregivers revealed something about themselves that made a personal connection...If I have learned anything, it is that we never know when, how, or whom a serious illness will strike. If and when it does, each one of us wants not simply the best possible care for our body but for our whole being." (Schwartz)

Schwartz speaks for most cancer patients when he describes the therapeutic effect of being treated with kindness and compassion.

A compassionate professional culture needs to be supportive of clinicians whose emotional wellbeing is threatened by constant exposure to loss and suffering. Andrea Watson, a pediatric oncologist, described her lived experience of caring for a child with incurable cancer. In her published essay, "Let it be hard", Dr. Watson writes:

"Caring for Kelly during the final days of her life was exhausting, challenging, and at times frustrating, yet there is nowhere in the world that I would rather have been… the dying process is unpredictable, and the desire to alleviate suffering can be overwhelming. At a time when parents desperately want control, our offerings feel inadequate…It takes wisdom and perspective not to see these events as personal failure. It is hard, but it is rich. When we embrace the richness, we find humility and courage. Walking with our patients and their families during those final weeks, days, and moments is some of the most important work we do." (Watson JCO 2015)

Dr. Watson is clear: it is difficult. A compassionate culture needs to recognize: mission-driven work is as sustaining as the importance of supporting clinicians through interventions designed to improve self-awareness and self-care (Meier, Shanafelt).

Clinicians working in under-resourced settings describe additional sources of frustration that result in demoralization. Dr. Gevorg Tamamyan articulates these dilemmas in "The Road Home", a thoughtful essay that describes the story of a young patient with relapsed Hodgkin's lymphoma who struggled terribly in the last months of life (Tamamyan). Tamamyan explains that in his native Armenia, not only is it difficult to obtain new cancer treatments, but many patients suffer from intractable pain because morphine and other palliative medications are widely inaccessible. He writes that despite a few initiatives underway to improve access to opioids, the *"plight of our patients remains dire"*. *End-of-life services are still largely unavailable so that nearly all patients are sent home with inadequate care once disease-modifying therapy is no longer an option… The endless stream of calls from desperate families is excruciating. The lack of adequate palliative care in Armenia and many other developing countries condemns hundreds of thousands of vulnerable patients to unnecessary pain, anguish, and fear."*

These perspectives illustrate the importance of compassion in care, and illustrate important themes that require the attention of those actively engaged in building palliative care programs across the world. Compassionate practice is rooted in mission, but it can only thrive when clinicians feel supported and valued by the organizations they are part of and represent. The expansion and success of palliative medicine requires an organizational culture that is open, flexible and quick to respond to the changing needs of the community of patients that it serves.

SHARING SOLUTIONS

Thinking Outside of the Box

We have identified several important questions and challenges for palliative care clinicians, researchers, and policymakers. The establishment of a recognized specialty with a growing research portfolio has paved the way for 'demonstration' projects that contributed to the acceptance by colleagues and payers of healthcare services. Still, many remaining challenges require resolve and imagination. Interestingly, some critical challenges exist in both high as well as poorly resourced settings, and both settings have much to gain from innovation and collaboration.

One of the major challenges is the need to provide a clear and consistent message to the lay public about the role of palliation in the care of patients with advanced and incurable cancer. A constantly expanding therapeutic armamentarium naturally engenders hopes for cure and life extension, but the facts remains that many patients still die of cancer despite cutting edge anticancer treatments. Improving public awareness of palliative care was named as a priority by the United States Institute of Medicine in 2014, but it is also a crucial need internationally.

One fascinating example of a grass roots movement dedicated to improve advance care planning is "The Conversation Project". This project started in 2010, when Pulitzer Prize-winning writer Ellen Goodman and a group of colleagues and concerned media, clergy, and medical professionals gathered to share stories of "good deaths" and "hard deaths" within their own circle of loved ones. This grew into a public engagement initiative with a goal that is simple and transformative: to have every person's wishes for end-of-life care expressed and respected (The Conversation Project).

These advocates believe it is time to "transform our culture so we shift from not talking about dying to talking about it. It's time to share the way we want to live at the end of our lives. And it's time to communicate about the kind of care we want and don't want for ourselves." The Conversation Project and its website and toolkits guide individuals to begin this conversation at the kitchen table by stating their own wishes before it is too late.

Translating the Conversation Project and similar efforts, trying innovative approaches, and learning from success and failure can also inform increasingly multi-cultural societies where gaps and needs for improved end of life care typify diverse communities of color.

Expanding Capacity

Once we identify the value of a service we need to find a mechanism for making it available to those who can benefit. In addition to the example of Dr. Anne Merriman in Uganda, Dr. Sanjeev Aurora's ECHO program was conceptualized as a movement to demonopolize knowledge and amplify the capacity to provide best practice care for underserved people all over the world (Arora). Project ECHO aims to improve access to treatment for various conditions and has expanded recently to encompass palliative care. Palliative Care Always and the Palliative Care-Promoting Access and Improvement of the Indian Cancer Experience (PC-PAICE) offer other examples of using technology to meet palliative needs (Kiss-Lane).

Conclusion

Palliative care is a crucial component of health systems, and there are many examples of innovation in meeting the profound needs for palliative care in lower resourced settings. As the examples above show, there are important lessons to be drawn from efforts to improve palliative care in regions of the world that have few resources. Through an expansion of research we will identify best practices and identify mechanisms that will guide implementation across cultures and according to local practice and resources. However, the degree to which lower and higher resourced efforts share common challenges in striking, and the care of cancer patients will be abetted by a continuous dialogue and mutual learning across these settings.

References

Arora S, Geppert CM, Kalishman S et al. Academic health center management of chronic diseases through knowledge networks: Project ECHO. *Acad Med.* 2007 Feb; 82(2):154-60.

Arora S, Smith T, Snead J et al. Project ECHO: an effective means of increasing palliative care capacity. *Am J Manag Care.* 2017 Jun;23.

Cleary J, Powell RA, Munene G et al. Formulary availability and regulatory barriers to accessibility of opioids for cancer pain in Africa: a report from the Global Opioid Policy Initiative (GOPI). *Ann Oncol.* 2013 Dec; 24 suppl 11.

Dying in America, Improving Quality and Honoring Individual Preferences near the End of Life. *IOM,* 2015. https://www.nap.edu.

Emanuel RH, Emanuel GA, Reitshculer EB et al. Challenges faced by informal caregivers of hospice patients in Uganda. *J Palliat Med* 2008 June; 11(5):746-50.

Ferrell BR, Temel JS, Temin S et al. Integration of Palliative Care Into Standard Oncology Care: American Society of Clinical Oncology Clinical Practice Guideline Update. *J Clin Oncol.* 2017 Jan;35(1):96-112.

Foley KM, Wagner JL, Joranson DE et al. Pain Control for People with Cancer and AIDS. In: *Disease Control Priorities in Developing Countries.* 2nd Edition. Jamison DR, Bremna JG, MEasham AR, et al., editors. *Washington (DC). The International Bank for Reconstruction and Development/The World Bank.* New York: Oxford University Press: 2006.

Jack BA, Kirton JA, Birakurataki J et al. The personal value of being a palliative care Community Volunteer Worer in Uganda: a qualitative study. *Palliat Med* 2012 Jul;26(5):753-9.

Kiss-Lane T, Spruijt O, Day T, et al. Palliative care clinicians and online education in India: a survey. *BMJ Supportive & Palliative Care*. Published Online First: 09 October 2018. doi: 10.1136/bmjspcare-2018-00154.

Kubler-Ross, E. *On Death and Dying.* New York, Mc Millan Co, 1989.

Meier DE, Back AL, Morrison RS. The Inner Life of Physicians and care of the seriously ill. *JAMA* 2001 Dec 19; 286 (23): 3007-14.

O'Brien M, Mwangi-Powell F, Adewole IF et al. Improving access to analgesic drugs for patients with cancer in sub-Saharan Africa. *Lancet Oncolgy* 2013, Vol 14, e176-182.

Osman H, Shrestha S, Temin S. Palliative Care in Global Setting: ASCO Resource-Stratified Practice Guideline. *J Glob Oncol* 2018 Jul (4):1-24.

Patel M, Sundaram V, Desai M et al. Effect of a Lay Health Worker Intervention on Goals-of-Care Documentation and on Health Care Use, Costs, and Satisfaction among Patients with Cancer: A Randomized Clinical Trial. *JAMA Onc* 01 Oct 2018, 4(10):1359-1366.

Schwartz K. *A Patient's Story.* https://www.bostonglobe.com/magazine/1995/07/16/patient-story/q8ihHg8LfyinPA25Tg5JRN/story.html.

Stulac S, Binagwaho A, Tapela NM et al. Capacity building for oncology programmes in sub-Saharan Africa: the Rwanda experience. *Lancet Oncol.* 2015 Aug; 16(8):e405-13.

Tamamyan G. The Road Home. *J Clin Onc* 2018 Sept 20, 36 (27).

The Conversation Project. https://theconversationproject.org/about/ellen-goodman.

Watson AM. Let it be hard. *J Clin Onc* 2015 Sept 1, vol 33 (25), 2821-2822.

West CP, Dyrbye LN, Shanafelt TD. Physician burnout: contributors, consequences and solutions. *J Intern Med.* 2018 Jun; 283(6):516-529.

BIOGRAPHICAL SKETCHES

Dr. Lidia Schapira, MD

Dr. Lidia Schapira, MD, is a medical oncologist and Director of the Cancer Survivorship Program at the Stanford Comprehensive Cancer Institute and an Associate Professor of Medicine at Stanford University. Dr. Schapira is an active clinician with a specialty in breast cancer and an investigator in a cohort study based at the Dana Farber in Boston, MA, of young women with breast cancer. Dr. Schapira serves as Editor-in-Chief of the American Society of Clinical Oncology's website for the public, Cancer.Net and has a long record of advocacy and leadership in fostering interventions to improve the experience of patients and families with cancer through better communication with healthcare professionals. Dr. Schapira serves as editorial consultant to the Journal of Clinical Oncology and has participated in many volunteer and professional efforts to strengthen palliative care in resource constrained settings through the education of clinicians.

Dr. Karl Lorenz, MD MSHS

Dr. Karl Lorenz, MD MSHS is a general internal medicine and palliative care physician, and Section chief of the VA Palo Alto-Stanford Palliative Care Program and a Professor of Medicine at Stanford University. Dr. Lorenz is a member of the Veterans Adminstration's (VA) national Hospice and Palliative Care Program (HPC) leadership team, director of the operational palliative care Quality Improvement Resource Center (QuIRC), and adjunct facility staff member at RAND. Dr. Lorenz's work and leadership has been influential to the field of palliative care research. Under Dr. Lorenz's leadership, since 2009 the Quality Improvement Resource Center (QuIRC) has served as one of three national leadership Centers responsible for strategic and operational support of the VA's national hospice and palliative care programs. QuIRC develops and implements provider facing electronic tools for the VA's national electronic medical record to improve the quality of palliative care. In that role, Dr. Lorenz participates with the national leadership team in strategic planning, policy development, and providing resources to support operational efforts. Dr. Lorenz has contributed to the field of global palliative care, serving the World Health Organization in its development of Palliative Care for Older People and leading methods for Palliative Care Essential Medications.

In: Palliative Care
Editor: Michael Silbermann

ISBN: 978-1-53616-199-1
© 2019 Nova Science Publishers, Inc.

Chapter 5

INTEGRATING PALLIATIVE CARE IN NON-ONCOLOGIC PATIENT POPULATIONS: THE CASE FOR RENAL SUPPORTIVE CARE

Emily Lu[1,*] and Craig D. Blinderman[2]

[1]Division of Nephrology and Department of Geriatrics and Palliative Medicine,
Icahn School of Medicine at Mount Sinai, New York, NY, US
[2]Department of Medicine, Columbia University Medical Center, New York, NY, US

ABSTRACT

Despite growing recognition of the importance of Palliative Care integration in non-oncologic practice, development and implementation of concrete, reproducible programs remain limited. Through a step-wise conceptual approach, we describe a proposed framework for building subspecialty embedded Palliative Care models in non-oncologic care. By applying these principles to the field of Nephrology and Chronic Kidney Disease, we explore the key features and unique challenges encountered in creating a sustainable Renal Supportive Care model. These concepts subsequently provide a guide for advancing management of Palliative Care in chronic disease.

Keywords: renal supportive care, chronic kidney disease, palliative care, model

INTRODUCTION

Over the past decade, the field of Oncology has come to embrace the integration of Palliative Care for patients with advanced cancer through the development of new and innovative models of care. While initial studies focused more heavily on the impact of Palliative Care in alleviating distress of patients and families at the end of life (EoL), more recently, early integration of Palliative Care has developed as an increasingly prominent,

---

[*] Corresponding Author's E-mail: lu.emily@mssm.edu.

much-needed component of oncologic care that helps to provide supportive care needs in conjunction with chemotherapeutic and immunologic treatments throughout the course of illness.

As the emerging therapeutic options for many malignancies become increasingly adept at prolonging patient survival, the approach to cancer care must now also focus on addressing symptom management, quality of life (QoL), and goal-concordant approaches to treatment in order to provide comprehensive care to patients and families. Research has demonstrated improved outcomes in QoL, mood, symptom burden, prognostic understanding, and survival with early integration of Palliative Care in Oncology [1, 2, 3].

By logical extension, these Oncology Supportive Care outcomes have suggested a potential benefit of Palliative Care if applied to other specialties, most notably in chronic diseases such as chronic kidney disease (CKD) and heart failure, in which our current treatment and technologic advancements' ability to extend survival make not only living—but living *well*—a growing priority.

However, despite an increasing recognition of the need for Palliative Care in other non-oncologic specialties, the actual implementation of novel programs has been limited, not only due to the unique challenges and differences inherent to each specialty, but also because of the highly variable site- or center-specific resources that hinder the translation of these programs into replicable models.

How do we develop concrete, sustainable models that embed Palliative Care in other subspecialties?

We propose a step-wise conceptual approach to building a subspecialty embedded Palliative Care model, as follows: (1) Establish need for Palliative Care in the specific subspecialty, noting both key stakeholder concerns and specific areas of clinical need that may be more prominent than in other diseases (e.g., symptom management, hospice utilization); (2) Create a conceptual framework for subspecialty Supportive Care; (3) Identify and recognize disease-specific barriers, prognosis, and trajectory; (4) Understand strengths, weaknesses, and reproducibility of previous research interventions, implementation, or programs; (5) Identify and build upon key components of these prior studies; (6) Borrow, reframe, and reinvent strategies from other specialties or disciplines to make them applicable to this specific subspecialty model.

In this chapter, we aim to introduce Palliative Care through the lens of Nephrology, delving into the components critical to integrating Palliative Care into subspecialty care by looking specifically at the development of a reproducible Renal Supportive Care model.

ESTABLISHING THE NEED FOR RENAL SUPPORTIVE CARE: IS THERE A PALLIATIVE CARE "DEFICIENCY" IN NEPHROLOGY?

High Mortality Rate

One of the most challenging aspects of Nephrology care in the past decade has been addressing the aging population and the concomitant rise in number of individuals requiring advanced CKD care and dialysis. Currently, end stage renal disease (ESRD) affects greater than 700,000 individuals in the United States, 75% of which are treated with dialysis

(USRDS 2017). Of these patients, those age > 75 have the highest incident rates of initiating dialysis, closely followed by those age 65-74 years. Unfortunately, perhaps because dialysis is often viewed as a life-sustaining treatment, both clinicians and laypersons frequently fail to recognize that while dialysis can confer extended survival, it does not restore normal life expectancy, such that the life expectancy of dialysis patients in their 7th decade is approximately 1/3 that of the general population [4]. Thus, dialysis patients experience severely limited life expectancy after initiating long-term dialysis— approximately 50% of all patients are alive 3 years after the onset of ESRD (USRDS 2015). Survival is further diminished in the very elderly, with one study showing that one-year mortality for octogenarians and nonagenarians was 46% after dialysis initiation. In fact, dialysis mortality is at least comparable to—if not higher than—that of many types of cancer (USRDS 2017).

High Symptom Burden

Prior studies have led to an increasing recognition of significant symptom burden in patients with kidney disease, particularly those with advanced CKD or ESRD [6-9]. The majority of literature describes symptom burden in ESRD patients undergoing hemodialysis (HD) and at EoL, demonstrating high symptom burden associated with substantial impairment in health-related quality of life (HRQoL) [10-13].

For more than a decade, investigators have consistently established the marked prevalence of not only individually described symptoms in ESRD, but also the total range of symptoms experienced, with both the reported presence and moderate or severe intensity of symptoms well above 50% in multiple studies [14, 15]. Unsurprisingly, some of the most frequently reported symptoms include fatigue, pain, poor appetite, and pruritus; however, depression and anxiety are also common. Less frequently noted is that the magnitude of symptom burden in ESRD is comparable to that of cancer and other serious illnesses [16]. For example, one early systematic study showed that the number—eleven—and severity of both physical and mental symptoms were shared in both cancer and ESRD patients; fatigue, pain, and dyspnea were similarly present in > 50% of patients [17]. In addition, the estimated prevalence of depression in CKD and ESRD is approximately 20%, higher than for most chronic illnesses, including cancer [18]. Clearly, the prominent symptom burden experienced by ESRD patients should not be overlooked.

Although less is understood regarding the impact of high symptom burden in CKD 4 and 5 patients, a growing body of work suggests that symptom burden—both in terms of mean number (10.7) and severity—prevalence of depression, and poor QoL are also comparable in advanced CKD versus ESRD patients at baseline [19]. Furthermore, symptom burden and QoL may be similar for CKD 5 patients selecting non-dialysis care compared to ESRD patients managed with dialysis [13, 20, 21]. In a study comparing elderly (age > 70) CKD 4 and 5 patients selecting dialysis versus conservative management (non-dialysis care with palliative care), both groups experienced significant symptom burden, but those receiving conservative management experienced improved symptom scores over time [22].

The importance of this substantial symptom burden in advanced CKD and ESRD cannot be overemphasized. First, collectively, high symptom burden is known to negatively affect and significantly compromise all aspects of HRQoL in ESRD patients [23]. In a Canadian study of almost 600 patients measuring overall symptom burden and HRQoL, investigators identified independent predictors of both physical and mental HRQoL, including pain, tiredness, lack of well-being, depression, and shortness of breath [6]. Likewise, in a small pilot study conducted at a large, urban academic center, transplant-*in*eligible ESRD patients on HD—usually those of older age, multiple comorbid conditions, poor functional status, greater clinical complexity—also experienced greater symptom burden and decreased HRQoL across all domains compared to individuals who were transplant-eligible, suggesting that particular higher-risk subgroups may also be even more susceptible to the repercussions of insufficiently managed symptom burden [24].

Separately, individual symptoms such as pain and depression are also independently associated with decreased HRQoL. In fact, not only have several studies estimated that approximately 50% of CKD patients report presence of pain, but a recent large, scoping review of nearly 1000 studies confirmed that > 58% of CKD patients experience pain, of which 82% report as moderate to severe intensity [25]. Alarmingly, however, 74% of patients experienced ineffective pain management and 18% were believed to have multiple etiologies of pain. Similarly, multiple studies have shown that pain is inadequately treated in 75% of ESRD patients receiving dialysis [26-29]. Together, these findings suggest both a lack of awareness of the prevalence of pain in this population, as well as an underlying need for increased attention to pain management education for Nephrology clinicians.

Not only do these results indicate that management of symptoms in kidney disease patients has not been adequately addressed, but perhaps even more importantly, the consequences of these symptoms are inter-related and can have far-reaching consequences. For example, chronic pain in ESRD is associated with a multitude of effects, including: Reduced HRQoL; increased irritability and inability to cope with stress; increased perception of burden of disease; decreased perception of social support; and decreased life satisfaction [15, 25, 30, 31]. Specifically, moderate to severe pain (compared to mild or no pain) in ERSD patients is associated with a two-fold increase in the prevalence of both depression and insomnia, and an almost three-fold increase in withdrawal from dialysis [15]. Conversely, increased depression in ESRD is also associated with increased perception of pain, increased insomnia, and reduced HRQoL—all of which further compound their respective negative clinical effects on the patient [9, 19, 32]. Moreover, patients with advanced CKD have also identified focusing on symptom assessment and management as a priority in future research [33].

Ultimately, there is a significant cost associated with high symptom burden, not only to the patient, but also to the healthcare system. Pain and depression are both adversely associated with poor HRQoL, which in and of itself is of concern. However, pain and depression are also independently associated with poor outcomes including increased mortality, dialysis non-adherence (missed or abbreviated HD sessions), and health services utilization (Emergency department visits and hospitalizations) [34-39].

Thus, the need for improved symptom management in CKD and ESRD encompasses advancing assessment, diagnosis, and treatment approaches to alleviate both symptoms and sequelae.

Shared Decision Making and Advance Care Planning

It is now widely accepted that advanced CKD and ESRD patients require individualized decision-making processes to achieve goal-concordant care. Accordingly, Nephrology clinical practice guidelines also support the use of advance care planning (ACP) and shared decision-making, offering strategies and tools to better address patient and family wishes. The International Society of Nephrology (ISN) KDIGO consensus recommends shared decision-making and ACP as a key pillar in advancing kidney supportive care [7]. Similarly, the American Society of Nephrology (ASN) identifies shared decision-making as one of the top 5 priorities in its "Choosing Wisely" campaign and focuses on the role of Renal Palliative Care, including eliciting patients' goals and preferences; discussing prognosis prior to the initiation of chronic dialysis; and discussing expected benefits versus harms of dialysis within this context [40]. Similarly, the Renal Physicians Association (RPA) "Shared Decision-Making in the Appropriate Initiation of and Withdrawal from Dialysis" Clinical Practice Guideline offers recommendations for facilitating ACP and making decisions regarding withholding or withdrawing dialysis in appropriate clinical situations [41].

Furthermore, it is well known that dialysis patients and their families wish to be informed about treatment options and engage in ACP, relying largely on their nephrologists or physicians for medical information and guidance [42-44]. Regrettably, ACP appears to occur for only about 40% of CKD patients [42, 45]. In addition, there is a disparity between patient preferences for communication and nephrologists' clinical practice. An extensive survey of more than 580 patients with CKD Stage 4 or 5 or ESRD on dialysis showed that despite > 80% of respondents expressing that it is important to be informed about treatment options and at least 50% desiring EoL discussions with their nephrology providers, 90% had not discussed prognosis with their nephrologists and < 10% had had an EoL discussion with their nephrologist in the preceding year [42]. Even more jarringly, in this context, over 60% of patients regretted their decision to start dialysis, again emphasizing the need to re-examine our current approach to ACP and shared decision-making. This gap between patient and family wishes to engage in shared decision-making and the paucity of documented discussions is also seen in qualitative studies examining how Nephrology teams discuss ACP. As expected, one of the dominant themes elicited revealed that most patients and families welcomed the opportunity to discuss prognosis, life goals, and care options with their Nephrology providers; however, *no* patients or families reported actually discussing these issues [46]. For those patients with even greater comorbidity and limited functional status potentially limiting life expectancy on dialysis—for example, nursing home residents—multiple studies have additionally demonstrated that the documentation of any advance directives or treatment-limiting directives (used as an imperfect surrogate for ACP) remains persistently less for ESRD patients than for patients with other serious diseases over the past 10 years [47, 48]. These findings reinforce the concern that although most CKD and ESRD patients value the importance of ACP and believe it should begin early in the illness course, in practice, discussions rarely occur.

End of Life and Hospice Care

Since the early 2000s, we have long been aware that ESRD patients in the United States experience limited use of EoL care and hospice services. USRDS data from 2001-2002 showed that hospice services were dramatically underutilized in advanced CKD; not only was hospice referral infrequent and variable based on region, but it was uncommon even for patients who elected to withdraw from dialysis with very limited anticipated survival [49]. Of a two-year cohort of over 115,000 patients, only 13.5% used hospice, and of 21.8% who withdrew from dialysis, only 41.9% selected hospice. Of note, the utilization of hospice was significantly associated with decreased rate of death in hospital compared to non-hospice use (22.9% versus 69.0%), as well as an approximately 3-fold lower cost of patient care during the last week of life. These results subsequently prompted further analysis of EoL resource utilization in CKD.

However, in a widely quoted paper published several years later, the landscape of EoL and hospice care in ESRD remained unchanged. The investigators studied treatment intensity of older patients age > 65 receiving long-term dialysis during the final month of life based on Medicare and USRDS data between 2004-2007 and 2009 and compared these patterns with corresponding data for patients with cancer or heart failure [27]. They found that not only was the rate of hospice use (20.0%) in ESRD less than half that of cancer or heart failure, but the rates of ICU admission, intensive procedure use, and death in hospital were also very high—over two times greater in ESRD than in cancer or heart failure. Thus, there has been a discrepancy between focus of care for ESRD patients compared to those with other severe, life-limiting illnesses.

Currently, these trends in underutilization of hospice services coupled with higher treatment intensity appear to persist for kidney disease patients. Over the past decade, between 2000 and 2012, the frequency of use of invasive procedures in the last 6 months of life in ESRD patients has continued to rise; rates of artificial nutrition and tracheostomy placement have remained stable, but selection of mechanical ventilation and cardiopulmonary resuscitation has heightened [50, 51]. These more aggressive measures at EoL are also occurring in the context of decreased quality of EoL care in ESRD patients compared to those with other severe chronic illnesses. In a large Veterans Affairs study, ESRD patients had the lowest rates of Palliative Care consultation in the last 90 days of life; increased deaths in ICU; decreased deaths in inpatient hospice units; and fewer DNR orders at time of death [51]. Moreover, measures of family-reported quality of EoL care was also consistently lower in ESRD compared to other diseases. Thus, despite having some of the highest disease burden, ESRD patients continue to experience limited EoL and hospice care.

From a provider perspective, studies have also confirmed that clinicians similarly believe that needs for supportive and EoL care remain unmet for the ESRD population. In a recent survey conducted of dialysis center providers across the United States (including nephrologists, nurse practitioners, physician assistants, social workers, and dialysis center administrators), respondents identified "Bereavement support; spiritual support; and EoL discussions and planning among providers, patients, and family" as the top 3 areas of unmet need in dialysis units [52]. Given that patients, families, and providers recognize the need for greater focus on quality of EoL care, greater attention must be placed on addressing this disparity.

Generalist Level Palliative Care Skills and Education Opportunities

For over 15 years, the Nephrology community has progressively heard "a call to action" to address the gap in Palliative Care education in Nephrology training. However, little has changed with regard to either Palliative Care approaches and skills integrated into fellowship curricula, or to Nephrology fellows' self-perceived preparedness to care for patients at EoL.

In 2003, a group of investigators assessed the quality and quantity of Palliative Medicine in U.S. Nephrology fellowship programs, conducting a national survey of renal fellows to gain insight into the experiences and perceptions of these trainees regarding EoL training [53]. Overall, although about half of respondents believed that it was "very important" to learn how to care for dying patients, they reported receiving infrequent and significantly less teaching in Palliative and EoL care (for example, compared to managing distal renal tubular acidosis or hemodialysis therapy). Of all clinical areas, they felt least prepared to manage patients at EoL. Regarding communication skills, almost 1/3 of fellows had conducted 2 or less family meetings. However, fellows who had had some contact with Palliative Care specialists felt better educated on EoL topics and more prepared to provide this care.

A follow-up survey in 2013 sought to provide a closer look at updates in EoL training [54]. Compared to data from 2003, these findings revealed that despite a significant increase to 95% of respondents citing importance of providing EoL care, there remained both insufficient quantity and quality of teaching in EoL care, which had not significantly changed from a decade ago. Still, fellows agreed that introducing a Palliative Medicine rotation during fellowship would best improve their EoL education.

Similarly, another national survey of U.S. Nephrology fellows focusing specifically on the content and depth of their Palliative Care experience during training showed that 80% of fellowship programs did not offer formal training in Palliative Care despite the majority of respondents stating that a formal rotation in Palliative Care would be helpful [55].

In a recent small study of first-year Nephrology fellows in New York City looking at perceptions and practices regarding initiation of dialysis in elderly CKD patients (age > 75) compared to CKD patients in general, respondents were aware that the prognosis and outcomes may differ between groups. However, the direction of their responses was not uniform, suggesting that these distinctions did not translate into shared practice patterns [56].

In short, Nephrology trainees are not adequately trained to effectively identify and manage symptoms and EoL care in patients with advanced CKD and ESRD, nor do they feel prepared to undertake these issues. Given the well-established need to further symptom management, shared decision-making, and hospice and EoL planning—as described previously—improving Palliative Care education in Nephrology remains a major cornerstone of any attempts toward advancing CKD care.

CREATING A CONCEPTUAL FRAMEWORK FOR RENAL SUPPORTIVE CARE

Given the symptom burden, need for improved shared decision making and ACP, low rates of hospice use at the end of life, and limited education or exposure to palliative care among nephrologists, we can say that there is a deficiency of palliative care in this population. A Renal Supportive Care program may serve as the means to addressing these unmet needs among patients with advanced CKD and ESRD, and among their providers who care for them.

Renal Supportive Care can be regarded as a framework to introduce Palliative Care approaches to improve HRQoL for patients throughout the stages of CKD [7, 8, 57, 58]. Specifically, Renal Supportive Care is aimed at:

- Assessing, diagnosing, and treating both physical and emotional symptoms
- Aligning treatments with patients' goals through shared decision-making and ACP
- Sharing prognostication and understanding of anticipated illness trajectory
- Providing psychologic, spiritual, and family and social support
- Coordinating care amongst various treatment teams.

Of note, there are several important points to highlight in this context. First, Renal Supportive Care should not be misconstrued as encompassing only EoL or hospice care. It is intended not only for those with advanced CKD or ESRD, but also for patients in earlier stages of CKD. By moving access to Palliative Care upstream, the goal is to better guide patients toward goal-concordant treatment options and improve their quality of life, regardless of treatment choices. Secondly, Renal Supportive Care is provided together with therapies intended to prolong life—such as dialysis or transplantation—but may also include non-dialysis management. Thus, increasing patient access to Renal Supportive Care does *not* preclude their selection of other intensive treatments or life-sustaining measures, as long as the risks and benefits of these choices have been fully explored and understood by the patient. Lastly, a fully mature conceptualization of Renal Supportive Care encompasses an integrated model of both primary and specialty Palliative Care, as previously proposed by Quill and Abernathy [59]. Through gradual education and dissemination of core Palliative Care principles and skills to generalist clinicians and trainees, non-Palliative Care specialist Nephrology providers can begin to address basic symptom management and GOC conversations, while Palliative Care-trained Nephrologists can provide additional support in cases of refractory symptoms, inter-family or team conflicts, and other complex situations.

Having constructed the foundation for developing a Renal Supportive Care model, the next step is to closely examine the nuances of Nephrology care in advanced CKD, taking into account specific issues and challenges that might be encountered by patients, families, and clinicians.

WHY HAS RENAL SUPPORTIVE CARE BEEN SO CHALLENGING TO IMPLEMENT IN PRACTICE? RECOGNIZING NEPHROLOGY-SPECIFIC BARRIERS; IDENTIFYING GOALS

Despite consensus surrounding the potential benefits of Palliative Care approaches for patients with CKD and ESRD, limited data exists regarding modes of implementation. Although various institutions and centers have worked to create Renal Palliative Care programs, these initiatives remain either largely site- or clinician-specific, or highly resource-intensive, and thus have not been scaled.

Nephrology-specific barriers are likely playing a role in explaining the limited number of Renal Palliative Care programs. Perhaps most importantly, illness trajectory and prognosis are variable and difficult to predict in advanced CKD. Traditionally, if we consider the relative impact of various diseases on functional ability versus time of survival, we have a generalized view of patients with oncologic diseases (e.g., colon cancer) beginning at a fairly high functional status which is potentially sustained for a prolonged period of time, until disease burden acutely overwhelms this equilibrium and patients progress to death within a relatively short period of time. On the opposite end of the spectrum, patients with frailty and dementia start with low levels of functional ability at baseline, which gradually declines until death. In contrast, patients with ESRD or other chronic diseases (including congestive heart failure or chronic obstructive pulmonary disease) exhibit a third trajectory, such that they have an initially moderate functional status which inexorably declines over time, but is punctuated by intermittent marked declines in functional ability due to acute illness (e.g., dialysis-related infection, pneumonia, volume overload heart failure exacerbations) after which the patient never quite rebounds to his/her prior state of functional ability, until finally reaching death. More recently, however, in the growing era of non-dialysis management of advanced CKD, a fourth potential trajectory has emerged—studies have suggested that for CKD 5 patients undergoing non-dialysis care, although they may also begin with a moderate level of functional ability akin to that of ESRD patients, they may be actually be able to maintain this functional status for an extended period of time until the composite burden of uremia eventually results in death [60-63].

Prognostication in the setting of advanced CKD is additionally complicated by the fact that illness trajectory is largely impacted by the degree and severity of comorbid conditions, which are unique to each individual patient. For example, a patient with renal disease and concurrent malignancy may experience an illness trajectory that is markedly different from another patient with underlying dementia, depending on the relative contribution of other illness states to a patient's clinical condition.

Further exacerbating this conundrum is that for a subset of patients, their loss of renal function is so gradual that they often outlive their renal prognosis. This is particularly prominent in older adults with CKD, many of which may have stable renal function for many years [64-68]. Unfortunately, distinguishing these patients from those with more rapid rate of renal function decline can be difficult because such estimations assume linear reduction in estimated glomerular filtration rate and do not account for episodes of acute kidney injury or other clinical changes.

Various sources have proposed guidelines for use of validated prognostic tools and markers in the prevalent dialysis population to better anticipate survival. The RPA suggests that patients with 2 or more of the following are at high risk of poor outcomes with dialysis: Age over 75 years; high comorbidity index (e.g., Charlson Comorbidity Index); poor functional status or disability (e.g., Karnofsky Performance Status); and severe chronic malnutrition (e.g., serum albumin < 2.5g/dL) [41]. Other studies have demonstrated that patients with increased frailty, cognitive impairment, and falls are at higher risk of mortality, especially with advancing age [4]. Moreover, initiation of dialysis in older patients is associated with both decreased functional status and increased risk of falls leading to death [4, 69-73]. Models have been developed to help predict mortality for ESRD patients on hemodialysis, including the "Surprise Question" ("Would you be surprised if this patient died in the next 12 months?), REIN Prognosis Score (developed by the French Renal

Epidemiology and Information Network based on nine risk factors), and Integrated 6-month mortality tool (available on TouchCalc, incorporating the Surprise Question, age, albumin level, presence of dementia, and presence of PVD) [74-77]. However, for patients with advanced CKD deciding between treatment options, there are currently *no* tools available to predict survival with dialysis versus non-dialysis care.

When offering potential treatment options to patients with advanced CKD and ESRD, the ability to provide accurate or concrete prognostic information is also variable depending on the clinical scenario. For patients electing to withdraw from dialysis, survival after discontinuation of renal replacement therapy generally follows an anticipated trajectory; mean survival is approximately 1 week but can range from 0 - 46 days [79].This knowledge can provide patients and families with much-needed anticipatory guidance as they plan for what to expect in the coming days after dialysis withdrawal.

However, for CKD 5 patients contemplating dialysis initiation versus non-dialysis care, the relative benefit of dialysis therapy (i.e., prolonged survival weighed against possible disadvantages (e.g., vascular access surgeries, time spent in in-center hemodialysis units and on transportation, risk of repeated hospitalizations for infectious complications) may be less apparent, and again must be addressed in the context of patients' preferences, values, and goals. Nevertheless, it is now widely accepted in current literature that when compared to non-dialysis care, the survival advantage accrued from dialysis is *attenuated* by presence of elderly age, ischemic heart disease, frailty, poor functional status, and/or multiple comorbidities. In a landmark study conducted in 2007, investigators showed that when corrected for ischemic heart disease and high comorbidities, the survival advantage offered by dialysis was no longer statistically significant [78]. These results have subsequently been confirmed in several other studies, which additionally demonstrated a similar impact of decreased survival in elderly patients age > 75 years [22, 78-83]. In addition, those patients who selected dialysis treatment were also more likely to have significantly higher rates of hospitalization and death in hospital [80]. Therefore, greater understanding of the factors and influences that drive patients to select dialysis or non-dialysis care are needed to improve the shared decision-making process. In an ongoing qualitative study of CKD patients selecting non-dialysis care at a large, urban academic center in the United States, four emerging themes have been identified: (1) Choice of non-dialysis care remains ultimately fluid, provisional, or circumstance dependent—that is, although patients have currently selected non-dialysis care, there remain situations in which patients would still change their minds; (2) emphasis on importance of quality of life, as defined individually by each patient; (3) perception of current state of health as being good or acceptable—again, suggesting that if symptoms were to worsen, dialysis decision-making might fluctuate; and (4) gaps in knowledge of or discussion with Nephrologist regarding CKD care [84]. These themes provide further insight into the ongoing uncertainty that patients and families face, not only in dialysis decision-making, but also throughout the course of kidney disease progression.

Similar to patients with other serious or life limiting illnesses, uncertainty surrounding anticipated prognosis is a concern for clinicians and patients alike. The variability in CKD disease course can lead to a downward spiral effect: discomfort engaging in prognostic conversations with patients and families, who in turn are even more limited in their ability to anticipate their future clinical states and participate meaningfully in the shared decision-making process. Similar to other patients with advanced illness, nephrology patients' prognostic expectations affect treatment preferences and intensity, such that overly optimistic views of prognosis may lead to inappropriately aggressive treatment choices. This is perhaps best demonstrated in a study within the Veteran Affairs health system, in which ESRD patients on dialysis and their Nephrologists were asked to estimate 1- and 5-year survival and associated preferences for life-extending care [85]. The study revealed a marked discrepancy in anticipated prognosis; 81% of patients believed they had a > 90% 1-year likelihood of survival whereas their Nephrologists estimated only 25%, and only 6% of patients thought that they had a less than 50% chance of being alive at 5 years, when the actual survival was already 56% prior to 2-year follow-up. Furthermore, those patients who estimated greater survival were significantly more likely to elect life-extending care. Thus, our ability—or inability—to confer accurate prognoses can have far-reaching consequences for both patients and our healthcare system.

Compounding this issue of limited prognostic capability is our limited research on and knowledge of symptom management in advanced CKD. The generalizability of previous studies may be limited by differences in patient populations, cultural perceptions, and overall applicability of findings. The majority of these studies were conducted in the UK, Canada, or Australia. There are very few studies from the United States describing symptom burden and HRQoL in patients with advanced CKD, particularly those not receiving dialysis [19]. Currently, at least 8 validated global symptom assessment tools exist for use in CKD and ESRD patients [25]. However, these survey instruments are often extensive and of varying utility, making them better suited for research purposes than for use in clinical settings. In addition, symptom burden has not been assessed across the spectrum of CKD patients, i.e., CKD 3 to 5, using the same assessment tools. Furthermore, not only do few large-scale, randomized controlled trials exist to test for effectiveness of suggested interventions or treatments for symptoms such as pain or depression, but our ability to provide improved management options in advanced CKD are thus limited. A recent study of pharmacologic management of depression showed that despite frequent use of SSRIs in ESRD, use of Sertraline in CKD 3 to 5 non-dialysis patients demonstrated no significant difference in depression scores, suggesting that Sertraline may not be an effective treatment in non-dialysis-dependent CKD [86]. As a result, even when patients' symptoms are adequately assessed, clinicians may not have compelling strategies for treatment in advanced CKD.

As discussed previously, Nephrology providers receive little or no training in Palliative Care approaches to symptom management or communication skills, thereby adding an additional layer of uncertainty to any discussion of CKD management.

Finally, system-level factors—including the health care system, culture of medicine, and societal culture—further augment the challenges of dialysis decision-making. Nephrologists in both the United States and England shared that major barriers to foregoing or withdrawing dialysis were lack of EoL and prognostication training, perceived difficulty of initiating these conversations, and public or cultural expectations for aggressive treatments [87]. From a policy perspective, our current health care delivery model for advanced CKD and ESRD is also heavily based on dialysis practice, resulting in lack of measures focusing on ACP and presence of disincentives to incorporate or provide access to Palliative Care [88]. These system-level barriers then impede growth of programs or initiatives intended to expand the culture of dialysis decision-making in the United States.

In sum, barriers and uncertainty exist on multiple levels throughout advanced CKD care:

- Illness trajectory and prognosis are variable and difficult to predict

- Knowledge of symptom burden and methods for providing effective management are limited
- Nephrology providers receive little training in Palliative Care principles, symptom management, and communication techniques
- System-level barriers further impede communication between providers and patients and families and limit available resources.

By acknowledging and understanding the various Nephrology-specific challenges to implementing change in the context of advanced CKD care, we are better equipped to recognize how we may adapt clinical practice, communication techniques, and provider or patient perceptions to create a successful Renal Supportive Care model.

IDENTIFYING PRIOR RESEARCH INTERVENTIONS AND EXISTING PROGRAMS THAT CAN PROVIDE FURTHER INSIGHT INTO THE IMPLEMENTATION OF A RENAL SUPPORTIVE CARE MODEL

In order to create an embedded Palliative Care model, what types of innovations or programs are most instructive and best suited to actualize this goal? Here, we highlight some of the most robust or thought-provoking interventions in the field of Nephrology and Palliative Care to date, focusing on their specific strengths, weaknesses, and potential reproducibility.

Routine Palliative Care for CKD Patients Managed without Dialysis can Provide Stable Symptom Burden and QoL

In 2015, Brown et al. introduced the first interventional study integrating Palliative Care into the routine care of patients with advanced CKD managed without dialysis through the development of a "Renal Supportive Care Clinic" [22]. In this landmark prospective trial, 273 pre-dialysis patients receiving usual Nephrology care and 122 non-dialysis patients receiving Palliative Care through the Renal Supportive Care Clinic underwent survey measurement of symptom burden and QoL over 12 months. Although it is important to note that non-dialysis patients were on average of older age and had a greater number of symptoms and poorer QoL at baseline, there was no difference in the proportion of patients in either group with stable or improved outcomes.

However, there are several important caveats to this study. First, this model was developed in Australia, and may not be entirely applicable to the culture and demographics of CKD patients in other countries or settings. Secondly, the findings reported represent work accumulated over approximately a decade, during which shifts in patient and provider attitudes toward non-dialysis care may also have had an impact. Like many other interventional studies, the investigators sought to introduce the concept of Palliative Care but did not provide a structured format for how symptoms were managed or conversations were conducted in the Renal Supportive Care Clinic, such that the reproducibility of the overall intervention may also be limited. Lastly, in this study, Palliative Care was provided *only* for those patients selecting non-dialysis care pathway, which does not coincide with our current concept of Renal Supportive Care as an approach encompassing kidney disease care regardless of stage or treatment modality. Nevertheless, this study essentially proved that by integrating routine Palliative Care in CKD management, symptoms and QoL could be managed effectively for advanced CKD patients selecting non-dialysis care.

Embedded Palliative Care Consultation Can Increase Rate of Consults, Improve Symptoms, and Increase ACP for Dialysis Patients

As demonstrated in Oncology Supportive Care models, creating an embedded Palliative Care clinic has been thought to contribute to multiple positive outcomes. Likewise, Feely et al. described a pilot study conducted at the Mayo Clinic, in which more than 90 patients received outpatient Palliative Medicine consultation [89]. Through the use of an embedded structure (i.e., geographically on-site with Nephrology), the rate of Palliative Care consultation increased to 98% and patients experienced statistically significant improvements in symptom assessment scores and increased documentation of code status and goals of care. Although there was no control (i.e., non-embedded) group in this study and patient symptoms are already well-controlled prior to the intervention—making the small but statistically significant improvements of questionable clinical relevance—the study confirmed that co-localization of outpatient specialty and Palliative Care can yield improved outcomes.

Regular Symptom Assessment for Dialysis Patients May Improve Symptoms

In a prospective, multi-center, cluster randomized effectiveness trial, investigators at the University of Pittsburgh suggested that routine symptom assessment—regardless of management by physician- or nurse-led strategies—can result in better symptom management [90]. They compared 220 patients randomized to either a physician feedback or nurse management arm over a 12-month intervention phase, comparing effects on pain, erectile dysfunction, and depression. In general, both groups demonstrated statistically significant improvements in symptom scores, although it is unclear if these results were also clinically significant. Thus, ongoing, routine assessment may aid in providing better symptom management over time.

Intensified Renal Palliative Care for Advanced CKD Can Decrease Symptoms, Emergency Department and Acute Hospital Admissions

Despite its limited generalizability as a small pilot study in Hong Kong, Chan et al. showed that for 19 high-risk CKD 5 patients—defined by the trigger of more than 1 emergency department visit within 3 months—enrollment in an intensified, multidisciplinary "Renal Palliative Care Clinic" of nurses, social workers, and clinical psychologists with frequent, up to weekly follow-up resulted in a significant decrease in symptoms, emergency department attendance, and acute hospital admissions [91]. Unfortunately, given the high resource utilization, this model may not be advisable for many centers. However, it suggests that identifying certain high-risk subgroups with targeted measures or triggers may help allocate resources to these patients who may benefit substantially from closer follow-up.

Inpatient Palliative Care Consultation Improves Symptoms in Renal Disease Patients

To better evaluate the value of Palliative Care consultations in the inpatient (hospital) setting for kidney disease patients, Grubbs et al. reported results from a large observational study of data collected by the Palliative Care Quality network at multiple hospitals and states in the U.S [92]. From a cohort of over 33,000 patients, they found that the 3.2% of patients with renal disease as the primary reason for consultation exhibited similar symptom improvement with Palliative Care consultation as that of patients with other illnesses. In fact, anxiety was even more frequently improved in patients with kidney disease compared to other conditions. As expected, then, inpatient Palliative Care consultation is likely to alleviate symptom burden in CKD and ESRD patients, although again the specific management strategies must be clarified.

Educating Renal Supportive Care Teams May Increase Hospice Utilization in Dialysis Patients

Dialysis providers can face particular challenges in caring daily for patients at risk of high mortality while also having limited familiarity with EoL and hospice care options. In an early study, Cohen et al. designed a longitudinal, prospective cohort pilot study of 5 dialysis units (assigned to intervention versus control) to assess the development of a specialized Renal Supportive Care team that would encourage participation in ACP and provide information regarding hospice services [93]. Dialysis staff—including social workers, nurses, and some physicians—received education about hospice, Palliative Care, and EoL issues via a 1-day training program. After following patients for 17 months, investigators found that hospice services increased at sites utilizing these Renal Supportive Care teams, particularly for patients age >65. Interestingly, these Renal Supportive Care team members were mainly organized on a volunteer basis, suggesting bias towards providers who were already engaged in learning more about Palliative Care approaches. Regardless, this pilot study offers a promising example of how education of Nephrology staff can implement change.

A Novel ACP Intervention for Dialysis Patients and their Surrogates May Increase Preparedness for EoL Decision-Making

In a novel study spanning several years, Song et al. devised a well-designed protocol to both (1) educate Nephrology team members through a 3 1/2-day training program to ensure competency in communication skills and EoL care for ESRD patients; and (2) conduct ACP conversations with dialysis patients and their surrogates through a structured intervention guide [94]. Entitled "SPIRIT," this randomized controlled ACP intervention consisted of multiple sessions with dialysis patients and surrogates to help increase preparedness for EoL decision-making [95]. As a result of this intervention, they reported increased patient-surrogate congruence on goals of care; increased surrogate decision-making confidence; and decreased bereavement outcomes of surrogate anxiety, depression, and post-traumatic distress at 3 to 6 months after patient death. In order to translate this study into clinical practice, dedicated time for education and training of Nephrology team members would be necessary to achieve the desired level of proficiency; however, this study presents a feasible and reproducible method of improving ACP in ESRD.

Early Exposure to Palliative Care in Nephrology Training May Increase Preparedness for Future Conversations

In response to a growing interest in developing Palliative Care education and curricula in Nephrology fellowship, Schell et al. created "NephroTalk," a 4-hour communication skills workshop centered around teaching Nephrology trainees to deliver bad news, express empathy, explore and define patient goals of care, and elicit EoL preferences in the context of dialysis initiation and withdrawal [96]. Based on the structure of VitalTalk and using simulated patient and family members, this program demonstrated significantly increased preparedness of respondents in all core areas. Despite its success as a novel communication strategy, however, its relatively time- and resource-intensive design and need for dissemination through prior attendees may make it difficult to employ as a widespread approach.

Future and Ongoing Interventions

Over the next several years, ongoing research may be able to provide further much-anticipated insight into the development of innovative communication interventions and ambulatory models of Renal Supportive Care in the United States [97, 98]. Until then, the previously described studies portray valuable lessons in the implementation of Renal Supportive Care.

SELECTING KEY ELEMENTS FROM PREVIOUS STUDIES TO BUILD A CORE MODEL OF RENAL SUPPORTIVE CARE

Previous work by investigators in the United States, England, Australia, and Asia has helped to define a set of key elements that are most likely to contribute to a successful Renal Supportive Care model.

1. **Co-localized, "embedded," interdisciplinary Renal Supportive Care teams:** By creating a geographical identity linking Palliative Care specialists to Nephrology providers—physicians, nurses, dialysis providers, social workers, administrators—

we are able to build greater cross-dissemination of learning, increasing knowledge of both approaches to symptom management and communication techniques, as well as of the nuances and considerations specific to renal care. Furthermore, patients are more likely to receive Palliative Care consultation and benefit from expertise of the interdisciplinary team.

2. **Regular symptom assessment using validated tools:** By assessing patients' symptoms longitudinally over time—as an integral part of Routine Palliative Care—we create the opportunity not only to improve patients' symptom experience and HRQoL, but just as importantly, Nephrology providers are provided insight into individual patients' illness trajectory and anticipated prognosis (e.g., Is fatigue becoming acutely more prominent, suggesting more rapid loss of renal function?). In concert with these findings, patients' symptoms may also allow them insight into their own care goals, values, and preferences as the disease progresses (e.g., Is the ongoing pain—despite treatment—associated with dialysis and procedures compatible with my wishes for "good" or "acceptable" quality of life?). Together, regularly assessing and treating symptom burden can thereby lead to further conversations about care options, improve shared decision-making between patients, families, and their providers, and increase goal-concordant care.

3. **Upstream, targeted engagement in CKD care:** As demonstrated in prior studies, through identification of subgroups of patients who may benefit most from early and/or intensified access to Renal Supportive Care, we can offer stable or even improved symptom management and HRQoL. While Palliative Care is intended to accompany CKD patients throughout the spectrum of disease progression, triggers such as increased emergency room visits or hospital admissions may help risk-stratify those who may be most susceptible to uncontrolled symptoms and inadequate ACP.

4. **Routine prognostication and ACP throughout the disease course:** Like regular symptom assessment, a standardized approach to providing prognosis and discussing ACP can begin to minimize the difficulty of broaching these topics when patients are either clinically worsening or acutely ill. By normalizing these conversations and making them a routine part of advanced CKD care, patients and families are likely to experience greater preparedness to have EoL discussions.

5. **Structured communication training for Nephrology providers:** Patients frequently look to their Nephrologists for guidance regarding recommended treatments and care options. However, few Nephrologists have formal training in communication skills. Studies have indicated that conducting these ACP interventions is both teachable and replicable for Nephrology providers. It follows that by using these existing structured, formalized series of training modules and lectures from prior studies—or perhaps developing new materials—Nephrology providers can better guide patients as a part of the Renal Supportive Care team.

6. **Early exposure to Palliative Care in Nephrology training:** Nephrology fellowship programs typically offer very limited opportunities to gain exposure to Palliative Care, resulting in misconceptions or delayed understanding about the role of Renal Supportive Care. In order to further practice change, it is imperative for Nephrology trainees to have access to learning of Palliative Care principles and approaches, whether through rotation with specialist services or via training programs such as

NephroTalk. By integrating Palliative Care into core curricula of Nephology training programs, we can begin to resolve some of the uncertainty surrounding providers' comfort with providing symptom management and discussing shared decision-making.

7. **Advancing research in Renal Supportive Care:** One of the major impediments to developing a Renal Supportive Care model is the lack of evidence-based research in Nephrology and Palliative Care. Compared to other serious illness areas such as Oncology or Cardiology and heart failure, Nephrology has relatively scarce large-scale trials investigating either interventions or models for integrating Palliative Care approaches in clinical practice. Although several important studies were highlighted above, there is still very limited high-quality data with which we can construct even components of a reproducible model. Therefore, incorporating well-defined protocols and pathways for the implementation of Renal Supportive Care in future research will be essential to moving the field forward.

BORROWING FROM OUR COLLEAGUES: TRANSFORMING STRATEGIES FROM OTHER DISCIPLINES TO INCORPORATE NOVEL APPROACHES INTO A RENAL SUPPORTIVE CARE MODEL

By thinking beyond the immediate realm of Nephrology and Palliative Care, we also find innovative approaches from other specialties that can be translated into a Renal Supportive Care model.

At our own academic institution in the United States, the generalist Palliative Care team has incorporated the use of the "Best Case/Worst Case" communication framework initially introduced by surgeons to aid in decision-making conversations [99]. It has quickly become apparent that by providing a pictorial representation of most extreme and most likely outcomes in a given clinical scenario, both patients and clinicians are better equipped to comprehend potential implications for their functional status, survival, and other factors that may affect their expectations for achieving goal-concordant care [100]. Adapted for an advanced CKD audience, this tool would thus be able to provide prognostic information about likely outcomes and possible alternatives in the complex decision-making processes surrounding dialysis care.

In the area of Cardiology, our ICU-based Palliative Care team has developed new tools to advance both prognostic awareness and ACP. Using a semi-structured script, all patients eligible for left ventricular assist device (LVAD) therapy at our center underwent a conversation (PreVAD evaluation) designed to assess patient comfort, explore patient and family understanding of LVAD and its potential complications and benefits, and perhaps most importantly, elicit further information regarding any condition(s) which would be unacceptable to the patient [101]. Correspondingly, a "Pre-Dialysis" semi-structured script could be employed with the same aims, thereby giving not only Nephrology providers, but also patients and their families, more concrete understanding of how a similarly life-sustaining treatment—dialysis—might contribute to their current and future state of health.

In addition to focusing on physician trainee learning in Palliative Care, we have created an Interdisciplinary Palliative Care Resource Champion (IPRC) Program at our institution, introducing a year-long curriculum of Palliative Care training to nurses, nurse practitioners, physician assistants, and social workers [102]. Through lectures and interactive discussions, our goal is to provide primary Palliative Care skills that can subsequently become the foundation for improving patient-centered care. By translating this program to a Nephrology-focused context, renal interdisciplinary providers—central to the implementation of Renal Supportive Care—may also gain knowledge and techniques that help to advance CKD care.

IDENTIFYING AND BRIDGING THE GAPS: THE FUTURE OF THE SUBSPECIALTY-EMBEDDED PALLIATIVE CARE MODEL

Through this in-depth exploration of the conceptual development of a Renal Supportive Care model, we draw upon key principles in creating an integrated, non-oncologic subspecialty Palliative Care program, carefully examining the dominant features and challenges unique to the individual subspecialty. Using this proposed framework, consisting of educational and clinical interventions, we hope to advance and expand the role of Palliative Care in the support and management of other chronic diseases.

REFERENCES

[1] Bakitas, M; Lyons, KD; Hegel, MT; Balan, S; Brokaw, FC; Seville, J; Hull, JG; Li, Z; Tosteson, TD; Byock, IR; Ahles, TA. Effects of a palliative care intervention on clinical outcomes in patients with advanced cancer: the Project ENABLE II randomized controlled trial. *JAMA.*, 2009, Aug 19, 302(7), 741-9.

[2] Temel, JS; Greer, JA; Muzikansky, A; Gallagher, ER; Admane, S; Jackson, VA; Dahlin, CM; Blinderman, CD; Jacobsen, J; Pirl, WF; Billings, JA; Lynch, TJ. Early palliative care for patients with metastatic non-small-cell lung cancer. *N Engl J Med.*, 2010, Aug 19, 363(8), 733-42.

[3] Zimmermann, C; Swami, N; Krzyzanowska, M; Hannon, B; Leighl, N; Oza, A; Moore, M; Rydall, A; Rodin, G; Tannock, I; Donner, A; Lo, C. Early palliative care for patients with advanced cancer: a cluster-randomised controlled trial. *Lancet.*, 2014, May 17, 383(9930), 1721-30.

[4] Koncicki, HM; Schell, JO. Communication Skills and Decision Making for Elderly Patients with Advanced Kidney Disease: A Guide for Nephrologists. *Am J Kidney Dis.*, 2016 Apr, 67(4), 688-95.

[5] Kurella, M; Covinsky, KE; Collins, AJ; Chertow, GM. Octogenarians and nonagenarians starting dialysis in the United States. *Ann Intern Med.*, 2007 Feb, 6, 146(3), 177-83.

[6] Davison, SN; Jhangri, GS. Impact of pain and symptom burden on the health-related quality of life of hemodialysis patients. *J Pain Symptom Manage.*, 2010 Mar, 39(3), 477-85.

[7] Davison, SN; Levin, A; Moss, AH; Jha, V; Brown, EA; Brennan, F; Murtagh, FE; Naicker, S; Germain, MJ; O'Donoghue, DJ; Morton, RL; Obrador, GT. Kidney Disease: Improving Global Outcomes. Executive summary of the KDIGO

Controversies Conference on Supportive Care in Chronic Kidney Disease: developing a roadmap to improving quality care. *Kidney Int.*, 2015 Sep, 88(3), 447-59.

[8] Kane, PM; Vinen, K; Murtagh, FE. Palliative care for advanced renal disease: a summary of the evidence and future direction. *Palliat Med.*, 2013 Oct, 27(9), 817-21.

[9] Kimmel, PL; Emont, SL; Newmann, JM; Danko, H; Moss, AH. ESRD patient quality of life: Symptoms, spiritual beliefs, psychosocial factors, and ethnicity. *Am J Kidney Dis*, 42, 713-721, 2003.

[10] Almutary, H; Bonner, A; Douglas, C. Symptom burden in chronic kidney disease: a review of recent literature. *J Ren Care.*, 2013 Sep, 39(3), 140-50.

[11] Flythe, JE; Powell, JD; Poulton, CJ; Westreich, KD; Handler, L; Reeve, BB; Carey, TS. Patient-Reported Outcome Instruments for Physical Symptoms among Patients Receiving Maintenance Dialysis: A Systematic Review. *Am J Kidney Dis.*, 2015 Dec, 66(6), 1033-46.

[12] Jablonski, A. The multidimensional characteristics of symptoms reported by patients on hemodialysis. *Nephrol Nurs J.*, 2007 Jan-Feb, 34(1), 29-37, quiz 38.

[13] Murtagh, FE; Addington-Hall, JM; Edmonds, PM; Donohoe, P; Carey, I; Jenkins, K; Higginson, IJ. Symptoms in advanced renal disease: a cross-sectional survey of symptom prevalence in stage 5 chronic kidney disease managed without dialysis. *J Palliat Med.*, 2007 Dec, 10(6), 1266-76.

[14] Murtagh, FE; Addington-Hall, J; Higginson, IJ. The prevalence of symptoms in end-stage renal disease: a systematic review. *Adv Chronic Kidney Dis.*, 2007 Jan, 14(1), 82-99.

[15] Davison, SN; Jhangri, GS. The impact of chronic pain on depression, sleep, and the desire to withdraw from dialysis in hemodialysis patients. *J Pain Symptom Manage.*, 2005 Nov, 30(5), 465-73.

[16] Kelley, AS; Morrison, RS. Palliative Care for the Seriously Ill. *N Engl J Med.*, 2015, Aug 20, 373(8), 747-55.

[17] Solano, JP; Gomes, B; Higginson, IJ. A comparison of symptom prevalence in far advanced cancer, AIDS, heart disease, chronic obstructive pulmonary disease and renal disease. *J Pain Symptom Manage.*, 2006 Jan, 31(1), 58-69.

[18] Palmer, S; Vecchio, M; Craig, JC; et al. Prevalence of depression in chronic kidney disease, Systematic review and meta-analysis of observational studies. *Kidney International*, (2013a), 84, 179–191.

[19] Abdel-Kader, K; Unruh, ML; Weisbord, SD. Symptom burden, depression, and quality of life in chronic and end-stage kidney disease. *Clin J Am Soc Nephrol.*, 2009 Jun, 4(6), 1057-64.

[20] Noble, H; Meyer, PJ; Bridge, DJ; Johnson, DB; Kelly, DD. Exploring symptoms in patients managed without dialysis: a qualitative research study. *J Ren Care.*, 2010 Mar, 36(1), 9-15.

[21] O'Connor, NR; Kumar, P. Conservative management of end-stage renal disease without dialysis: a systematic review. *J Palliat Med.*, 2012 Feb, 15(2), 228-35.

[22] Brown, MA; Collett, GK; Josland, EA; Foote, C; Li, Q; Brennan, FP. CKD in elderly patients managed without dialysis: survival, symptoms, and quality of life. *Clin J Am Soc Nephrol.*, 2015, Feb 6, 10(2), 260-8.

[23] Soni, RK; Weisbord, SD; Unruh, ML. Health-related quality of life outcomes in chronic kidney disease. *Curr Opin Nephrol Hypertens.*, 2010 Mar, 19(2), 153-9.

[24] Berman, N; Christianer, K; Roberts, J; Feldman, R; Reid, MC; Shengelia, R; Teresi, J; Eimicke, J; Eiss, B; Adelman, R. Disparities in symptom burden and renal transplant eligibility: a pilot study. *J Palliat Med.*, 2013 Nov, 16(11), 1459-65.

[25] Davison, SN; Koncicki, H; Brennan, F. Pain in chronic kidney disease: a scoping review. *Semin Dial.*, 2014 Mar, 27(2), 188-204.

[26] Moss, AH. Integrating Supportive Care Principles into Dialysis Decision Making: A Primer for Palliative Medicine Providers. *J Pain Symptom Manage.*, 2017 Mar, 53(3), 656-662.

[27] Wong, SP; Kreuter, W; O'Hare, AM. Treatment intensity at the end of life in older adults receiving long-term dialysis. *Arch Intern Med*, 2012, 172, 661e663, discussion 3e4.

[28] USRD System. 2015 USRDS annual data report: Epidemiology of kidney disease in the United States. Bethesda, MD: *National Institutes of Health, National Institute of Diabetes and Digestive and Kidney Diseases*, 2015.

[29] Wong, SP; Kreuter, W; O'Hare, AM. Healthcare intensity at initiation of chronic dialysis among older adults. *J Am Soc Nephrol*, 2014, 25, 143e149.

[30] Davison, SN. Pain in hemodialysis patients: prevalence, cause, severity, and management. *Am J Kidney Dis.*, 2003 Dec, 42(6), 1239-47.

[31] Koncicki, HM; Unruh, M; Schell, JO. Pain Management in CKD: A Guide for Nephrology Providers. *Am J Kidney Dis.*, 2017 Mar, 69(3), 451-460.

[32] Weisbord, SD; Fried, LF; Arnold, RM; Fine, MJ; Levenson, DJ; Peterson, RA; Switzer, GE. Prevalence, severity, and importance of physical and emotional symptoms in chronic hemodialysis patients. *J Am Soc Nephrol.*, 2005 Aug, 16(8), 2487-94.

[33] O'Hare, AM; Armistead, N; Schrag, WL; Diamond, L; Moss, AH. Patient-centered care: an opportunity to accomplish the "Three Aims" of the National Quality Strategy in the Medicare ESRD program. *Clin J Am Soc Nephrol.*, 2014, Dec 5, 9(12), 2189-94.

[34] Weisbord, SD; Mor, MK; Sevick, MA; Shields, AM; Rollman, BL; Palevsky, PM; Arnold, RM; Green, JA; Fine, MJ. Associations of depressive symptoms and pain with dialysis adherence, health resource utilization, and mortality in patients receiving chronic hemodialysis. *Clin J Am Soc Nephrol.*, 2014, Sep 5, 9(9), 1594-602.

[35] Farrokhi, F; Abedi, N; Beyene, J; Kurdyak, P; Jassal, SV. Association between depression and mortality in patients receiving long-term dialysis: a systematic review and meta-analysis. *Am J Kidney Dis.*, 2014 Apr, 63(4), 623-35.

[36] Harris, TJ; Nazir, R; Khetpal, P; Peterson, RA; Chava, P; Patel, SS; Kimmel, PL. Pain, sleep disturbance and survival in hemodialysis patients. *Nephrol Dial Transplant.*, 2012 Feb, 27(2), 758-65.

[37] Hedayati, SS; Bosworth, HB; Briley, LP; Sloane, RJ; Pieper, CF; Kimmel, PL; Szczech, LA. Death or hospitalization of patients on chronic hemodialysis is associated with a physician-based diagnosis of depression. *Kidney Int.*, 2008 Oct, 74(7), 930-6.

[38] Hedayati, SS; Minhajuddin, AT; Afshar, M; Toto, RD; Trivedi, MH; Rush, AJ. Association between major depressive episodes in patients with chronic kidney disease and initiation of dialysis, hospitalization, or death. *JAMA.*, 2010, May 19, 303(19), 1946-53.

[39] Lopes, AA; Bragg, J; Young, E; Goodkin, D; Mapes, D; Combe, C; Piera, L; Held, P; Gillespie, B; Port, FK. Dialysis Outcomes and Practice Patterns Study (DOPPS).

Depression as a predictor of mortality and hospitalization among hemodialysis patients in the United States and Europe. *Kidney Int.*, 2002 Jul, 62(1), 199-207.

[40] Williams, AW; Dwyer, AC; Eddy, AA; Fink, JC; Jaber, BL; Linas, SL; Michael, B; O'Hare, AM; Schaefer, HM; Shaffer, RN; Trachtman, H; Weiner, DE; Falk, AR. American Society of Nephrology Quality, and Patient Safety Task Force. Critical and honest conversations: the evidence behind the "Choosing Wisely" campaign recommendations by the American Society of Nephrology. *Clin J Am Soc Nephrol.*, 2012 Oct, 7(10), 1664-72.

[41] Renal Physicians Association. *Shared Decision-Making in the Appropriate Initiation of and Withdrawal from Dialysis*, 2nd ed., Rockville, MD: Renal Physicians Association, 2010.

[42] Davison, SN. End-of-life care preferences and needs: perceptions of patients with chronic kidney disease. *Clin J Am Soc Nephrol.*, 2010 Feb, 5(2), 195-204.

[43] Saini, T; Murtagh, FE; Dupont, PJ; et al. Comparative pilot study of symptoms and quality of life in cancer patients and patients with end stage renal disease. *Palliat Med*, 2006, 20, 631e636.

[44] Solano, JP; Gomes, B; Higginson, IJ. A comparison of symptom prevalence in far advanced cancer, AIDS, heart disease, chronic obstructive pulmonary disease and renal disease. *J Pain Symptom Manage*, 2006, 31, 58e69.

[45] Kurella Tamura, M; Goldstein, MK; Pérez-Stable, EJ. Preferences for dialysis withdrawal and engagement in advance care planning within a diverse sample of dialysis patients. *Nephrol Dial Transplant.*, 2010 Jan, 25(1), 237-42.

[46] Goff, SL; Eneanya, ND; Feinberg, R; Germain, MJ; Marr, L; Berzoff, J; Cohen, LM; Unruh, M. Advance care planning: a qualitative study of dialysis patients and families. *Clin J Am Soc Nephrol.*, 2015 Mar, 6, 10(3), 390-400.

[47] Kurella Tamura, M; Montez-Rath, ME; Hall, YN; Katz, R; O'Hare, AM. Advance Directives and End-of-Life Care among Nursing Home Residents Receiving Maintenance Dialysis. *Clin J Am Soc Nephrol.*, 2017, Mar 7, 12(3), 435-442.

[48] Kurella Tamura, M; Liu, S; Montez-Rath, ME; O'Hare, AM; Hall, YN; Lorenz, KA. Persistent Gaps in Use of Advance Directives among Nursing Home Residents Receiving Maintenance Dialysis. *JAMA Intern Med.*, 2017, Aug 1, 177(8), 1204-1205.

[49] Murray, AM; Arko, C; Chen, SC; Gilbertson, DT; Moss, AH. Use of hospice in the United States dialysis population. *Clin J Am Soc Nephrol.*, 2006 Nov, 1(6), 1248-55.

[50] Eneanya, ND; Hailpern, SM; O'Hare, AM; Kurella Tamura, M; Katz, R; Kreuter, W; Montez-Rath, ME; Hebert, PL; Hall, YN. Trends in Receipt of Intensive Procedures at the End of Life Among Patients Treated With Maintenance Dialysis. *Am J Kidney Dis.*, 2017 Jan, 69(1), 60-68.

[51] Wachterman, MW; Pilver, C; Smith, D; Ersek, M; Lipsitz, SR; Keating, NL. Quality of End-of-Life Care Provided to Patients With Different Serious Illnesses. *JAMA Intern Med.*, 2016, Aug 1, 176(8), 1095-102.

[52] Culp, S; Lupu, D; Arenella, C; Armistead, N; Moss, AH. Unmet Supportive Care Needs in U.S. Dialysis Centers and Lack of Knowledge of Available Resources to Address Them. *J Pain Symptom Manage.*, 2016 Apr, 51(4), 756-761, e2.

[53] Holley, JL; Carmody, SS; Moss, AH; Sullivan, AM; Cohen, LM; Block, SD; Arnold, RM. The need for end-of-life care training in nephrology: national survey results of nephrology fellows. *Am J Kidney Dis.*, 2003 Oct, 42(4), 813-20.

[54] Combs, SA; Culp, S; Matlock, DD; Kutner, JS; Holley, JL; Moss, AH. Update on end-of-life care training during nephrology fellowship: a cross-sectional national survey of fellows. *Am J Kidney Dis.*, 2015 Feb, 65(2), 233-9.

[55] Shah, HH; Adams, ND; Mattana, J; Kadiyala, A; Jhaveri, KD. Nephrology elective experience during medical residency: a national survey of US nephrology fellowship training program directors. *Ren Fail.*, 2015 Jul, 37(6), 999-1006.

[56] Lu, E; et al. American Society of Nephrology (ASN) Conference 2017. Initiation of Dialysis in the Elderly Patient: A Survey of Nephrology Trainee Perceptions and Practices. Emily Lu, Manney Carrington Reid, Ronald D. Adelman, Mark S Lachs, Brian M Eiss, Clara Oromendia, Phyllis August, Jeffrey I. Silberzweig and Nathaniel E. Berman. Nephrology & Hypertension, Weill Cornell Medicine/New York Presbyterian Hospital (WC/NYPH); Geriatrics & Palliative Medicine, WC/NYPH and Biostatistics, Healthcare Policy & Research, WC/NYPH.

[57] Moss, AH. Chapter 19: Palliative care in patients with kidney disease and cancer. *Onco-nephrology Curriculum, American Society of Nephrology.*, 2016.

[58] Noble, H; Kelly, D; Rawlings-Anderson, K; Meyer, J. A concept analysis of renal supportive care: the changing world of nephrology. *J Adv Nurs.*, 2007 Sep, 59(6), 644-53.

[59] Quill, TE; Abernethy, AP. Generalist plus specialist palliative care--creating a more sustainable model. *N Engl J Med.*, 2013, Mar 28, 368(13), 1173-5.

[60] Holley, JL. Advance care planning in CKD/ESRD: an evolving process. *Clin J Am Soc Nephrol.*, 2012 Jun, 7(6), 1033-8.

[61] Murtagh, FE; Addington-Hall, JM; Higginson, IJ. End-stage renal disease: a new trajectory of functional decline in the last year of life. *J Am Geriatr Soc.*, 2011 Feb, 59(2), 304-8.

[62] Murtagh, FE; Sheerin, NS; Addington-Hall, J; Higginson, IJ. Trajectories of illness in stage 5 chronic kidney disease: a longitudinal study of patient symptoms and concerns in the last year of life. *Clin J Am Soc Nephrol.*, 2011 Jul, 6(7), 1580-90.

[63] Murtagh, FE; Murphy, E; Sheerin, NS. Illness trajectories: an important concept in the management of kidney failure. *Nephrol Dial Transplant.*, 2008 Dec, 23(12), 3746-8.

[64] Rosansky, SJ; Schell, J; Shega, J; Scherer, J; Jacobs, L; Couchoud, C; Crews, D; McNabney, M. Treatment decisions for older adults with advanced chronic kidney disease. *BMC Nephrol.*, 2017, Jun 19, 18(1), 200.

[65] Rosansky, SJ. Renal function trajectory is more important than chronic kidney disease stage for managing patients with chronic kidney disease. *Am J Nephrol.*, 2012, 36, 1–10. PMID: 22699366.

[66] Conway, B; Webster, A; Ramsay, G; Morgan, N; Neary, J; Whitworth, et al. Predicting mortality and uptake of renal replacement therapy in patients with stage 4 chronic kidney disease. *Nephrol Dial Transplant.*, 2009, 24, 1930–7. PMID: 19181760.

[67] Demoulin, N; Beguin, C; Labriola, L; Jadoul, M. Preparing renal replacement therapy in stage 4 CKD patients referred to nephrologists: a difficult balance between futility and insufficiency. A cohort study of 386 patients followed in Brussels. *Nephrol Dial Transplant.*, 2011, 26, 220–6. PMID: [20610526].

[68] Levin, A; Djurdjie, O; Beaulieu, M; Er, L. Variability and risk factors for kidney disease progression and death following attainment of stage 4 CKD in a referred cohort. *Am J Kidney Dis.*, 2008, 52, 661–71. PMID: 18805347.

[69] Kurella Tamura, M; Covinsky, KE; Chertow, GM; Yaffe, K; Landefeld, S; McCulloch, CE. Functional status of elderly adults before and after initiation of dialysis. *N Engl J Med.*, 2009, 361, 1539-1547.

[70] Jassal, SV; Chiu, E; Hladunewich, M. Loss of independence in patients starting dialysis at 80 years of age or older. *N Engl J Med.*, 2009, 361, 1612-1613.

[71] Berger, JR; Hedayatti, SS. Renal replacement therapy in the elderly population. *Clin J Am Soc Nephrol.*, 2012, 7, 1029-1046.

[72] Roberts, R; Jeffrey, C; Carlisle, G; Brierley, E. Prospective investigation of the incidence of falls, dizziness and syncope in haemodialysis patients. *Int Urol Nephrol.*, 2007, 39, 275-279.

[73] Li, M; Tomlinson, G; Naglie, G; Cook, WL; Jassal, SV. Geriatric comorbidities, such as falls, confer an independent mortality risk to elderly dialysis patients. *Nephrol Dial Transplant.*, 2008, 23, 1396-1400.

[74] Salat, H; Javier, A; Siew, ED; Figueroa, R; Lipworth, L; Kabagambe, E; Bian, A; Stewart, TG; El-Sourady, MH; Karlekar, M; Cardona, CY; Ikizler, TA; Abdel-Kader, K. Nephrology Provider Prognostic Perceptions and Care Delivered to Older Adults with Advanced Kidney Disease. *Clin J Am Soc Nephrol.*, 2017, Nov 7, 12(11), 1762-1770.

[75] Couchoud, C; Labeeuw, M; Moranne, O; Allot, V; Esnault, V; Frimat, L; Stengel, B. French Renal Epidemiology and Information Network (REIN) registry. A clinical score to predict 6-month prognosis in elderly patients starting dialysis for end-stage renal disease. *Nephrol Dial Transplant.*, 2009 May, 24(5), 1553-61.

[76] Cohen, LM; Ruthazer, R; Moss, AH; Germain, MJ. Predicting six-month mortality for patients who are on maintenance hemodialysis. *Clin J Am Soc Nephrol.*, 2010 Jan, 5(1), 72-9.

[77] Couchoud, C; Hemmelgarn, B; Kotanko, P; Germain, MJ; Moranne, O; Davison, SN. Supportive Care: Time to Change Our Prognostic Tools and Their Use in CKD. *Clin J Am Soc Nephrol.*, 2016, Oct 7, 11(10), 1892-1901.

[78] Murtagh, FE; Marsh, JE; Donohoe, P; Ekbal, NJ; Sheerin, NS; Harris, FE. Dialysis or not? A comparative survival study of patients over 75 years with chronic kidney disease stage 5. *Nephrol Dial Transplant.*, 2007 Jul, 22(7), 1955-62.

[79] O'Connor, NR; Dougherty, M; Harris, PS; Casarett, DJ. Survival after dialysis discontinuation and hospice enrollment for ESRD. *Clin J Am Soc Nephrol.*, 2013 Dec, 8(12), 2117-22.

[80] Carson, RC; Juszczak, M; Davenport, A; Burns, A. Is maximum conservative management an equivalent treatment option to dialysis for elderly patients with significant comorbid disease? *Clin J Am Soc Nephrol.*, 2009 Oct, 4(10), 1611-9.

[81] Chandna, SM; Da Silva-Gane, M; Marshall, C; Warwicker, P; Greenwood, RN; Farrington, K. Survival of elderly patients with stage 5 CKD: comparison of conservative management and renal replacement therapy. *Nephrol Dial Transplant.*, 2011 May, 26(5), 1608-14.

[82] O'Connor, NR; Kumar, P. Conservative management of end-stage renal disease without dialysis, a systematic review. *J Palliat Med.*, 2012 Feb, 15(2), 228-35.

[83] Foote, C; Kotwal, S; Gallagher, M; Cass, A; Brown, M; Jardine, M. Survival outcomes of supportive care versus dialysis therapies for elderly patients with end-stage kidney disease: A systematic review and meta-analysis. *Nephrology (Carlton)*, 2016 Mar, 21(3), 241-53.

[84] Lu, E; et al. Why select medical management without dialysis? *Poster. American Society of Nephrology (ASN) Conference*, 2017.

[85] Wachterman, MW; Marcantonio, ER; Davis, RB; Cohen, RA; Waikar, SS; Phillips, RS; McCarthy, EP. Relationship between the prognostic expectations of seriously ill patients undergoing hemodialysis and their nephrologists. *JAMA Intern Med.*, 2013, Jul 8, 173(13), 1206-14.

[86] Hedayati, SS; Gregg, LP; Carmody, T; Jain, N; Toups, M; Rush, AJ; Toto, RD; Trivedi, MH. Effect of Sertraline on Depressive Symptoms in Patients With Chronic Kidney Disease Without Dialysis Dependence: The CAST Randomized Clinical Trial. *JAMA.*, 2017, Nov 21, 318(19), 1876-1890.

[87] Grubbs, V; Tuot, DS; Powe, NR; O'Donoghue, D; Chesla, CA. System-Level Barriers and Facilitators for Foregoing or Withdrawing Dialysis: A Qualitative Study of Nephrologists in the United States and England. *Am J Kidney Dis.*, 2017 Nov, 70(5), 602-610.

[88] Tamura, MK; O'Hare, AM; Lin, E; Holdsworth, LM; Malcolm, E; Moss, AH. Palliative Care Disincentives in CKD, Changing Policy to Improve CKD Care. *Am J Kidney Dis.*, 2018 Jun, 71(6), 866-873.

[89] Feely, MA; Swetz, KM; Zavaleta, K; Thorsteinsdottir, B; Albright, RC; Williams, AW. Reengineering Dialysis: The Role of Palliative Medicine. *J Palliat Med.*, 2016 Jun, 19(6), 652-5.

[90] Weisbord, SD; Mor, MK; Green, JA; Sevick, MA; Shields, AM; Zhao, X; Rollman, BL; Palevsky, PM; Arnold, RM; Fine, MJ. Comparison of symptom management strategies for pain, erectile dysfunction, and depression in patients receiving chronic hemodialysis: a cluster randomized effectiveness trial. *Clin J Am Soc Nephrol.*, 2013 Jan, 8(1), 90-9.

[91] Chan, KY; Cheng, HW; Yap, DY; Yip, T; Li, CW; Sham, MK; Wong, YC; Lau, WK. Reduction of acute hospital admissions and improvement in outpatient attendance by intensified renal palliative care clinic follow-up: the Hong Kong experience. *J Pain Symptom Manage.*, 2015 Jan, 49(1), 144-9.

[92] Grubbs, V; O'Riordan, D; Pantilat, S. Characteristics and Outcomes of In-Hospital Palliative Care Consultation among Patients with Renal Disease Versus Other Serious Illnesses. *Clin J Am Soc Nephrol.*, 2017, Jul 7, 12(7), 1085-1089.

[93] Cohen, LM; Ruthazer, R; Germain, MJ. Increasing hospice services for elderly patients maintained with hemodialysis. *J Palliat Med.*, 2010 Jul, 13(7), 847-54.

[94] Song, MK; Unruh, ML; Manatunga, A; Plantinga, LC; Lea, J; Jhamb, M; Kshirsagar, AV; Ward, SE. SPIRIT trial: A phase III pragmatic trial of an advance care planning intervention in ESRD. *Contemp Clin Trials.*, 2018 Jan, 64, 188-194.

[95] Song, MK; Ward, SE; Fine, JP; Hanson, LC; Lin, FC; Hladik, GA; Hamilton, JB; Bridgman, JC. Advance care planning and end-of-life decision making in dialysis: a randomized controlled trial targeting patients and their surrogates. *Am J Kidney Dis.*, 2015 Nov, 66(5), 813-22.

[96] Schell, JO; Green, JA; Tulsky, JA; Arnold, RM. Communication skills training for dialysis decision-making and end-of-life care in nephrology. *Clin J Am Soc Nephrol.*, 2013 Apr, 8(4), 675-80.

[97] Eneanya, ND; Goff, SL; Martinez, T; Gutierrez, N; Klingensmith, J; Griffith, JL; Garvey, C; Kitsen, J; Germain, MJ; Marr, L; Berzoff, J; Unruh, M; Cohen, LM. Shared decision-making in end-stage renal disease: a protocol for a multi-center study of a communication intervention to improve end-of-life care for dialysis patients. *BMC Palliat Care.*, 2015, Jun 12, 14, 30.

[98] Scherer, JS; Wright, R; Blaum, CS; Wall, SP. Building an Outpatient Kidney Palliative Care Clinical Program. *J Pain Symptom Manage.*, 2018 Jan, 55(1), 108-116.e2.

[99] Taylor, LJ; Nabozny, MJ; Steffens, NM; Tucholka, JL; Brasel, KJ; Johnson, SK; Zelenski, A; Rathouz, PJ; Zhao, Q; Kwekkeboom, KL; Campbell, TC; Schwarze, ML. A Framework to Improve Surgeon Communication in High-Stakes Surgical Decisions: Best Case/Worst Case. *JAMA Surg.*, 2017, Jun 1, 152(6), 531-538.

[100] Kruser, JM; Taylor, LJ; Campbell, TC; Zelenski, A; Johnson, SK; Nabozny, MJ; Steffens, NM; Tucholka, JL; Kwekkeboom, KL; Schwarze, ML. "Best Case/Worst Case", Training Surgeons to Use a Novel Communication Tool for High-Risk Acute Surgical Problems. *J Pain Symptom Manage.*, 2017 Apr, 53(4), 711-719.e5.

[101] Nakagawa, S; Yuzefpolskaya, M; Colombo, PC; Naka, Y; Blinderman, CD. Palliative Care Interventions before Left Ventricular Assist Device Implantation in Both Bridge to Transplant and Destination Therapy. *J Palliat Med.*, 2017 Sep, 20(9), 977-983.

[102] Broglio, K; Pandey, S; Eicholz Heller, F; Blinderman, C. First Responders: Educating Interdisciplinary Champions to Provide Primary Palliative Care. *J Pain Symptom Manage*, 2018, 55(2), 701.

BIOGRAPHICAL SKETCHES

Dr. Emily Lu

Dr. Emily Lu is an Assistant Professor at the Icahn School of Medicine at Mount Sinai.

She received her undergraduate degree from Harvard University, concentrating in Biology with a secondary field in the History of Art and Architecture. She earned her medical degree from Emory University School of Medicine and subsequently completed a residency in Internal Medicine and a fellowship in Nephrology and Hypertension at Weill Cornell Medical Center. She then completed a fellowship in Hospice and Palliative Medicine at Columbia University Medical Center.

Dr. Lu's clinical and research interests focus on the integration of Palliative Care in chronic kidney disease management and Nephrology education. She has also developed museum programs designed to engage individuals with Alzheimer's disease and dementia in the visual arts within a supportive community.

Dr. Craig D. Blinderman

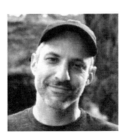

Dr. Craig D. Blinderman is the director of the Adult Palliative Medicine Service at Columbia University Medical Center/New-York Presbyterian Hospital and Co-Director of the *Center for Supportive Care and Clinical Ethics*, and an Associate Professor of Medicine in the Department of Medicine, Columbia University, College of Physicians & Surgeons. He was previously an attending physician on the Palliative Care Service at the Massachusetts General Hospital and co-directed the MGH Cancer Pain Clinic from 2007-2010.

Dr. Blinderman received his undergraduate degree in chemistry (Boston University) and a M.A. in philosophy (Columbia University) before earning his medical degree from Ben Gurion University in Israel. He completed both a residency in Family Medicine and a fellowship in Hospice and Palliative Medicine at Beth Israel Medical Center in NY. He then went on to complete a Medical Ethics fellowship at Harvard Medical School.

Dr. Blinderman has published numerous original articles, reviews and chapters in the following areas: early palliative care in lung cancer patients (Temel et al. NEJM 2010), comfort care for the dying patient (NEJM, 2015), medical ethics, existential distress, symptom assessment and quality of life in chronic lung and heart failure patients, as well as cancer pain management, and the management of pain in patients with a history of substance abuse. He currently is the section editor for *Case Discussions* in the Journal of Palliative Medicine. Dr. Blinderman also serves on the advisory board and teaches at the *New York Zen Center for Contemplative Care*.

His academic interests include: decision-making at the end of life, the role of palliative care in public health, palliative care in developing countries, medical ethics, and the integration of contemplative care, narrative tools, and meditation in medical practice. He also has a strong interest in teaching and developing programs to improve students' and residents' skills in communication and care for the dying.

In: Palliative Care
Editor: Michael Silbermann

ISBN: 978-1-53616-199-1
© 2019 Nova Science Publishers, Inc.

Chapter 6

PALLIATIVE CARE RESEARCH: INCREASING THE AWARENESS, DELIVERY AND QUALITY OF PALLIATIVE CARE

Egidio Del Fabbro[∗]*, MD and J. Brian Cassel, PhD*

Division of Hematology, Oncology, and Palliative Care,
Massey Cancer Center, Virginia Commonwealth University,
Richmond, VA, US

ABSTRACT

Palliative Care research is important for the integration of palliative care into mainstream medicine and for improving clinical care. Important research in symptom intervention, quality of life, clinical model effectiveness, and health utilization over the last two decades has contributed to practice changes in palliative care. Securing funding and the establishing collaborative research groups, particularly at the national level, remain important factors in the development of an effective structure and process for palliative care research. Most research has been conducted in patients with cancer, and additional research is necessary on outcomes in other disease states. Challenges to research persist in the form of data access, health care disparities, and variation of clinical models and health care systems.

Keywords: early palliative care, landmark clinical trials, collaborative research groups, heterogeneity of health systems and clinical models

1. INTRODUCTION

Palliative Care (PC) Research has proven to be a crucial factor for the integration of PC into mainstream medicine and for improving clinical care. The influence of research is identifiable ever since the 1950's [1], gaining momentum with the founding of the modern

---
∗ Corresponding Author's E-mail: egidio.delfabbro@vcuhealth.org.

Hospice movement, and then underscored by several landmark studies over the past decades affirming the importance of Palliative Medicine in improving the care experienced by patients and their families. These accomplishments have been realized in spite of formidable research challenges related to insufficient funding, an underdeveloped organizational structure, clinical complexities that are specific to palliative care, and differences internationally in how PC is defined, operationalized, and funded.

2. SIGNIFICANT PC RESEARCH

PC research has contributed to improving care of the individual patient and in making the case for increasing the availability and access of PC to all patients with life-limiting illnesses. Although most PC studies involve observational research, an increasing number of randomized controlled trials (RCT) have contributed to the literature. Practice-changing research over the past 20 years has included studies on symptom intervention and quality of life, the development of effective clinical models, and the evaluation of PC's impact on health utilization. The following are some examples of important research contributing to practice changes.

2.1. Early Palliative Care

Few trials in PC have gained more public attention from the mass media than the 2010 RCT comparing early palliative care to usual oncology care in patients with lung cancer. This single-center trial showed early palliative care improved quality of life, reduced depressive symptoms, and prolonged survival, compared to a control group of patients receiving only oncological care [2]. A subsequent large, cluster-randomized trial in Canada showed improved symptoms and quality of life but not survival in oncology patients receiving early concurrent palliative care [3]. Following the evidence from these PC trials, the American Society of Clinical Oncology practice guidelines recommended that patients with advanced cancer should receive specialist PC services early in the disease course, concurrent with active treatment [4]. An RCT using a nursing intervention has also been identified as potentially practice changing research. The ENABLE ("Educate, Nurture, Advise Before Life Ends") study, showed the addition of a telephone-based, nurse-led palliative care intervention was associated with better quality of life compared to usual care alone [5]. This intervention is one of the few supportive care studies endorsed by the National Cancer Institute (NCI) Research-Tested Intervention Programs (RTIPs).

2.2. Clinical Models

Studies have evaluated the effects of particular clinical models of palliative care on quality and cost. Most but not all of the research has focused on patients in the oncology setting. Surprisingly, a survey of cancer centers and their PC programs revealed a relative lack of outpatient clinics and palliative care units, even in large Academic Centers [6], highlighting the need to expand and integrate PC into the daily oncological care of patients in all settings and throughout their illness. There may be a number of reasons for the absence of palliative care units (PCUs) and outpatient clinics. Palliative care units are resource intensive, requiring continuous staffing and an interdisciplinary team with special skill sets in order to manage patients and families with high symptom burden and psychosocial or spiritual distress. Despite being resource intensive, recent research has indicated that PCUs should be considered as important components of the PC clinical model, since they improve quality and also appear to be cost effective. A large Veterans Administration (VA) study found bereaved family members rated care provided by dedicated palliative care units more highly than care by PC consultation teams [7], and a report from a single institution showed lowered costs compared to the consult service [8].

2.3. Symptoms

Palliative Care research has revealed insights into the assessment and management of important symptoms and conditions that burden PC patients. Symptoms such as delirium, fatigue [9], neuropathic pain [10], opioid induced constipation [11], nausea, dyspnea [12], and depression [13] are better controlled because of knowledge gained through clinical trials and observational studies. Several retrospective studies have shown that opioid rotation is a useful strategy for managing tolerance, decreasing opioid side effects, and reducing opioid doses, in the inpatient and outpatient [14] settings. The concept of opioid rotation is unlikely to be tested in a prospective RCT because the practice is so well established that there would be ethical concerns about harm to participants in a control arm. Some areas of research are fortunate to have several trials addressing the issue – in these cases, systematic reviews are possible. For example, systematic reviews revealed the potential harm of interventions such as tube feedings in severely cognitively impaired elderly nursing home residents [15] and showed the benefit of exercise for cancer-related fatigue [16].

2.4. Goals of Care

Research including randomized trials and systematic reviews have highlighted the importance of effective, compassionate [17], and candid discussions between clinicians and patients [18] regarding prognosis, the benefits and risks of chemotherapy [19], and Advance Directives [20]. Having these discussions earlier appears to be beneficial with regard to patients receiving less aggressive care [21]. Surveys in the United States [22] and Canada [23] have been important in determining the issues patients, families, physicians, and other care providers consider important at the end of life.

3. STRUCTURE AND PROCESS FOR PALLIATIVE CARE RESEARCH

The development of an effective structure and process for PC research is dependent on several factors including adequate funding by academic departments, institutions, and governments. The creation of collaborative partnerships between researchers (within and outside the PC field) and institutions are equally important so that multicenter trials are possible and their findings generalizable.

3.1. Funding

Funding of research is important in every part of the world; however, nowhere is the complexity of funding resources illustrated more vividly than the wealthiest nation, the United States. Funding has increased in the 21st century in the U.S. However, funding since 2001 has remained fairly static, with the major contributors being the National Institutes of Health, with cancer (NCI), aging (NIA), and nursing (NINR) leading the way. Importantly, < 1% of all grants awarded by the National Institutes of Health (NIH), were awarded to palliative medicine researchers, with some NIH institutes having never funded PC research, despite their focus on life-limiting illnesses such as end-stage renal disease. Although funding for PC has been relatively stagnant for more than a decade, a recent report identified some encouraging trends, including a doubling of early stage career development funding and of NIH-funded original palliative medicine research articles [24].

Other organizations funded by philanthropy, such as the National Palliative Care Research Center (NPCRC), have been important promoters through pilot grants of many early and midcareer researchers. Finally, the support of individual health care institutions is crucial for creating robust palliative care programs that can support researchers with salaries, internal grants, and allowing time for mentoring of junior faculty.

3.2. Collaborative Research Groups

PC is able to improve symptom control, increase family satisfaction, decrease health care utilization, and prolong survival. In spite of these remarkable outcomes, many studies are from single institutions or have small sample sizes and should therefore be repeated at other institutions or in multi-center studies before they can be considered to be generalizable. This is especially important in a relatively young specialty such as PC, where the scope and integration of PC services varies, even among large centers. The ability to conduct multicenter PC trials has improved with the establishment of cooperative consortiums such as the Palliative Care Research Cooperative (PCRC) and the National Clinical Trials Network (NCTN) groups including the Alliance for Clinical Trials in Oncology. Other difficulties inherent in PC trials, such as the potential for progression of disease and inability to continue trial participation, support the creation of a platform for multisite trials that would encourage optimal accrual.

3.3. National Collaborative Initiatives

National or Federal initiatives to increase cooperation among clinicians and researchers in measuring outcomes and improving clinical care have been implemented in Europe, Canada, Australia, and the Veteran's Administration (VA) within the United States. These programs stemming from developed nations may serve as models for illustrating both the successes and deficiencies of national initiatives. Ideally, programs should have common patient-reported outcomes, and there should be national benchmark standards, collection, and analysis of aggregated data with feedback to the individual services.

A recent white paper developed by the European Association for Palliative Care (EAPC) taskforce recommended introduction of several outcome measures into practice that would also allow for national and international comparisons [25]. The task force noted that outcome measures needed to be free in order to encourage widespread use, and should be specific to palliative care. Examples of these outcome and quality of life measures included the Palliative care Outcome Scale (POS) (www.pos-pal.org) [26], the Edmonton Symptom Assessment Scale (ESAS), and the European Organization for Research and Treatment of Cancer Quality of Life Questionnaire Core 15 Palliative (EORTC QLQ-C15-PAL) [27]. In addition to providing a guidelines and a forum for exchange of ideas, the EAPC provides an established infrastructure for collaborative research and data handling, the ability to conduct multicenter trials, accessibility to wide range of experts, and mentorship for junior researchers including a palliative care PhD program.

Canada has a standard for administration of the ESAS, a patient-reported outcome (PRO) measuring symptom intensity that is commonly used use in daily clinical practice and as an outcome measure in multiple studies. However, these data need to be routinely collected from all centers and reported to allow for comparisons and improvements [28]. The Canadian Partnership against Cancer's (CPAC) initiative in conjunction with others to increase standardized screening for cancer patients, develop benchmarks, and analyze data could be expanded to include the non-cancer palliative patients in future. Nevertheless, despite some imperfections, a province-wide initiative adopted the ESAS as a standardized symptom screening tool in the province of Ontario, Canada, and generated important studies describing the temporal nature of symptom intensity in patients with advanced cancer [29]. The routine collection of the ESAS also provided preliminary evidence that implementation of such a measure may have a positive effect on health utilization [30].

Australia has a federally funded program, the Palliative Care Outcomes Collaborative (PCOC). The program's goals are to improve palliative care by measuring symptom outcomes, analyzing the data and reporting back to individual palliative care services. This national collaborative reported patient-centered, statistically significant improvements in all domains of patient- and clinician-reported outcomes except for pain [31]. Unfortunately, the United States does not have a federally supported PC strategy; however, the Veterans Administration (VA) has a program designed to implement PC into all VA hospitals. The Veterans Health Administration (VA) Comprehensive End-of-Life Care Initiative (CELCI) (2009-2012) was designed to enable reliable access to hospice and palliative care services at all VA facilities and build an infrastructure to ensure sustainable high quality end-of-life care [32]. Unlike other insurers in the U.S., the VA also has the advantage of allowing concurrent hospice services and disease-specific treatment, with about 1 in 4 patients receiving concurrent care by 2012 [33]. Despite this initiative, a retrospective study of 719 patients with cancer in the VA found a number of care gaps, particularly in the outpatient setting [34].

4. COLLABORATION BETWEEN PC RESEARCHERS AND OTHERS

Collaboration between Palliative Care researchers, behavioral scientists, art researchers, and pre-clinical translational scientists may be an effective approach to address resistant conditions or unmet symptom needs such as fatigue, weight loss, neuropathic pain, existential suffering, and psychological and spiritual distress.

Good examples of this multidisciplinary approach to particular symptoms include the approaches to cachexia and neuropathic pain. Cachexia, a condition common to a number of seemingly disparate serious illnesses is the focus of a professional organization that organizes yearly symposiums, publishes a scientific journal devoted to the condition [35], and provides a forum for clinical and translational scientists to exchange ideas which may prove to be beneficial for both groups. In neuropathic pain, for example, current animal models and assays may not be ideal strategies to explore a symptom that is typically based on patient-reported outcomes. Collaborative efforts between PC research and pre-clinical scientist could facilitate translational research from bench to bedside and back again.

5. SCOPE OF RESEARCH

Overall, the scope of PC research is broad, aimed at diverse disease states, and uses a variety of quantitative and qualitative methods. Although most research has been conducted in patients with cancer, a systematic review of 124 randomized controlled trials (the majority from the U.S.) concluded that PC also improves selected outcomes in other life-limiting illnesses such as Heart Failure (HF), Chronic Obstructive Pulmonary Disease and Dementia. Improvements were reported in communication and planning, psychosocial health, and the experience of patients and their caregivers [36]. While the preliminary evidence for PC intervention is especially promising in HF [37], more disease-specific research needs to be done since the framework of palliative care used in oncology may not be ideal for patients with other chronic life-limiting illnesses, such as HF [38]. A systematic review and meta-analysis of PC interventions in HF found team-based interventions improved patient-centered outcomes, documentation of preferences, and lowered the risk of re-hospitalization.

The incorporation of PC into guidelines from professional organizations such as the American Heart Association and the American College of Surgeons is a necessary first step in raising awareness of palliative care needs within these subspecialties. However, an endorsement should be followed by active, substantive support of PC research. Oncology has been at the forefront of PC research for many years, and in particular, the American Cancer Society has been instrumental in developing the careers of many PC researchers.

6. RESEARCH CHALLENGES

6.1. Access to Data

Palliative care should be accessible to all patients with life-limiting illness and in any setting, whether at home, in the outpatient clinic, or in a hospital. Over the past two decades, home hospice care has expanded in the United States, with bereaved family members reporting higher satisfaction and fewer unmet needs than patients without hospice care. More recent research shows a concerning trend for more burdensome transitions of care [39] in the last month of life and increased ICU admission despite increased hospice enrollment. These findings would not be possible without access to Medicare federal data. Unfortunately, using Medicare administrative data to measure health utilization in younger patients is not possible, and obtaining utilization data on palliative care (rather than hospice) is more challenging in the US [40]. In addition to lack of access, there are few institutions that consistently collect useful patient-reported outcomes. Access to all these data are important since health utilization coupled with patient-reported outcomes may produce powerful research findings that could influence models of care.

6.2. Variation in Palliative Care Models and Delivery

Currently PC clinical models vary widely depending on resources, befitting the still-evolving nature of the field. While clinical innovation is valuable, it can also hobble efforts to produce research on large-scale implementation akin to phase IV studies in clinical therapies. This is particularly true when seeking to understand the impact of palliative care across non-cancer diseases and in less-often studied populations such as non-elderly patients. Research and outcome measures may also be facilitated by national strategies for PC which would promote standardization of services and data points collected [41]. In the meantime it is crucial that clinical innovations be applied and assessed systematically.

7. WORKFORCE SHORTAGE AND DISPARITIES

A worldwide shortage of PC clinicians and researchers is likely with an aging population, especially in developed countries. A 2010 study estimated that 6,000 to 18,000 additional physicians are needed to meet the current demand in the U.S. for the inpatient setting alone [42]. In addition, the needs of a rapidly growing racially and ethnically diverse population of older adults with life-limiting illness needs to be anticipated. This will require additional research into the racial and ethnic disparities in PC, such as decreased access and poorer clinical outcomes. Research support, training of researchers, and national and institutional attention will be necessary in order to develop effective models, allocate necessary resources, and provide ongoing analysis and dissemination of outcomes. Given that it is unlikely that sufficient numbers of specialists will be trained in palliative care, further research into the most effective means of disseminating evidence-based palliative care practices among generalists is much needed. The relatively new area of "dissemination and implementation" science is applicable in this regard.

REFERENCES

[1] Clark D. From margins to centre: a review of the history of palliative care in cancer. *Lancet Oncol.* 2007 May;8(5):430-8.

[2] Temel JS, Greer JA, Muzikansky A, Gallagher ER, Admane S, Jackson VA, Dahlin CM, Blinderman CD, Jacobsen J, Pirl WF, Billings JA, Lynch TJ. Early palliative care for patients with metastatic non-small-cell lung cancer. *N Engl J Med.* 2010 Aug 19;363(8):733-42.

[3] Zimmermann C, Swami N, Krzyzanowska M, Hannon B, Leighl N, Oza A, Moore M, Rydall A, Rodin G, Tannock I, Donner A, Lo C. Early palliative care for patients with advanced cancer: a cluster-randomised controlled trial. *Lancet.* 2014 May 17;383(9930):1721-30.

[4] Ferrell BR, Temel JS, Temin S, Alesi ER, Balboni TA, Basch EM, Firn JI, Paice JA, Peppercorn JM, Phillips T, Stovall EL, Zimmermann C, Smith TJ. Integration of Palliative Care Into Standard Oncology Care: American Society of Clinical Oncology Clinical Practice Guideline Update. *J Clin Oncol.* 2017 Jan;35(1):96-112.

[5] Bakitas M, Lyons KD, Hegel MT, Balan S, Brokaw FC, Seville J, Hull JG, Li Z, Tosteson TD, Byock IR, Ahles TA. Effects of a palliative care intervention on clinical outcomes in patients with advanced cancer: the Project ENABLE II randomized controlled trial. *JAMA.* 2009 Aug 19;302(7):741-9.

[6] Hui D, Elsayem A, De la Cruz M, Berger A, Zhukovsky DS, Palla S, Evans A, Fadul N, Palmer JL, Bruera E. Availability and integration of palliative care at US cancer centers. *JAMA.* 2010 Mar 17;303(11):1054-61. PMC3426918.

[7] Casarett D, Johnson M, Smith D, Richardson D. The optimal delivery of palliative care: a national comparison of the outcomes of consultation teams vs inpatient units. *Arch Intern Med.* 2011 Apr 11;171(7):649-55.

[8] May P, Garrido MM, Del Fabbro E, Noreika D, Normand C, Skoro N, Cassel JB. Does modality matter? Palliative care unit associated with more cost-avoidance than consultations. *J Pain Symptom Manage.* 2018 Mar;55(3):766-774.e4.

[9] Yennurajalingam S, Frisbee-Hume S, Palmer JL, Delgado-Guay MO, Bull J, Phan AT, Tannir NM, Litton JK, Reddy A, Hui D, Dalal S, Massie L, Reddy SK, Bruera E. Reduction of cancer-related fatigue with dexamethasone: A double-blind, randomized, placebo-controlled trial in patients with advanced cancer. *J Clin Oncol.* 2013 Sept 1;31(25):3076-82.

[10] Smith EM, Pang H, Cirrincione C, Fleishman S, Paskett ED, Ahles T, Bressler LR, Fadul CE, Knox C, Le-Lindqwister N, Gilman PB, Shapiro CL; Alliance for Clinical Trials in Oncology. Effect of duloxetine on pain, function, and quality of life among patients with chemotherapy-induced painful peripheral neuropathy: a randomized clinical trial. *JAMA.* 2013 Apr 3;309(13):1359-67. PMC3912515.

[11] Thomas J, Karver S, Cooney GA, Chamberlain BH, Watt CK, Slatkin NE, Stambler N, Kremer AB, Israel RJ. Methylnaltrexone for opioid-induced constipation in advanced illness. *N Engl J Med.* 2008 May 29;358(22):2332-43.

[12] Bruera E, Macmillan K, Pither J, MacDonald RN. Effects of morphine on the dyspnea of terminal cancer patients. *J Pain Symptom Manage.* 1990 Dec;5(6):341-4.

[13] Mitchell AJ, Chan M, Bhatti H, Halton M, Grassi L, Johansen C, Meader N. Prevalence of depression, anxiety, and adjustment disorder in oncological, haematological, and palliative-care settings: A meta-analysis of 94 interview-based studies. *Lancet Oncol.* 2011 Feb;12(2):160-74.

[14] Reddy A, Yennurajalingam S, Pulivarthi K, Palla S, Wang X, Kwon J, Frisbee-Hume S, Bruera E. Frequency, Outcome and Predictors of Success within 6 weeks of an Opioid Rotation Among Outpatient with Cancer Receiving Strong Opioids. *Oncologist.* 2013;18(2):212-20. PMC3579606.

[15] Finucane TE, Christmas C, Travis K. Tube feeding in patients with advanced dementia: A review of the evidence. *JAMA.* 1999 Oct 13;282(14):1365-70.

[16] Cramp F, Byron-Daniel J. Exercise for the management of cancer-related fatigue in adults. *Cochrane Database Syst Rev.* 2012 Nov 14;11:CD006145.

[17] Tanco K, Rhondall W, Perez-Cruz P, et al. Patient perception of physician compassion after a more optimistic vs a less optimistic message: a randomized clinical trial. *JAMA Oncol.* 2015 May;1(2):176-83.

[18] Wright AA, Zhang B, Ray A, Mack JW, Trice E, Balboni T, Mitchell SL, Jackson VA, Block SD, Maciejewski PK, Prigerson HG. Associations between end-of-life discussions, patient mental health, medical care near death, and caregiver bereavement adjustment. *JAMA.* 2008 Oct 8;300(14):1665-73. PMC2853806.

[19] Weeks JC, Catalano PJ, Cronin A, Finkelman MD, Mack JW, Keating NL, Schrag D. Patients' expectations about effects of chemotherapy for advanced cancer. *N Engl J Med.* 2012 Oct 25367(17):1616-25. PMC3613151.

[20] Teno JM, Gruneir A, Schwartz Z, Nanda A, Wetle T. Association between advance directives and quality of end-of-life care: a national study. *J Am Geriatr Soc.* 2007 Feb;55(2): 189-94.

[21] Mack JW, Cronin A, Keating NL, Taback N, Huskamp HA, Malin JL, Earle CC, Weeks JC. Associations between end-of-life discussion characteristics and care received near death: A prospective cohort study. *J Clin Oncol.* 2012 Dec 10; 30(35):4387-95. PMC3675701.

[22] Steinhauser KE, Christakis NA, Clipp EC, McNeilly M, McIntyre L, Tulsky JA. Factors considered important at the end of life by patients, family, physicians, and other care providers. *JAMA.* 2000 Nov 15;284(19):2476-82.

[23] Singer PA, Martin DK, Kelner M. Quality end-of-life care: Patients' perspectives. *JAMA.* 1999 Jan 13;281(2):163-8.

[24] Brown E, Morrison RS, Gelfman LP. An Update: NIH Research Funding for Palliative Medicine, 2011-2015. *J Palliat Med.* 2018 Feb;21(2):182-187. PMC5797329.

[25] Bausewein C, Daveson BA, Currow DC, Downing J, Deliens L, Radbruch L, Defilippi K, Lopes Ferreira P, Costantini M, Harding R, Higginson IJ. EAPC White Paper on outcome measurement in palliative care: Improving practice, attaining outcomes and delivering quality services - Recommendations from the European Association for Palliative Care (EAPC) Task Force on Outcome Measurement. *Palliat Med.* 2016 Jan;30(1):6-22.

[26] Hearn J, Higginson IJ. Development and validation of a core outcome measure for palliative care: the palliative care outcome scale. Palliative Care Core Audit Project Advisory Group. *Qual Health Care.* 1999 Dec;8(4): 219-227. PMC2483665.

[27] Groenvold M, Petersen MA, Aaronson NK, Arraras JI, Blazeby JM, Bottomley A, Fayers PM, de Graeff A, Hammerlid E, Kaasa S, Sprangers MA, Bjorner JB; EORTC Quality of Life Group. The development of the EORTC QLQ-C15-PAL: a shortened questionnaire for cancer patients in palliative care. *Eur J Cancer.* 2006 Jan; 42(1): 55-64.

[28] Dudgeon D. The Impact of Measuring Patient-Reported Outcome Measures on Quality of and Access to Palliative Care. *J Palliat Med.* 2018 Jan;21(S1):S76-S80. PMC5733646.

[29] Seow H, Barbera L, Sutradhar R, Howell D, Dudgeon D, Atzema C, Liu Y, Husain A, Sussman J, Earle C. Trajectory of performance status and symptom scores for patients with cancer during the last six months of life. *J Clin Oncol.* 2011 Mar 20;29(9):1151-8.

[30] Barbera L, Sutradhar R, Howell D, Sussman J, Seow H, Dudgeon D, Atzema C, Earle C, Husain A, Liu Y, Krzyzanowska MK. Does routine symptom screening with ESAS decrease ED visits in breast cancer patients undergoing adjuvant chemotherapy? *Support Care Cancer.* 2015 Oct;23(10):3025-32.

[31] Currow D, Allingham S, Yates P, Johnson C, Clark K, Eagara K. Improving national hospice/palliative care service symptom outcomes systematically through point-of-care data collection, structured feedback and benchmarking. *Support Care Cancer* 2015 Feb;23(2):307-15. PMC4289012.

[32] Edes T, Shreve S, Casarett D. Increasing access and quality in Department of Veterans Affairs care at the end of life: a lesson in change. *J Am Geriatr Soc.* 2007 Oct;55(10):1645-9.

[33] Mor V, Joyce NR, Coté DL, Gidwani RA, Ersek M, Levy CR, Faricy-Anderson KE, Miller SC, Wagner TH, Kinosian BP, Lorenz KA, Shreve ST. The rise of concurrent care for veterans with advanced cancer at the end of life. *Cancer.* 2016 Mar 1;122(5):782-90.

[34] Walling AM, Tisnado D, Asch SM, Malin JM, Pantoja P, Dy SM, Ettner SL, Zisser AP, Schreibeis-Baum H, Lee M, Lorenz KA. The quality of supportive cancer care in the veterans affairs health system and targets for improvement. *JAMA Intern Med.* 2013 Dec 9-23;173(22):2071-9.

[35] Anker SD, von Haehling S, Coats AJS. More variety with the Journal of Cachexia, Sarcopenia and Muscle: JCSM Clinical Reports and JCSM Rapid Communications have both gone live. *J Cachexia Sarcopenia Muscle.* 2018 Apr;9(2):217-219. PMC5879971.

[36] Singer AE, Goebel JR, Kim YS, Dy SM, Ahluwalia SC, Clifford M, Dzeng E, O'Hanlon CE, Motala A, Walling AM, Goldberg J, Meeker D, Ochotorena C, Shanman R, Cui M, Lorenz KA. Populations and Interventions for Palliative and End-of-Life Care: A Systematic Review. *J Palliat Med.* 2016 Sep;19(9):995-1008. PMC5011630.

[37] Diop MS, Rudolph JL, Zimmerman KM, Richter MA, Skarf LM. Palliative Care Interventions for Patients with Heart Failure: A Systematic Review and Meta-Analysis. *J Palliat Med.* 2017 Jan;20(1):84-92.

[38] Kavalieratos D, Gelfman LP, Tycon LE, Riegel B, Bekelman DB, Ikejiani DZ, Goldstein N, Kimmel SE, Bakitas MA, Arnold RM. Palliative Care in Heart Failure: Rationale, Evidence, and Future Priorities. *J Am Coll Cardiol.* 2017 Oct 10;70(15):1919-1930. PMC5731659.

[39] Teno JM, Gozalo PL, Bynum JP, Leland NE, Miller SC, Morden NE, Scupp T, Goodman DC, Mor V. Change in end-of-life care for Medicare beneficiaries: site of death, place of care, and health care transitions in 2000, 2005, and 2009. *JAMA*. 2013 Feb 6;309(5):470-7. PMC3674823.

[40] May P, Cassel JB. Economic outcomes in palliative and end-of-life care: current state of affairs. *Ann Palliat Med*. 2018 Oct;7(Suppl 3):S244-S248.

[41] Meier DE, Back AL, Berman A, Block SD, Corrigan JM, Morrison RS. A National Strategy For Palliative Care. *Health Aff* (Millwood). 2017 Jul 1;36(7):1265-1273.

[42] Lupu D; American Academy of Hospice and Palliative Medicine Workforce Task Force. Estimate of current hospice and palliative medicine physician workforce shortage. *J Pain Symptom Manage*. 2010 Dec;40(6):899-911.

BIOGRAPHICAL SKETCH

Egidio Del Fabbro, MD

Egidio Del Fabbro, MD, is the Palliative Care Endowed Chair and Program Director at Virginia Commonwealth University Massey Cancer Center. Dr. Del Fabbro also serves as an Associate Professor of Internal Medicine within the Division of Hematology, Oncology and Palliative Care of the Department of Internal Medicine at the VCU School of Medicine.

Dr. Del Fabbro received his medical degree from the University of the Witwatersrand in Johannesburg, South Africa in 1990. In 1998, he completed his residency in Internal Medicine at Barnes-Jewish Hospital, Washington University, St. Louis and palliative care fellowship at MD Anderson Cancer Center in 2004. He joined the Palliative Care and Rehabilitation department in 2005. He was director of the Cachexia clinic from 2005 to 2011. He assumed his role as Director of Palliative Care at Virginia Commonwealth University in 2012 and as Endowed Chair in 2015.

His clinical research is focused on therapeutic interventions for symptoms in patients with cancer, and opioid related side-effects. He was the Principal Investigator of two randomized, placebo-controlled trials for poor appetite and cancer-related fatigue in patients with advanced cancer. He has published more than 100 peer-reviewed papers, abstracts and book chapters related to Palliative Care and symptom management. He has received funding from the American Cancer Society to explore the effect of testosterone replacement in male patients with advanced cancer. He is also Editor of the Oxford University textbook *Nutrition and the Cancer Patient*, and an Associate Editor for the Journal of Cachexia Sarcopenia and Muscle.

Part II. Western Europe

In: Palliative Care
Editor: Michael Silbermann

ISBN: 978-1-53616-199-1
© 2019 Nova Science Publishers, Inc.

Chapter 7

STRATEGIES FOR THE PROMOTION OF HOME PALLIATIVE CARE – WHAT IS STILL TO BE LEARNED AND HOW?

Manuel Luís Capelas[*], PhD, Sílvia Patrícia Coelho, PhD and Tânia Sofia Afonso

Universidade Católica Portuguesa, Institute of Health Sciences (Lisbon),
Center for Interdisciplinary Research in Health, Portuguese Observatory
for Palliative Care, Porto, Portugal

ABSTRACT

Home palliative care (HPC) is one of the most important strategies to achieve universal health coverage in patients at end-of-life. In this chapter, we explore how this kind of care can be promoted and delivered in different realities, and what its impact will be on health care costs and on the use of health resources. For these purposes, human resources in quality and quantity, funding, quality improvement strategies and programs, outcomes and continuous evaluation play a very important role. E-health seems to be promising and useful for achieving the HPC expected outcomes.

Keywords: palliative care, home palliative care teams, organization of services, e-health, outcomes, costs

BACKGROUND

Today, we know that the majority of patients prefer to be cared for and to die at home [1–9], but the real congruence with this desire is too low [3, 8, 10], and this preference is not always the best or even a possible option [11].

---

[*] Corresponding Author's E-mail: luis.capelas@ucp.pt.

One of the most important factors to increase the fulfilment of these preferences is the availability of and accessibility to good quality primary care, including good home palliative care [3, 10–12]. To achieve that, it is strongly necessary to have a funded team work in the home palliative care team, which must include not only social workers, psychologists, volunteers, physio- and occupational therapists, but also a strong liaison to palliative hospital based teams and general practitioners [10].

Reinforcing this issue, the 67th World Health Assembly approved the recommendation: "Strengthening of palliative care as a component of comprehensive care throughout the life course" [13] which aims *"to develop, strengthen and implement, where appropriate, palliative care policies to support the comprehensive strengthening of health systems to integrate evidence-based, cost-effective and equitable palliative care services in the continuum of care, across all levels, with emphasis on* **primary care, community and home-based care***, and* **universal coverage schemes***"* [13].

Also the conceptual transitions in palliative care in this century imply an early identification with the community and all settings that people need for palliative care, as well as a community approach instead of an institutional one.

To identify palliative needs and life-threatening illnesses there are some important and useful tools, which when associated with a defined patient complexity tool like IDC-PAL [20], help health care professionals to allocate the necessary resources to patients. Some of the most used are the "Proactive Identification Guidance at the Gold Standards Framework (PIG)" [15], the "Supportive and Palliative Care Indicator Tool (SPICT)" [16], the "NECesidades PALiativas (NECPAL-CCOMS-ICO)" [17], the "RADPAC" [18], the "Residential Care Homes Steps End of Life Care Tool Kit" [19] and "The CARING criteria" [20].

After the patients in need of this care are identified, the community-based or generalist palliative care teams in primary care have a unique role and position to achieve the best quality of life possible for patients with palliative care needs. This is because they can reach these patients early in the course of life-threatening disease, meet all dimensions of need (physical, social, psychological and spiritual), provide care in clinics, care homes and at home, thus preventing unnecessary hospital admissions, supporting family caregivers and providing bereavement care [21].

DEFINITION AND HUMAN RESOURCES

The European Association for Palliative Care (EAPC) defines the home palliative care team (HPCT) as *"a multiprofessional team that, in the first place, supports people at home or in a nursing home"* [22]. The HPCT aims are not restricted to patient care, but also provide an advisory and mentoring role alongside the other primary care teams or professionals, namely in symptom control, palliative care and psychosocial spiritual care [22, 23].

In order to achieve the aims of HPCT work, human resources play a central role. We can estimate its needs by two strategies. One is based on full-time equivalent (FTE) by patients, and the other strategy is a population based approach. The first requires one nurse for every five patients on daily service, one physician for every 25 patients on service, and in addition other health professionals, such as social workers, psychologists, therapists, drivers or home care aides (one FTE of other clinical services for every 10 patients). For the second strategy, three physicians, 12 nurses and six other clinical staff are needed per 100,000 inhabitants [24].

These teams have as common activities patient care; family care; bereavement follow-up; ethical decision-making and advance care planning; continuing care and case management; liaison of resources; team work (meetings, roles, support, relations, climate); registration and documentation; evaluation of results; internal and external training; research and publications; volunteering; advocacy and links to society [25].

Four major outcomes are expected to ensue through their work: the effectiveness (emotional impact, adjustment to the situation, reducing suffering, symptom control, quality of life and reducing the risk of complicated bereavement), efficiency (reducing acute hospital and emergency use, procedures, therapeutics and costs), satisfaction (patients, family, other professionals and services, stakeholders) and added value (person or family centered-care, ethical issues, compassion, and a multidisciplinary approach to the care of vulnerable people) [26].

As we wrote above it is very important for the success of these teams that they have a solid connection with other care settings and non-palliative care health professionals. For this purpose it will be important to set down in advance the criteria for intervention (either early intervention or that based on patient complexity and degree of suffering); the mechanisms of intervention (identification, assessment, role in the follow up, shared decision-making and information systems, and so on); the mechanisms of shared decision-making, coordination and integrated-care (meetings, joint clinical processes and so on) and shared care, flexible patterns of intervention and joint policies [26].

DEVELOPMENT AND QUALITY IMPROVEMENT

According to the Toolkit for the Development of Palliative Care in the Community, developed by the EAPC Task Force in Primary Palliative Care in 2014 [21], five steps should be taken to develop HPCT and community palliative care:

1) Identify key individuals or organizations interested in this development;
2) Organize a meeting or working group to identify and discuss local challenges and solutions;
3) Contact experts who may be able to provide some specific guidance on relevant issues;
4) Seek to establish improvements in each of the four domains of the public health model in order to create a balanced system of provision;
5) Collate data supporting the need for and potential outcomes of palliative care in the community.

After that, crucial measures must be taken to establish HPCT, which provides high quality care. These are an institutional commitment, context analysis, leadership, targeting patients, mission, vision, principles and values, internal consensus, models of care and intervention, team building, training, starting clinical activities, external consensus, quality indicators, standards and quality improvement, budgeting, follow up and review [25].

Budgeting is a forgotten issue, but a crucial one considering the development of all health care services, so HPCT must take it into account.

Most or more than 70 percent of health care costs refer to care provided in the last six months of life. These costs are mainly due to hospitalizations, emergency room visits, treatments, diagnostic exams and an increase in the need for health care [27]. On the other hand, more so than in other healthcare fields, in palliative care most expenses (about 70 percent) involve health professionals [27].

Health care services can be funded through a payment of one fee for service, by day, by patient, by month, by admission, by structure, by capitative model or using combined methods using public and/or private funding. Out of these, the capitative model seems to be the most appropriate, because it favors equity, efficiency and cost control; promotes quality assessment and improvement of health care, facilitates the development of alternative resources, and encourages networking with community resources and civil society [27].

Quality improvement is one of the basic tools and key principles of palliative care [14]. It's the reason why in the last decade we have seen an increased concern about the quality of this care, which has been under strong scrutiny [28].

Recently, in 2014, the European Declaration on Palliative Care that appeals to the recognition of palliative care as a public health priority was published, and as such should be approached under this perspective; to the development of national palliative care policies and programs integrated in all settings of national health systems with clear referral criteria and accessibility in useful time; patient services and health professionals' education must be focused on patient and family needs; improvement of the population awareness about palliative care, educating and training the volunteers and caregivers; the increase of research and its funding, as well as the promotion of a quality improvement process [29–32].

High quality care requires a multidisciplinary team, well-coordinated and trained, with good communicational skills, capable of assessment and control of symptoms and problems, and engaging in research, as well as a systematic and regular outcome evaluation [33–39].

Geoff Mitchel and colleagues suggest some actions to improve the quality of palliative home care, which include the establishment and documentation of a formal policy that guarantees total accessibility to palliative care; identification and assessment of staff needed for palliative care while using validated tools; establishment of protocols, registers and tools to assess patients' needs; education and training of all health professionals; identification, support and caregivers' care; an increased multidisciplinary team approach; coordination and integrated care; evaluation of the palliative approach results; addressing the ethical challenges and involvement of patients and society in its design and evaluation [40].

In 2015 the EAPC developed 12 recommendations which identify the key elements to be evaluated [41]:

1) Use of Patient-Reported Outcome Measures that are clear, brief, sufficiently direct and validated to palliative care patients;
2) Use of multidimensional assessment tools that assess physical, psychological, social and spiritual suffering;
3) Use of assessment tools to evaluate outcomes in caregivers regarding their needs and the impact of patient care;

4) Use of measures with good psychometric properties;
5) Use of measures adjusted to both clinical practice and care goals;
6) Use of valid and reliable research measures that are relevant to research and take into account the patient overload of their use;
7) Incorporate outcome measurement into routine clinical practice and evaluate the implementation of a process of change;
8) Associate the outcomes measure to quality indicators;
9) Development and use of a quality improvement system to sustain clinical practice;
10) Use of measures that allow comparisons between different care modalities and with other programs;
11) Promote national and international benchmarking;
12) Increase quality and amount of clinical data records.

After all, there are important barriers to high quality palliative primary care, such as the lack of professional or specialist support structure, financial systems not permitting reimbursement for palliative care, competing demands in primary care, limited public understanding of palliative care, poor identification of patients requiring palliative care, and lack of knowledge and skills within primary care [40].

OUTCOMES AND USE OF RESOURCES

If high quality care is provided, HPCT can promote the decrease of:

- The number of patients in need of hospitalization (almost 50 percent) and the length of hospital stay [42–44];
- The number of hospital deaths [43, 45];
- The use of emergency department at end of life [43, 45];
- The use of health resources in general [46];
- 30-days hospital readmissions [44, 45].

Conversely, it can increase:

- The odds of the patient dying at home (OR: 2.21; $CI^2_{95\%}$: 1.31-3.71) [47];
- Patient satisfaction [46];
- Symptom control and quality of life [46];
- Survival [46].

ECONOMIC IMPACT

One inpatient-based palliative care case is 71 percent more expensive than one community-based program [48].

---

2 Confidence Interval

In the United States of America (USA) the HPCT can decrease the average daily cost per patient by $273/day [49]. Also, providing palliative care with the patients in their homes in the last three months of life decreases costs by $5,000 per patient [50].

In South Africa, these teams generate a daily average savings of 50 percent in patient costs in comparison with other palliative care teams [51].

One study made in Japan showed a reduction of 16.7 percent in health costs when compared with acute care settings [52]. This study is similar to another, made in Australia, which shows a decrease of 4,827-6,155 A$ while making the same comparisons [53].

An interesting study which includes patients with heart failure showed a cost savings of 50,000 euros per patient in the last six months of life [54].

E-HEALTH IN HOME PALLIATIVE CARE

In the highly technological world of today, use of the new technologies in palliative care provision should be thought out carefully, because there are now new and important ways of communication and promoting relationships [55].

Among the various technologies used in health care, the most used and studied in palliative care are remote self-monitoring and videoconferences or teleconsultations [56]. However, Podcast technology is now emerging, especially at information, education and training levels [57].

Several authors [58–65] have described how its use, namely in videoconferencing or teleconsultations, increases accessibility to palliative care, and the achievement of human rights through the improvement of integrated care, together with its accessibility by those living in remote areas or with fewer human resources [56].

Although the use of these technologies is short-lived, the results are very promising. Some of the most important achieved outcomes are:

1) Better communication between health care professionals and patient or family [66, 67];
2) Regular symptom self-assessment, where and when the patients wish, which allows access to data by HPCT in real time, which in turn promotes the continuity of care [66, 68];
3) Improvement and promotion of patient involvement [62];
4) Promotion of the maintenance of patients at home, where continuity of care can be achieved [69];
5) Increasing the safety and confidence of patients, families and caregivers, who feel more supported and informed [63, 68, 70, 71];
6) Promotion of contact between patients, family and friends, at any time, thus avoiding social isolation [72, 73];
7) Better quality of life and decrease of the caregiver burden [74, 75];
8) Increased care satisfaction by patients, family and caregivers [68, 76];
9) Decrease of both hospital and emergency department admissions [63, 77];
10) Better integrated care and interprofessional communication [78–80];

11) Better symptom control, quality of life, shared information and decision-making process [63, 67, 68, 75, 81–83];
12) More privacy in the transmission of very personal and intimate information [68];
13) Better quality of care [65, 67, 84];
14) Better quality clinical data records with less effort by health care professionals [67, 83, 84];
15) Better conditions for patient self-care through psychoeducational videos and other strategies [66, 85];
16) Family meetings promotion [78].

CONCLUSION

In summary, to meet patient preferences and choices about the place of care at end-of-life, as well as the place of death, home palliative care performs a key role in health care for these patients. However, to reach universal health coverage, it is not only necessary to guarantee access but also to deliver this care with enough quality to improve health and quality of life of patients and their families. If quality improvement is assumed as a home palliative care team key function, good outcomes will be achieved for the patients, families, health services and systems, in addition to society.

Therefore, there is a lot to do to achieve universal home palliative care coverage. It will be a challenge but also an opportunity to make a difference in the quality of life of these patients and their families and also within society.

REFERENCES

[1] Gomes B, Higginson IJ, Calanzani N, Cohen J, Deliens L, Daveson BA, et al. Preferences for place of death if faced with advanced cancer: A population survey in England, Flanders, Germany, Italy, The Netherlands, Portugal and Spain. *Ann Oncol.* 2012;23(8):2006–15.

[2] Capelas ML, Coelho SP. Local de prestação de cuidados no final da vida e local de morte : preferências dos portugueses [Place of end-of-life care and place of death: Portuguese preferences]. *Cad saúde.* 6(único):7–18.

[3] De Roo ML, Miccinesi G, Onwuteaka-Philipsen BD, Van Den Noortgate N, Van Den Block L, Bonacchi A, et al. Actual and preferred place of death of home-dwelling patients in four European countries: Making sense of quality indicators. *PLoS One.* 2014;9(4):6–10.

[4] Chung RYN, Wong ELY, Kiang N, Chau PYK, Lau JYC, Wong SYS, et al. Knowledge, Attitudes, and Preferences of Advance Decisions, End-of-Life Care, and Place of Care and Death in Hong Kong. A Population-Based Telephone Survey of 1067 Adults. *J Am Med Dir Assoc* [Internet]. 2017;18(4):367.e19-367.e27. Available from: http://dx.doi.org/10.1016/j.jamda.2016.12.066.

[5] Higginson IJ, Sen-Gupta GJA. Place of care in advanced cancer: A qualitative systematic literature review of patients preferences. *J Palliat Med.* 2000;3:287–300.

[6] Rainsford S, Macleod RD, Glasgow NJ. Place of death in rural palliative care: A systematic review. *Palliat Med.* 2016;30(8):745–63.
[7] Neergaard MA, Jensen AB, Sondergaard J, Sokolowski I, Olesen F, Vedsted P. Preference for place-of-death among terminally ill cancer patients in Denmark. *Scand J Caring Sci.* 2011;25(4):627–36.
[8] Howell DA, Wang HI, Roman E, Smith AG, Patmore R, Johnson MJ, et al. Preferred and actual place of death in haematological malignancy. *BMJ Support Palliat Care.* 2017;7(2):150–7.
[9] Skorstengaard MH, Neergaard MA, Andreassen P, Brogaard T, Bendstrup E, Løkke A, et al. Preferred Place of Care and Death in Terminally Ill Patients with Lung and Heart Disease Compared to Cancer Patients. *J Palliat Med* [Internet]. 2017;20(11): jpm.2017.0082. Available from: http://online.liebertpub.com/doi/10.1089/jpm.2017.0082.
[10] O'Neill B, Rodway a. ABC of palliative care. Care in the community. *BMJ.* 1998;316(7128):373–7.
[11] Macleod U. Place of death: is home always best? *Br J Hosp Med* (Lond). 2011;72(8):441–3.
[12] Cohen J, Pivodic L, Miccinesi G, Onwuteaka-Philipsen B, Naylor WA, Wilson DM, et al. International study of the place of death of people with cancer: a population-level comparison of 14 countries across 4 continents using death certificate data. *Br J Cancer* [Internet]. 2015;113(9):1397–404. Available from: http://dx.doi.org/10.1038/bjc.2015.312.
[13] The World Health Organization. *Strengthening of palliative care as a component of integrated treatment within the continuum of care.* 2014;2014(January):1–6.
[14] Gómez-Batiste X, Connor S, Murray S, Krakauer E, Radbruch L, Luyirika E, et al. Principles, Definitions and Concepts. In: Gómez-Batiste X, Connor S, editors. *Building Integrated Palliative Care Programs and Services.* Barcelona: Chair of Palliative Care; WHO Collaboration Centre Public Health Palliative Care Programmes; Worldwide Hospice Palliative Care Alliance; "la Caixa" Banking Foundation; 2017. p. 45–62.
[15] The Gold Standards Framework. *The GSF Prognostic Indicator Guidance* [Internet]. 4th ed. 2011. Available from: http://www.goldstandarsframework.org.uk.
[16] Highet G, Crawford D, Murray SA, Boyd K. Development and evaluation of the Supportive and Palliative Care Indicators Tool (SPICT): a mixed-methods study. *BMJ Support Palliat Care* [Internet]. 2014;4(3):285–90. Available from: https://www.ncbi.nlm.nih.gov/pubmed/24644193.
[17] Gómez-batiste X, Martínez-Muñoz M, Blay C, Amblàs J, Vila L, Costa X, et al. Identifying patients with chronic conditions in need of palliative care in the general population: development of the NECPAL tool and preliminary prevalence rates in Catalonia. *BMJ Support Palliat Care.* 2013;3(3):300–8.
[18] Thoonsen B, Engels Y, van Risjwijk E, van Weel C, Groot M. Early identification of palliative care patients in general practice: development of RADbound indicators for Palliative Care Needs (RADPAC). *Bristish J Gen Pract* [Internet]. 2012;62(602):e625–31. Available from: https://www.ncbi.nlm.nih.gov/pubmed/22947583.
[19] *St. Cristopher's. Residential Care Homes Steps End of Life Care Tool Kit* [Internet]. 2016 [cited 2017 Aug 1]. Available from: http://www.stchristophers.org/steps.

[20] Fischer SM, Gozansky WS, Sauaia A, Min SJ, Kutner JS, Kramer A. A Practical Tool to Identify Patients Who May Benefit from a Palliative Approach: The CARING Criteria. *J Pain Symptom Manage* [Internet]. 2006;31(4):285–92. Available from: https://www.ncbi.nlm.nih.gov/pubmed/16632076.

[21] Murray S a, Firth A, Schneider N, Van den Eynden B, Gomez-Batiste X, Brogaard T, et al. Promoting palliative care in the community: Production of the primary palliative care toolkit by the European Association of Palliative Care Taskforce in primary palliative care. *Palliat Med.* 2015;29(2):101–11.

[22] Radbruch L, Payne S, Bercovitch M, Caraceni A, Vlieger T De, Firth P, et al. White paper on standards and norms for hospice and palliative care in Europe: part 2. *Eur J Palliat care*. 2010;17(1):22–33.

[23] Doyle D. Getting Started: Guidelines and Suggestions for those Starting a Hospice/*Palliative Care Service* [Internet]. 2009. 1-76 p. Available from: papers2://publication/uuid/A6277469-9B86-4691-A217-7BFD0DFBB714.

[24] Connor S, Gómez-Batiste X. Assessing the Need for Palliative Care in Populations and Contexts. In: Gómez-Batiste X, Connor S, editors. *Building Integrated Palliative Care Programs and Services.* Barcelona: Chair of Palliative Care; WHO Collaboration Centre Public Health Palliative Care Programmes; Worldwide Hospice Palliative Care Alliance; "la Caixa" Banking Foundation; 2017. p. 79–92.

[25] Gómez-Batiste X, Connor S. Design and Implementation of Specialized Palliative Care Services. In: Gómez-Batiste X, Connor S, editors. *Building Integrated Palliative Care Programs and Services.* Barcelona: Chair of Palliative Care; WHO Collaboration Centre Public Health Palliative Care Programmes; Worldwide Hospice Palliative Care Alliance; "la Caixa" Banking Foundation; 2017. p. 103–22.

[26] Luyirika E, Gómez-Batiste X, Connor S. Models and Levels of Organization. In: Gómez-Batiste X, Connor S, editors. *Building Integrated Palliative Care Programs and Services*. Barcelona: Chair of Palliative Care; WHO Collaboration Centre Public Health Palliative Care Programmes; Worldwide Hospice Palliative Care Alliance; "la Caixa" Banking Foundation; 2017. p. 93–102.

[27] Connor S, Mosoiu D, Gómez-Batiste X, Herrera E. Cost, Funding and Reimbursement Models for Palliative Care. In: Gómez-Batiste X, Connor S, editors. *Building Integrated Palliative Care Programs and Services*. Barcelona: Chair of Palliative Care; WHO Collaboration Centre Public Health Palliative Care Programmes; Worldwide Hospice Palliative Care Alliance; "la Caixa" Banking Foundation; 2017. p. 175–84.

[28] Rosenfeld K, Wenger NS. Measuring Quality in End-of-Life Care. *Clin Geriatr Med.* 2000;16(2):387–400.

[29] IMPACT, EURO IMPACT. 2014 European Declaration on Palliative Care [Internet]. *Palliative Care* 2020. 2014 [cited 2017 Apr 17]. Available from: http://www.palliativecare2020.eu/declaration/.

[30] Lohman D, Wilson D, Marston JM. Advocacy and Human Rights Issues. In: Gómez-Batiste X, Connor S, editors. *Building Integrated Palliative Care Programs and Services*. Barcelona: Chair of Palliative Care; WHO Collaboration Centre Public Health Palliative Care Programmes; Worldwide Hospice Palliative Care Alliance; "la Caixa" Banking Foundation; 2017. p. 185–205.

[31] Gómez-Batiste X, Connor S, Foley K, Callaway M, Kumar S, Luyirika E. The Foundations of Palliative Care Public Health Programs. In: Gómez-Batiste X, Connor

S, editors. *Building Integrated Palliative Care Programs and Services*. Barcelona: Chair of Palliative Care; WHO Collaboration Centre Public Health Palliative Care Programmes; Worldwide Hospice Palliative Care Alliance; "la Caixa" Banking Foundation; 2017. p. 63–78.

[32] Gómez-Batiste X, Connor S, Luyrika E, Kumar S, Krakauer E, Ela S, et al. The Techinical Advisory Group (TAG) Supporting the WHO Palliatve Care Initiative. In: Gómez-Batiste X, Connor S, editors. *Building Integrated Palliative Care Programs and Services*. Barcelona: Chair of Palliative Care; WHO Collaboration Centre Public Health Palliative Care Programmes; Worldwide Hospice Palliative Care Alliance; "la Caixa" Banking Foundation; 2017. p. 21–42.

[33] National Quality Forum. *A National Framework and Preferred Practices for Palliative and Hospice Care Quality*. Washington: National Quality Forum; 2006. 11-14 p.

[34] National Consensus Project for Quality Palliative Care. *Clinical Practice Guidelines for Quality Palliative Care*. Practice. 2009.

[35] Gómez-Batiste X. Evaluación y mejora continua de calidad, planificación estratégica, organización de la formación y de la investigación en servicios de cuidados paliativos. In: Gómez-Batiste X, Porta J, Tuca A, Stjernsward J, editors [Evaluation and continuous improvement of quality, strategic planning, organization of training and research in palliative care services]. *Organización de Servicios y Programas de Cuidados Paliativos*. Madrid: Arán Ediciones; 2005. p. 81–98.

[36] Sancho MG. Enfermedad terminal y Medicina Paliativa [Terminal Illness and Palliative Medicine]. In: Sancho MG, editor. *Medicina Palliativa en la Cultura Latina*. Madrid: Arán Ediciones; 1999. p. 153–72.

[37] Ferris FD, Balfour HM, Bowen K, Farley J, Hardwick M, Lamontagne C, et al. A model to guide patient and family care: Based on nationally accepted principles and norms of practice. *J Pain Symptom Manage*. 2002;24(2):106–23.

[38] Capelas ML, Neto IG, Coelho SP. Organização de Serviços [Service Organization]. In: Barbosa A, Pina PR, Tavares F, Neto IG, editors. *Manual de Cuidados Paliativos*. 3{ª}. Lisboa: Faculdade de Medicina de Lisboa; 2016. p. 915–36.

[39] Mount BM. International group issues proposal for standards for care of terminally ill. *C Can Med Assoc J*. 1979;120(November 1974):1280–2.

[40] Mitchell G, Gómez-Batiste X, Murray S. Implementing a Palliative Care Approach in the Communituy and all Settings of Care. In: Gomez-Batiste X, Connor S, editors. Building Integrated Palliative Care Programs and Services. Barcelona: Chair of Palliative Care; WHO Collaboration Centre Public Health Palliative Care Programmes; Worldwide Hospice Palliative Care Alliance; "la Caixa" Banking Foundation; 2017. p. 123–36.

[41] Bausewein C, Daveson BA, Currow DC, Downing J, Deliens L, Radbruch L, et al. EAPC White Paper on outcome measurement in palliative care: Improving practice, attaining outcomes and delivering quality services - Recommendations from the European Association for Palliative Care (EAPC) Task Force on Outcome Measurement. *Palliat Med*. 2016;30(1):6–22.

[42] Fernandes, Braun K, Ozawa, Compton, Guzman, Somogyi-Zalud. Home-based palliative care services for underserved populations. *J Palliat Med* [Internet]. 2010;13(4):41. Available from: http://search.ebscohost.com/login.aspx?direct=true

&amp%5Cndb=cin20&amp%5CnAN=2010628288&amp%5Cnlang=es&amp%5Cnsite =ehost-liv.

[43] Alonso-Babarro A, Astray-Mochales J, Domínguez-Berjón F, Gènova-Maleras R, Bruera E, Díaz-Mayordomo A, et al. The association between in-patient death, utilization of hospital resources and availability of palliative home care for cancer patients. *Palliat Med* [Internet]. 2013;27(1):68–75. Available from: http://www.ncbi.nlm.nih.gov/pubmed/22492481.

[44] Lukas L, Foltz C, Paxton H. Hospital outcomes for a home-based palliative medicine consulting service. *J Palliat Med* [Internet]. 2013;16(2):179–84. Available from: http://www.ncbi.nlm.nih.gov/pubmed/23308377.

[45] Seow H, Brazil K, Sussman J, Pereira J, Marshall D, Austin PC, et al. Impact of community based, specialist palliative care teams on hospitalisations and emergency department visits late in life and hospital deaths: a pooled analysis. *BMJ* [Internet]. 2014;348(June):g3496. Available from: http://www.pubmedcentral.nih.gov/articlerender.fcgi?artid=4048125&tool=pmcentrez&rendertype=abstract.

[46] Rabow M, Kvale E, Barbour L, Cassel JB, Cohen S, Jackson V, et al. Moving upstream: a review of the evidence of the impact of outpatient palliative care. *J Palliat Med* [Internet]. 2013;16(12):1540–9. Available from: http://online.liebertpub.com/doi/abs/10.1089/jpm.2013.0153.

[47] Gomes B, Calanzani N, McCrone P, Higginson IJ. Effectiveness and cost-effectiveness of home palliative care services for adults with advanced illness and their caregivers (Review) Effectiveness and cost-effectiveness of home palliative care services for adults with advanced illness and their caregiv. *Cochrane Database Syst Rev.* 2013;(6):1–279.

[48] Serra-Prat M, Gallo P, Picaza JM. Home palliative care as a cost-saving alternative: evidence from Catalonia. *Palliat Med* [Internet]. 2001;15(4):271–8. Available from: http://www.ncbi.nlm.nih.gov/pubmed/12054144.

[49] McGrath S, Foote Gargis D, Frith H, Hall Michael W. Cost Effectiveness of a Palliative Care Program in a Rural Community Hospital. *Nurs Econ* [Internet]. 2013;31(4):176–83. Available from: http://search.ebscohost.com/login.aspx?direct=true&db=ccm&AN=107964016&site=ehost-live.

[50] Blackhall LJ, Read P, Stukenborg G, Dillon P, Barclay J, Romano A, et al. CARE Track for Advanced Cancer: Impact and Timing of an Outpatient Palliative Care Clinic. *J Palliat Med* [Internet]. 2015;19(1):57–63. Available from: http://www.ncbi.nlm.nih.gov/pubmed/26624851.

[51] Hongoro C, Dinat N. A cost analysis of a hospital-based palliative care outreach program: Implications for expanding public sector palliative care in South Africa. *J Pain Symptom Manage* [Internet]. 2011;41(6):1015–24. Available from: http://dx.doi.org/10.1016/j.jpainsymman.2010.08.014.

[52] Kinjo K, Sairenji T, Koga H, Osugi Y, Yoshida S, Ichinose H, et al. Cost of physician-led home visit care (Zaitaku care) compared with hospital care at the end of life in Japan. *BMC Health Serv Res* [Internet]. 2017;17(1):40. Available from: http://www.ncbi.nlm.nih.gov/pubmed/28095906%0A;http://www.pubmedcentral.nih.gov/articlerender.fcgi?artid=PMC5240473.

[53] Youens D, Moorin R. The Impact of Community-Based Palliative Care on Utilization and Cost of Acute Care Hospital Services in the Last Year of Life. *J Palliat Med*

[Internet]. 2017;20(7):jpm.2016.0417. Available from: http://www.ncbi.nlm.nih.gov/pubmed/28437201%5Cnhttp://online.liebertpub.com/doi/10.1089/jpm.2016.0417.

[54] Sahlen K-G, Boman K, Brännström M. A cost-effectiveness study of person-centered integrated heart failure and palliative home care: Based on a randomized controlled trial. *Palliat Med* [Internet]. 2016;30(3):296–302. Available from: http://journals.sagepub.com/doi/10.1177/0269216315618544.

[55] van Gurp J, van Selm M, van Leeuwen E, Hasselaar J. Transmural palliative care by means of teleconsultation: a window of opportunities and new restrictions. *BMC Med Ethics* [Internet]. 2013;14(1):1–12. Available from: http://www.pubmedcentral.nih.gov/articlerender.fcgi?artid=3608168&tool=pmcentrez&rendertype=abstract.

[56] Bates BM. Innovation Comes to Palliative Care. *IEEE Pulse*. 2016;(november/december):25–9.

[57] Nwosu AC, Monnery D, Reid VL, Chapman L. Use of podcast technology to facilitate education, communication and dissemination in palliative care: the development of the AmiPal podcast. *BMJ Support Palliat Care*. 2017;7(2):212–7.

[58] Wade VA, Taylor AD, Kidd MR, Carati C. Transitioning a home telehealth project into a sustainable, large-scale service: a qualitative study. *BMC Health Serv Res* [Internet]. 2016;16(1):183. Available from: http://bmchealthservres.biomedcentral.com/articles/10.1186/s12913-016-1436-0.

[59] Donnem T, Ervik B, Magnussen K, Andersen S, Pastow D, Andreassen S, et al. Bridging the distance: A prospective tele-oncology study in Northern Norway. *Support Care Cancer*. 2012;20(9):2097–103.

[60] Liptrott S, Bee P, Lovell K. Acceptability of telephone support as perceived by patients with cancer: A systematic review. *Eur J Cancer Care* (Engl) [Internet]. 2017;([Epub ahead of print]):1–28. Available from: http://doi.wiley.com/10.1111/ecc.12643.

[61] Van Gurp J, Soyannwo O, Odebunmi K, Dania S, VanSelm M, Van Leeuwen E, et al. Telemedicine's potential to support good dying in Nigeria: A qualitative study. *PLoS One* [Internet]. 2015;10(6):1–15. Available from: http://dx.doi.org/10.1371/journal.pone.0126820.

[62] Van Gurp J, Van Selm M, Vissers K, Van Leeuwen E, Hasselaar J. How outpatient palliative care teleconsultation facilitates empathic patient-professional relationships: A qualitative study. *PLoS One* [Internet]. 2015;10(4):1–13. Available from: http://dx.doi.org/10.1371/journal.pone.0124387.

[63] Hennemann-Krause L, Lopes AJ, Araújo JA, Petersen EM, Nunes RA. The assessment of telemedicine to support outpatient palliative care in advanced cancer. *Palliat Support Care* [Internet]. 2015;13:1025–30. Available from: http://www.ncbi.nlm.nih.gov/pubmed/25159308.

[64] Tieman JJ, Swetenham K, Morgan DD, To TH, Currow DC, Wiencek C, et al. Using telehealth to support end of life care in the community: a feasibility study. *BMC Palliat Care* [Internet]. 2016;15(1):94. Available from: http://bmcpalliatcare.biomedcentral.com/articles/10.1186/s12904-016-0167-7.

[65] Johnston B. UK telehealth initiatives in palliative care: a review. *Int J Palliat Nurs*. 2011;17(6):301–8.

[66] Dy SM, Roy J, Ott GE, McHale M, Kennedy C, Kutner JS, et al. Tell Us: A web-based tool for improving communication among patients, families, and providers in hospice and palliative care through systematic data specification, collection, and use. *J Pain*

Symptom Manage [Internet]. 2011;42(4):526–34. Available from: http://dx.doi.org/10.1016/j.jpainsymman.2010.12.006.

[67] Capurro D, Ganzinger M, Perez-Lu J, Knaup P. Effectiveness of ehealth interventions and information needs in palliative care: A systematic literature review. *J Med Internet Res.* 2014;16(3):1–15.

[68] Abernethy AP, Currow DC. Patient self-reporting in palliative care using information technology: Yes, there is hope! *Palliat Med.* 2011;25(7):673–4.

[69] Lutz BJ, Chumbler NR, Roland K. Care coordination/home-telehealth for veterans with stroke and their caregivers: addressing an unmet need. *Top Stroke Rehabil* [Internet]. 2007;14(2):32–42. Available from: http://www.ncbi.nlm.nih.gov/pubmed/17517572.

[70] Munck B, Sandgren A. The impact of medical technology on sense of security in the palliative home care setting. *Bristish J Community Nurs.* 2017;22(3):130–5.

[71] Slev VN, Mistiaen P, Pasman HRW, Leeuw IMV de, Uden-Kraan CF van, Francke AL. Effects of eHealth for patients and informal caregivers confronted with cancer: A meta-review. *Int J Med Inform.* 2016;87(2016):54–67.

[72] Guo Q, Cann B, McClement S, Thompson G, Chochinov HM. Keep in touch (KIT): perspectives on introducing internet-based communication and information technologies in palliative care. *BMC Palliat Care* [Internet]. 2016;15(1):66. Available from: http://bmcpalliatcare.biomedcentral.com/articles/10.1186/s12904-016-0140-5.

[73] Brecher DB. The Use of Skype in a Community Hospital Inpatient Palliative Medicine Consultation Service. *J Palliat Med.* 2012;16(1):110–2.

[74] Zheng Y, Head BA, Schapmire TJ. A Systematic Review of Telehealth in Palliative Care: Caregiver Outcomes. *Telemed J E Health* [Internet]. 2015;22(4):1–7. Available from: http://online.liebertpub.com/doi/abs/10.1089/tmj.2015.0090.

[75] Jones J. Using Skype to Support Palliative Care Surveillance. *Nurs Older People.* 2014;26(1):16–9.

[76] Kilbourn KM, Costenaro A, Madore S, DeRoche K, Anderson D, Keech T, et al. Feasibility of a Telephone-Based Counseling Program for Informal Caregivers of Hospice Patients. *J Palliat Med.* 2011;14(11):1200–5.

[77] Harrison JD, Durcinoska I, Butow PN, White K, Solomon MJ, Young JM. Localized versus centralized nurse-delivered telephone services for people in follow up for cancer: Opinions of cancer clinicians. *Asia Pac J Clin Oncol.* 2014;10(2):175–82.

[78] Menon PR, Stapleton RD, McVeigh U, Rabinowitz T. Telemedicine as a Tool to Provide Family Conferences and Palliative Care Consultations in Critically Ill Patients at Rural Health Care Institutions: A Pilot Study. *Am J Hosp Palliat Med* [Internet]. 2015;32(4):448–53. Available from: http://ajh.sagepub.com/content/32/4/448.abstract.

[79] Esterle L, Mathieu-Fritz A. Teleconsultation in geriatrics: Impact on professional practice. *Int J Med Inform* [Internet]. 2013;82(2013):684–95. Available from: http://dx.doi.org/10.1016/j.ijmedinf.2013.04.006.

[80] Van Gurp J, Van Selm M, Van Leeuwen E, Vissers K, Hasselaar J. Teleconsultation for integrated palliative care at home: A qualitative study. *Palliat Med.* 2016;30(3):257–69.

[81] Strasser F, Blum D, von Moos R, Ribi K, Aebi S, Betticher D, et al. The effect of real-time electronic monitoring of patient-reported symptoms and clinical syndromes in outpatient workflow of medical oncologists.pdf. *Ann Oncol.* 2015;27(2):324–32.

[82] Steel JL, Geller DA, Kim KH, Butterfield LH, Spring M, Grady J, et al. Web-based collaborative care intervention to manage cancer-related symptoms in the palliative care setting. *Cancer*. 2016;122(8):1270–82.

[83] Larsen AC. Trappings of technology: Casting palliative care nursing as legal relations. *Nurs Inq*. 2012;19(4):334–44.

[84] Abernethy AP, Wheeler JL, Bull J. Development of a health information technology-based data system in community-based hospice and palliative care. *Am J Prev Med* [Internet]. 2011;40(5 SUPPL. 2):S217–24. Available from: http://dx.doi.org/10.1016/j.amepre.2011.01.012.

[85] O'Halloran P, Scott D, Reid J, Porter S. Multimedia psychoeducational interventions to support patient self-care in degenerative conditions: A realist review. *Palliat Support Care* [Internet]. 2015;13(5):1473–86. Available from: http://www.ncbi.nlm.nih.gov/pubmed/25336040.

BIOGRAPHICAL SKETCHES

Manuel Luís Vila Capelas

Degree in Nursing, Master in Palliative Care, Doctorate (PhD) in Health Sciences-Palliative Care in 2013. Assistant Professor in Institute of Health Sciences of Universidade Católica Portuguesa, where coordinates the courses and research in the palliative care field. Is, also, a codiretor of the Portuguese Observatory for Palliative Care. Published 41 papers in scientific journals and 59 abstracts in proceedings congresses. Has 4 books and 9 chapters published. Also, have 285 communications (conferences, free communications and and posters) in national and international conferences/scientific meetings. Supervised 15 and cosupervised 30 master dissertations.

Patrícia Coelho

Assistant Professor of the Universidade Católica Portuguesa, Institute of Health Sciences, Porto. PhD in Nursing and Master in Medical-Surgical Nursing. Post-Graduate in Health Quality Management, Post-Graduation in Bioethics, and Post-Graduation in Palliative Care. Collaborator of the European Association for Palliative Care Nursing Task Force and the Portuguese Palliative Care Observatory

Tânia Afonso

Tânia Afonso is a Specialist Nurse who works in a Palliative Care Team of a Public Hospital in Portugal. Born in Lisbon, Portugal in 1989, she graduated from the Universidade Católica Portuguesa with Master's degree in Nursing. She lives in Sintra and has important participatory community intervention in some projects - environmental and animal welfare are the more relevant issues - and is a Volunteer Health Teacher at a Senior University.

Palliative Care starts as a major subject in her life, since the pre-training formative period. Passionate about the response to the human needs and the development of quality of care she starts studying this scientific area. That led to the conclusion of a Master in Palliative Care in the University of Lisbon - Faculdade de Medicina de Lisboa in 2015.

Her primary interests include the Palliative Care study, the research and teaching.

She is currently working on a Nursing's PhD at the Universidade Católica Portuguesa since 2015 where she's also a Research Assistant in the Portuguese Observatory for Palliative Care developing numerous projects with great enthusiasm.

For the future, she hopes to contribute to improving the knowledge and development of Palliative Care and Nursing care in Portugal.

In: Palliative Care
Editor: Michael Silbermann

ISBN: 978-1-53616-199-1
© 2019 Nova Science Publishers, Inc.

Chapter 8

COPING WITH DEATH COMPETENCE IN PEDIATRIC NURSES

*Amparo Oliver[1], Laura Galiana[1], Noemí Sansó[2] and Juan Manuel Gavala[3]**

[1]Faculty of Psychology, Universitat de Valencia, Valencia, Spain
[2]Department of Nursing & Physiotherapy, University of Balearic Island, Palma de Mallorca, Spain
[3]Hospital Son Espases, Palma de Mallorca, Spain

ABSTRACT

Palliative care professionals are continually dealing with death, a process that escapes one's control and produces great concern, fear, and anxiety. To access professionals' skills in facing this process, Bugen developed the Coping with Death Competence Scale. This 30-item instrument assesses a wide range of skills for facing death, as well as beliefs and attitudes about these capacities. Due to its length, the scale has only been used in broad survey studies. The aim of the current research is to test the psychometric properties of a short version of the scale in a sample of pediatric palliative care nurses. In all, 171 pediatric palliative care nurses participated in the study. Analyses included a confirmatory factor analysis to test the a priori unidimensional structure and estimates of reliability. The structure was successfully tested: $\chi^2(27) = 58.199$, $p < .001$; CFI = .972; RMSEA = .083[.053,.112]. Estimates of reliability were also adequate, with a Cronbach's alpha of .869. Thus, the results pointed out the good properties of a short version of Bugen's Coping with Death Scale. Implications of this short version in palliative care research are discussed.

Keywords: competence with death, validity, reliability, pediatric nurses

---

* Corresponding Author's E-mail: amparo.oliver@uiv.es

1. Background

Health professionals establish helping relationships with patients and their relatives to help them through the illness process. This relationship is especially relevant when caring for patients who cope with life threatening diseases, such as cancer. In this context, professionals try to reduce suffering as much as possible.

1.1. Death and Suffering in the Helping Relationship

Developing a proper helping relationship involves empathic, intense, and continuous communication with patients and their families, and being intimately in touch with their emotions. Working in an environment with intense and potentially stressful factors, such as contact with other people's pain, feelings of loss, suffering, and death, undoubtedly turns the helping relationship into an intense experience that can have negative consequences for the professional, but also stimulate the development of coping strategies (Puchalski, 2013).

Fear of death is an ancestral and universal fear. However, for health professionals, daily contact with death and suffering surpasses their control and can generate great concern and anxiety (Puchalski, 2012). In fact, evidence reveals that attending to pain, suffering, and death is one of professionals' main stressors (Cumplido and Molina, 2011, Benbunan et al., 2007). This is especially true in the field of oncology, where most healthcare professionals have stated that they experience grief when their patients die (Granek et al., 2015; Plante & Cry, 2011). This stressor is even greater when the patient is a child (Pascual MC, 2011). Taking care of a child during the treatment for a life-threatening disease, or even during the process of dying, has a high emotional impact on both the family and caregivers (Martino R, 2014). Despite this fact, the research on coping with the death of a child has focused almost entirely on family members' experiences, rather than on professional caregivers (Barrera et al., 2013; Granek et al., 2013).

Professionals' attitudes in dealing with emotional situations can modulate both the quality of care and professionals' quality of life (Grundfeld et al., 2005; Samson & Schvartzman, 2017). In fact, evidence shows that occupational exposure to patient death is related to fear of death and death avoidance, a decline in empathy and compassion satisfaction, and an increase in secondary traumatic stress and burnout (Liney & Joseph, 2005; McFarland, Malone, & Roth, 2016; Sansó et al., 2015). Therefore, it is important for health professionals to develop competence in coping with death, in order to keep their own fears from influencing the patient's suffering (Puchalski, 2012).

1.2. Professionals' Competence with Death

The coping with death competence is a construct that represents a wide range of skills, beliefs, and attitudes about facing death (Schmidt, 2007). Furthermore, it is especially relevant because competence in coping with death has been related to improved work performance (Robbins, 1992; Schmidt, 2007) and a lower risk of experiencing the negative effects of caring, such as burnout or compassion fatigue (Holland & Neimeyer, 2005; Sansó et al., 2015).

Death anxiety, death attitudes, or coping with death are interrelated constructs, and in the literature, they have led to a wide range of measurement instruments, including the Collett-Lester Fear of Death Scale (CL-FODS; Collett & Lester, 1969), the Revised Profile of Attitudes toward Death (Wong, Rever & Gesser, 1997), the Death Anxiety Inventory (DAI) (Tomás-Sábado, Gómez-Benito, & Limonero, 2005), the Death Attitude Profile-Revised (DAP-R; Wong, Reker, & Gesser, 1997), the Death Anxiety Scale (DAS; Templer, 1970), or the Coping with Death Scale (CDS; Bugen, 1980-81). Among them, the first scale for assessing coping with death, Bugen's Scale (1980-1981), was designed in the palliative care field.

Bugen developed the scale with the objective of assessing the effect of a training program on death competence (Bugen 80-81; 1977). It is a 30-item questionnaire that, as far as we know, is the only instrument created specifically for staff working in the hospice and palliative care field. The Bugen scale has been used by many researchers to measure the level of coping with death in different groups, such as university students (Colell, 2005; Robbins, 1991), hospice volunteers (Bugen 1980-1981; Brysiewicz & McInerney, 2004; Claxton-Oldfield et al., 2007; Robbins, 1992), volunteers in a religious context (Robbins, 1997), and healthcare professionals (Galiana et al., 2017).

A few studies have focused on how to improve this competence. In a control trial study with palliative care volunteers, Robbins (1992) showed that the more experience in palliative care they had, the higher their coping with death competence was, although no evidence was gathered about changes in anxiety. Claxton-Oldfield et al. (2007) studied the effect of a training program on palliative care volunteers, showing that participants felt significantly more capable of coping with death and dying after the training program than before it. Furthermore, the team led by Schmidt-Riovalle (2012) used quasi-experimental research to successfully show the impact of a palliative care training program on death competence in 87 health sciences students.

From a more statistical perspective, few studies have focused on the Coping with Death Scale's psychometric properties. Schmidt (2007), for example, was the first to carry out an exploratory study of its psychometric properties in the Spanish context. Results showed a one-factor structure and identified validity and reliability problems with some items. In the Portuguese context, the work by Forte and Gomes (2015) also focused on Bugen's scale using exploratory factor analysis. This study again found several items with psychometric problems and a two-factor structure. More recently, Galiana et al. (2017) also studied the scale's functioning in the Spanish context, with evidence of a one-factor structure in the context of structural equation modeling (confirmatory factor analysis). Again, several items showed poor reliability estimates and non-statistically significant factor loadings. In 2019, and with the aim of developing a short version of Bugen's Coping with Death Scale, Galiana et al. (2019) presented a 9-item version in Spanish and Argentinian palliative care professionals. This short version of the scale showed appropriate psychometric properties.

1.3. Aim of the Study

Taking into account these issues and the advantages of having brief measures in demanding work contexts such as pediatric services, the aim of the present study is to validate the short version of Bugen's Coping with Death Scale (Galiana et al., 2019). For this purpose, a brief, simpler questionnaire was studied, using some of the original items. Construct validity and reliability estimates of this new version have been gathered from a sample of pediatric nurses on the Balearic Islands.

2. METHOD

2.1. Design and Procedure

A cross-sectional survey was presented in Spanish to pediatric nurses on the Balearic Islands. The sample was recruited through the Head of nurses in each Service. Nurses who were caring for children in the end of life phase were invited to participate. After giving their informed consent, they filled out the on-line self-administered survey. The study focused on the following services: Pediatric Oncology Services, Neonatal Intensive Care Units, Pediatric Intensive Care Units, and Pediatric Emergency Services.

2.2. Participants

In all, 171 pediatric nurses participated in the study. 90% were women. Their mean number of years of experience was 4.05 ($SD = 1.49$).

2.3. Measurement Outcomes

The instrument used in the present study was the short version of the Coping with Death Scale (Bugen, 1980–1981), developed by the authors (Galiana et al., 2019). In order to choose the best items from Bugen's Coping with Death Scale, a two-step procedure was carried out. First, those items with valid content from the original scale were chosen by experts on coping with death. Second, among these chosen items, those that had shown greater reliability in previous research (Galiana et al., 2017) made up the new short version. Table 1 shows the items and their descriptive statistics.

2.4. Data Analyses

Statistical analyses included a Confirmatory Factor Analysis (CFA). A unifactorial structure, in which a factor of Coping with death competence explained items 6, 9, 15, 10, 20, 22, 26, 27 and 28, was hypothesized, estimated, and tested in the sample. In order to assess the model's fit, several fit criteria were used: the chi-square, CFI, TLI, SRMR, and RMSEA. The following cut-off points were used to determine good fit: CFI above .90 (even better, above .95) and SRMR or RMSEA below .08 (even better, below .05).

Additionally, reliability estimates were also calculated using Cronbach's alpha and the Composite Reliability Index (CRI).

3. RESULTS

Results of the confirmatory factor analysis revealed an excellent overall fit of the model: $\chi^2_{SB}(27) = 58.199$, $p < .001$; CFI = .972; RMSEA = .083[.053,.112]. With regard to the analytical fit, all the factor loadings were statistically significant and high (above .50). Estimates of reliability were also adequate, with a Cronbach's alpha of .869 for the scale. Results appear in Table 1.

Table 1. Items' descriptive statistics and standardized factor loadings for the short version of Bugen's Coping with Death Scale

Items	M	SD	λ	α if item deleted
6. I am aware of the full array of emotions that characterize human grief	4.81	1.75	.565	.863
9. I feel prepared to face my dying process	3.46	1.86	.514	.863
15. I can put words to my gut-level feelings about death and dying	4.74	1.60	.574	.860
19. I know who to contact when death occurs	4.57	1.87	.631	.855
20. I will be able to cope with future losses	4.12	1.74	.552	.858
22. I know how to listen to others, including the terminally ill	5.09	1.61	.631	.855
26. I can help someone with their thoughts and feelings about death and dying	4.36	1.55	.747	.843
27. I would be able to talk to a friend or family member about their death	4.78	1.68	.687	.850
28. I can lessen the anxiety of those around me when the topic is death and dying	4.31	1.53	.684	.849

Notes: M = Mean; SD = standard deviation; λ = factor loading. All factor loadings were statistically significant ($p < .001$).

4. DISCUSSION

The aim of this study was to test the psychometric properties of a new short version of Bugen's Scale in a sample of pediatric nurses from the Balearic Islands (Spain).

Evidence gathered in this study shows that the tool is appropriate and effective for measuring competence with death in professionals working in high emotionally demanding environments, such as pediatric oncology, the ICU, and emergency services. The short version of the Bugen Scale shows appropriate factorial validity and excellent estimates of reliability.

A lack of the coping with death competence can lead to emotional distress and burnout (Sansó et al, 2015, Holland & Neimeyer, 2005). Thus, it is important to monitor this skill in healthcare professionals who work in highly emotionally demanding environments. This is even more important when the professionals are caring for children, where the emotional impact is even greater. We also know that this competence can be improved through training (Bugen 1980-1981; Brysiewicz & McInerney, 2004; Claxton-Oldfield et al., 2007; Robbins, 1992). Thus, the outcome of the present study is valuable because it provides a psychometrically sound, short tool with suitable psychometric properties and length to adequately and easily assess this competence.

The main strength of this study is the sample's uniqueness. There is little available research about the coping with death competence in pediatric nurses, or about a validated scale specifically for this collective. However, as a study limitation is that the findings from this research are limited to a regional sample of pediatric nurses. Another limitation would be the absence of external validity evidence. Further research is needed in other regions or countries to assess the validity and reliability of the scale and include additional variables to test the convergent and discriminant validity of this new version.

Future studies could study the impact of specific training programs on the coping with death competence, compare the levels of these skills across different disciplines, or even analyze the relationship between this competence and the quality of care.

4.1. Practical Implications

The ability to cope with death is related to burnout syndrome and compassion fatigue (Holland & Neimeyer, 2005; Sansó et al., 2015). Therefore, this variable should be taken into account in occupational health services for healthcare professionals as an indicator that directly impacts the professional quality of life and indirectly affects the quality of care provided by professionals. Having a useful tool facilitates the incorporation of psychological variables, such as the competence of coping with death, in monitoring and preventing the risks involved in caring for suffering children and their families.

REFERENCES

Barrera, M., Granek, L., Shaheed, J., Nicholas, D., Beaune, L., D'Agostino, N. M., & Antle, B. (2013). The tenacity and tenuousness of hope: Parental experiences of hope when their child has a poor cancer prognosis. *Cancer Nursing, 36*(5), 408–416. doi:10.1097/NCC.0b013e318291ba7d.

Benbunan-Bentata, B., Alfaya Góngora, M. M., Chocrom, S., Cruz Quintana, F., Villaverde Gutiérrez, C. & Roa Venegas, J. M. (2007). El impacto emotivo del hospital, Implicaciones en la formación universitaria de los estudiantes de Enfermería [The emotional impact of the hospital. Implications in Nursing students' university curricula]. *Revista ROL Enfermería, 28,* 675-682.

Brysiewicz, P. & McInerney, P. A. (2004). A pilot study of competency amongst health workers in the Uthukela District in Kwazulu-Natal. *Curationis, 27*(3), 43-48.

Bugen, L. A. (1977). Human grief: a model for prediction and intervention. *American Journal of Orthopsychiatry, 47*(2), 196-206.

Bugen, L. A. (1980-81). Coping: Effects of death education. *Journal of Death and Dying, 11,* 175-183.

Claxton-Oldfield, S., Crain, M., & Claxton-Oldfield, J. (2007). Death anxiety and death competency: the impact of a palliative care volunteer training program. *American Journal of Hospice and Palliative Care, 23*(6), 464-468.

Colell, R. (2005). *Análisis de las actitudes ante la muerte y el enfermo al final de la vida en estudiantes de enfermería de Andalucía y Cataluña* [Attitudes towards death and the end-of-life paitent in nursing students from Andalusia and Catalonia]. Doctoral Thesis, Universidad Autónoma de Barcelona.

Collet, L. J., & Lester, D. (1969), The fear of death and the fear of dying. *Journal of Psychology, 72*, 179-181.

Cumplido, R., & Molina, C. (2011). Aproximación cualitativa al afrontamiento de la muerte en profesionales de cuidados intensivos [Qualitative approach to coping with the death in intensive care professionals]. *Medicina Paliativa, 18*(4), 141-148.

Forte, A. P., & Rodrigues, S. M. (2015). Translation and validation of the coping with death scale: A study with nurses. *Journal of Nursing Referência, 4*, 113-121.

Galiana, L., Oliver, A., Sansó, N., Pades, A., & Benito, E. (2017). Validación confirmatoria de la Escala de Afrontamiento de la Muerte en profesionales de cuidados paliativos [Confirmatory validation of the Coping with Death Scale in palliative care professionals]. *Medicina Paliativa, 24*(3), 126-135.

Galiana, L., Olivrer, A., de Simone, G., Linzitto, J. P., Benito, E., & Sansó, N. (2019). A Brief Measure for the Assessment of Competence in Coping With Death: The Coping With Death Scale Short Version. *Journal of Pain and Symptom Management, 57*(2), 209-215.

Granek, L., Barrera, M., Shaheed, J., Nicholas, D., Beaune, L., D'Agostino, N., & Antle, B. (2013). Trajectory of parental hope when a child has difficult to treat cancer: A prospective qualitative study. *Psycho-Oncology, 22*(11), 2436–2444.

Granek, L., Bartels, U., Scheinemann, K., Labrecque, M., & Barrera, M. (2015). Grief reactions and impact of patient death on pediatric oncologists. *Pediatric Blood & Cancer, 62*(1), 134-142.

Grundfeld, E., Zitzelsberger, L., Coristine, M., Whelan, T. J., Aspelund, F., & Evans, W. K. (2005). Job stress and job satisfaction of cancer care workers. *Psychoonology, 14*, 61-69.

Holland, J. M., & Neimeyer, R. A. (205). Reducing the risk of burnout in end-of-life care settings: the role of daily spiritual experiences and training. *Palliative and Supportive Care, 3*, 173-181.

Liney, P. A., & Joseph, S. (2005). Positive and negative changes following occupational death exposure. *Journal of Traumatic Stress, 18*(6), 751-758.

Martino, R. (2014). *Cuidados paliativos pediátricos en el Sistema Nacional de Salud: Criterios de Atención* [Pediatric palliative care in the National Health System: Care criteria]. Ministerio de Sanidad, Servicios Sociales e Igualdad. Gobierno de España.

McFarland, D. C., Malone, A. K., & Roth, A. (2016). Acute empathy decline among resident physician trainees on a hematology-oncology award: An exploratory analysis of house staff empathy, distress, and patient death exposure. *Psycho-Oncology, 26*(5), 698-703.

Pascual, M. C. (2011). Ansiedad del personal de enfermería ante la muerte en las unidades de críticos en relación con la edad de los pacientes [Anxiety of nursing staff in the face of death in critical care units and its relationship with the patients' age]. *Enfermería Intensiva, 22*(3), 96-103.

Plante, J., & Cyr, C. (2011). Health care professionals' grief after the death of a child. *Pediatrics & Child Health, 16*(4), 213–216.

Puchalski, C. M. (2012). Spirituality in the cancer trajectory. *Annals of Oncology, 23*(3), 49-55.

Puchalski, C. M. (2013). Integrating spirituality into patient care: an essential element of person-centered care. *Polish Archives of Internal Medicine, 123*(9), 491-7.

Robbins, R. A. (1991). Death anxiety, death competency and self-actualization in hospice volunteers. *The Hospice Journal, 7*(4), 24-35.

Robbins, R. A. (1992). Death competency: a study of hospice volunteers. *Death Studies, 16*(6), 557-569.

Robbins, R. A. (1997). Competencia ante la muerte: escala de Bugen de afrontamiento de la muerte y escala de autoeficacia frente a la muerte[Competency towards death: Bugen's coping with death scale and self-efficacy towards death scale]. En R. A. Neimeyer (Ed.), *Métodos de evaluación de la ansiedad ante la muerte* (pp. 159-174). Barcelona: Paidós.

Samson, T., & Shvartzman, P. (2017). Association between level of exposure to death and dying and profesional quality of life among palliative care workers. Palliative and Supportive Care, 1-10.

Sansó, N., Galiana, L., Oliver, A., Pascual, A., Sinclair, S., & Benito, E. (2015). Palliative care professionals' inner life: Exploring the relationships among awareness, self-care and compassion satisfaction and fatigue, Burnout and coping with death. *Journal of Pain and Symptom Management, 50* (2), 200-207.

Schmidt, J. (2007). *Validación de la versión española de la escala Bugen de afrontamiento de la muerte y del perfil revisado de actitudes hacia la muerte. Estudio comparativo y transcultural. Puesta en marcha de un programa de intervención* [Validation of the Spanish versión of the Bugen's coping with death scale and the attitudes towards death profile reviewed. Implementation of an intervention program]. Doctoral Thesis, University of Granada.

Schmidt, J., Montoya, R., Campos, C. P., García, M. P., Prados, D., Cruz, F. (2012). Efectos de un programa de formacion en cuidados paliativos sobre el afrontamiento de la muerte [The effects of a training program on coping with death in palliative care]. *Medicina Paliativa, 19*(3), 113-20.

Templer, D. (1970). The construction and validation of a death anxiety scale. *Journal of General Psychology, 82*, 165-177.

Tomás-Sábado, J., Gómez-Benito, J., & Limonero, J. T. (2005). The Death Anxiety Inventory: a revision. *Psychological Reports, 97*(3), 793-6.

Wong, P., Reker, G. & Gesser, G. (1997). Perfil revisado de actitudes hacia la muerte: un instrumento de medida multidimensional [Attitudes towards death profile reviewed: a multidimensional measurement instrument]. En R. A. Neimeyer (Ed.), *Métodos de Evaluación de la ansiedad ante la muerte* (pp. 131-158). Barcelona: Paidós.

BIOGRAPHICAL SKETCH

Amparo Oliver, PhD

Full Professor in Quantitative Methods Applied to Behavioral Sciences at University of Valencia, SPAIN. Head of ARMAQoL interdisciplinar research group (Advanced Research Methods Applied to Quality of Life, GIUV-2017-359) and co-leader of the Biogender Medicine Unit, pionnering with CIPF (Centro de Investigación Príncipe Felipe) this research topic in Spain. Head of the interdisciplinary PhD program in Promotion of Autonomy and Socio-Sanitary Care addressed to national and international PhD students from Psychology, Nursing, Social Work, Medicine, Phisiotherapy.

Research in advanced statistical models applied to quality of life and welfare promotion. Some particular fields with relevant gender perspective: successful aging; dignity & quality at the end of life (palliative care patients and professional's inner CV); gender violence (diagnostic and intervention); equity and entrepreneurship from education.

https://orcid.org/0000-0002-1207-4088
Twitter: @ARMAQoL
LinkedIN: Amparo Oliver

In: Palliative Care
Editor: Michael Silbermann

ISBN: 978-1-53616-199-1
© 2019 Nova Science Publishers, Inc.

Chapter 9

THE NEED FOR A RESEARCH ORIENTED PSYCHO-ONCOLOGY IN PALLIATIVE CARE

Simone Cheli[*]

School of Human Health Sciences, University of Florence, Florence, Italy
Department of Human Sciences, Guglielmo Marconi University, Rome, Italy

ABSTRACT

Palliative care may be considered a frontier of research in psycho-oncology. Although a few standardized protocols have been developed, the available studies are frequently biased. Ethical concerns, sampling and methodological biases, and unstructured delivery settings have affected the quality of clinical research. The aim of this chapter is to summarize and grade the evidence of the most popular interventions, and to suggest relevant trends for future research. I maintain that a research-oriented psycho-oncology in palliative care would entail balancing an empathetic personalization with rigorous standardization.

1. TOWARDS A RESEARCH-ORIENTED PSYCHO-ONCOLOGY

All therapists remember a few patients who significantly changed their way of providing therapeutic care. If we assume that learning involves trial and error, we may serenely accept the mistakes we made when working with such unforgettable patients. For me, this patient was Lidia. She was a 22 year-old woman diagnosed with a pleomorphic osteosarcoma, who asked for psycho-oncology support and died in less than six months. I committed, session by session, the most common errors a psychotherapist can make in a palliative care setting. I assumed the exigency was just death anxiety, but it was not. I confused spiritual care with psycho-oncology care, and the guidelines with unethical obstacles. I alternatively shifted from being scared to yearning to take responsibility for her. I am grateful for my supervisor's support and for my thirst for knowledge.

---

[*] Corresponding Author's E-mail: simone.cheli@unifi.it.

Finally, I realized, or came to assume, that being a psychotherapist in palliative care means rigorously trying to apply evidence and to promote the implementation of psycho-oncology interventions in this targeted setting. The existing literature seems to support this assumption, by highlighting that on the one hand "psychosocial care is underdeveloped in home care generally "(Connor, 2015, p. 250), while on the other hand noting that this kind of care specifically emerged when multi-professional teams started to become a best practice in Western countries (Jeffrey, 2003). Thus, psychosocial care evolved into two connected paths: (i) psychosocial approaches aimed at supporting patients, families and professional caregivers to express their own feelings, thoughts and concerns about the illness; (ii) a set of specific psychosocial interventions meant to improve the psychological and emotional wellbeing of the same targets (Breitbart & Alici, 2014; Chochinov & Breitbart, 2000; Lloyd-Williams, 2003). More specifically, the role of a psycho-oncologist includes multiple essential interventions: (i) support of the team's pain and symptom management; (ii) diagnosis and treatment of comorbid psychiatric disorders; (iii) support for existential and/or spiritual issues; (iv) bereavement management; (v) facilitation of decision-making processes and patient-physician communication; (vi) psycho-education and training for patients, families and professional caregivers (Breitbart & Alici, 2014, pp. 15-16).

Given these factors, we must acknowledge that any metasynthesis of existing literature will be highly biased. Indeed, very few systematic reviews or meta-analyses about psycho-oncology interventions in palliative care exist. On one hand, many ecological, ethical and sampling constraints may limit the number of unbiased studies (e.g., randomized controlled trials (RCT); cohort studies, and so on) to be included in a meta-analysis. Search engines such as MEDLINE, PsychInfo and Cochrane report just a few protocols that are grounded on significant effect size. We maintain that early integrated palliative care interventions (Prescott et al., 2017) and specific psychotherapeutic treatments (Akechi, Okuyama, Onishi, Morita & Furukawa, 2010) are effective in reducing psychopathological symptoms such as depression and anxiety. That said, the subgroup of interventions aimed at supporting the patients themselves are the most difficult to operationalize. Most of the studies' samples are very small and RCTs are rather rare, even though a growing body of evidence supports the need to review recently developed protocols such as Meaning Centered Group Psychotherapy (Breitbart, 2017), Dignity Therapy (Martinez et al., 2017) and Managing Cancer and Living Meaningfully (Lo et al., 2016).

The present and future of psycho-oncology in palliative care should perhaps be shaped by a double effort: (i) to collect and assess the existing studies to be included in meta-analyses and evidence-based guidelines; (ii) to promote the development of new research studies, and the systematic uptake of research findings into routine practice. The patient's trajectory across cancer and palliative care is a complex experience we have to support by constantly delivering, testing and revising the best evidence-based practices we have. The role of research in palliative care may be so pivotal that we might consider each and every case as a new study within an unknown area of investigation.

The aim of this chapter is to summarize the existing evidence and explore the methodological biases and challenges of a research oriented psycho-oncology in supporting palliative care patients.

2. EVIDENCE-BASED INTERVENTIONS IN PALLIATIVE CARE

As I previously reported, very few systematic reviews and meta-analyses explore the effectiveness of psycho-oncology interventions on palliative care patients. In considering existing literature, we can go a step further by preliminarily grading the quality of evidence and consequently summarizing the strength of their findings (see Table 1; GRADE Working Group, 2004).

The most relevant studies report that standard interventions significantly reduce depression, anxiety and death anxiety (Akechi, Okuyama, Onishi, Morita, & Furukawa, 2010; Fulton, Newins, Porter, & Ramos, 2018; Grossman, Brooker, Michael, & Kissane, 2017; moderate evidence). On the other hand, psychosocial treatments do not affect fatigue and quality of life (QoL; Poort et al., 2017; very low evidence). Furthermore, because crucial outcomes, such as suicidal ideation (Goelitz, 2003), and specific populations, such as minors (Wiener, Viola, Koretski, Perper, & Patenaude, 2015), are understudied, it is difficult to grade these studies' evidence robustly. However, reviewed trials define a specific range of convenience of psychosocial interventions: (i) therapeutic treatments may be effective for highly-to-moderately distressed patients, by significantly reducing depressive and anxious symptoms; (ii) recommended interventions intended to reduce fatigue and improve QoL refer to multidisciplinary strategies, so these psychosocial interventions are ultimately single components of wider protocols.

Table 1. Grade of evidence of psychosocial interventions

Outcome	Sample	Intervention	Evidence	Note	Reference
Anxiety	Adults (≥18 years) of either sex with any primary diagnosis of incurable cancer.	CBT; EI; TW	Moderate	CBT and TW report higher evidence. Such interventions also show moderate evidence in reducing depression.	Fulton et al. 2018
Death Anxiety	Adults (≥18 years) of either sex with any primary diagnosis of incurable cancer	EI; SP	Moderate	Different meaning centered and spiritually oriented interventions. Significant improvement in spiritual well-being and existential distress.	Grossman et al. 2017
Depression	Adults (≥18 years) of either sex with any primary diagnosis of incurable cancer.	CBT; PSP; SP	Moderate	SP and CBT report higher evidence. Recent studies confirm the results (Okuyama et al. 2017)	Akechi et al. 2010
Fatigue	Adult patients (≥18 years) with a diagnosis of incurable cancer, receiving some form of disease-focused treatment.	PSI	Very Low	Different and often overlapped PSIs were delivered. Very low evidence for quality of life.	Poort et al. 2017

Legend: CBT = Cognitive Behavioral Therapy; EI = Existential Interventions; PSI = Psychosocial Interventions; PSP = Problem-Solving Therapy; SP = Supportive Psychotherapy; TW = Third Wave of Cognitive Behavioral Therapy.

Table 2. Relevant treatments in the light of future research

	Model Development	Theoretical Framework	Types of Intervention	Existing Evidence
Managing Cancer And Living Meaningfully (CALM)	Gary Rodin and colleagues developed CALM (Rodin et al. 2016) in 2010. An exploratory RCT has been concluded and a confirmatory RCT is ongoing(Lo et al., 2017).	CALM focuses on 4 domains of disease experience that were empirically identified in metastatic cancer, and aims to foster metallization and attachment security.	CALM is a brief, individual, supportive expressive psychotherapy that focuses on practical and psychological problems contributing to distress in advanced cancer.	An RCT reports a significant decrease of depression. A moderate effect is expected in a confirmatory RCT.
Dignity Therapy (DT)	Harvey Chochinov developed DT in 2002 (hCochinov, 2002). A recent systematic review on the existing RCT report promising results (Martínez et al., 2017).	DT is based on an empirical model of dignity that begins with a reflection on why some patients with advanced disease wish to die, while others find serenity.	DT is a brief, individualized psychotherapy that aims to relieve psycho-emotional and existential distress.	A few RCTs exist, reporting a reduction of anxiety and distress. Patients with high levels of distress seem to benefit more from DT
Family Narrative Therapy (FNT)	During the last 20 years, Lea Baider (2008) and colleagues developed a psycho-oncology model that is focused on family narratives and tested in palliative care (Baider, Cooper & Kaplan De-Nour, 2000).	FNT extensively refers to different family therapy models and techniques and to narrative and communication approaches to cancer care (patients, families, professionals, etc.).	Different and specific interventions have been developed in an integrative manner, always focused on narrative dynamics and processes that shape the family's adaptation to cancer.	Scarce RCTs on specific protocols exist. There is consistent evidence from many observational and case series studies.
Meaning Centered Therapy (MCT)	William Breitbart and colleagues (Breitbart, 2017; Breitbart & Poppito, 2014a & 2017b) developed MCT at Memorial Sloan Kettering and progressively tested it on diverse targets (patients, caregivers) and settings (individual, group).	MCT is overtly rooted in existential tradition and is intended to alleviate existential distress (i.e., spiritual despair and loss of meaning) which often arises in patients with advanced disease.	MCT addresses existential distress by helping patients to sustain or enhance their sense of meaning by re-experiencing and recreating meaning, and thus identifying sources of meaning in a patient's life.	A few RCTs report benefits for spiritual and existential suffering. The group format has collected higher evidence than the individual one. Scarce data on caregivers' samples.
Third Wave of Cognitive Behavioral Therapy (TW-CBT)	Standard CBT reported low evidence in palliative care (Campbell & Campbell, 2012). In the last 10 years, TW-CBT interventions such as MBI, ACT, CFT, have reported promising results with advanced cancer patients.	TW-CBT is defined as an evolution of standard CBT that is defined by a process oriented and contextualized look at human experience. In palliative care, TW-CBT aims to promote acceptance and mindfulness.	Even if TW-CBT is a very complex and recent field, MBI are usually group interventions, whereas ACT and CFT individual ones.	A few RCTs report a significant decrease of anxiety for standard CBT (e.g., Greer et al., 2012). We are accumulating consistent evidence from many observational and case series studies for TW-CBT (e.g., Lotorraca et al., 2017).

Legend: ACT = Acceptance and Commitment Therapy; CFT = Compassion Focused Therapy; MBI = Mindfulness Based Interventions.

Despite meta-analysis' methodology being reputedly a highly effective option when outlining guidelines and recommendations, many biases and limitations can limit such effectiveness (Lyman & Kuderer, 2005). When dealing with fields of knowledge where data are scarcely available, publication bias and small study effect may significantly contort our method of planning future research (Greco, Zangrillo, Biondi-Zoccai, & Landoni, 2013). Because outlining an RCT in palliative care is methodologically difficult, available recommendations (i.e., with moderate or high grade of evidence) may be significantly biased. A better course would be to integrate the results of existing RCTs with available observational and/or cohort studies, so as to balance the strength and quality of evidence (GRADE Working Group, 2004). This methodological caveat is pivotal for the research-oriented framework of the present work.

To integrate existing guidelines with relevant areas of current research, I summarize in Table 2 a narrative review of relevant psychosocial treatments that seem to shape present and future palliative care. In the last 15 years, we have seen a proliferation of explorative and confirmatory studies about psychosocial interventions (Breitbart & Alici, 2014). As reported (Table 2), we may consider at least five relevant types of interventions that foster psycho-oncology development. In terms of grade of evidence, MCT is collecting the strongest evidence through RCTs for both the individual and the group formats (Breitbart, 2017; Breitbart & Poppito, 2014a & 2017b). DT (Chochinov, 2002; Martínez et al., 2017) and CALM (Lo et al., 2017; Rodin et al. 2016), may be considered at lower levels of evidence than MCT, though DT and CALM are standardized interventions that are expected to increase in popularity and validity. FNT (Baider, 2008; Baider, Cooper,& Kaplan De-Nour, 2000) and TW-CBT (Greer et al., 2012; Lotorraca et al., 2017) refer to two wide ranges of interventions that provide strong long-lasting evidence in different fields of psychotherapy, which cannot be excluded when determining the future of palliative care. Although they are mainly characterized by observational and cohort studies (rather than RCTs), they have shown crucial achievements in terms of improving the quality of interventions.

The inclusion criteria of the reported narrative review (Table 2) are defined by attempts to balance strength and quality of existing evidence (GRADE Working Group, 2004), and, especially, to overcome methodological biases of psycho-oncology research in palliative care in order to promote its future. I maintain that CALM, DT, FNT, MCT, and TW-CBT clearly fit such criteria, thus stimulating and extending our research horizon.

3. FROM METHODOLOGICAL BIASES TO RESEARCH CHALLENGES

All of the reviewed studies (see Tables 1 and 2) highlight how existing theoretical approaches include different types (psychotherapy; counseling; psycho-education; etc.) and formats (individual; group; couple; etc.) of interventions. Therefore, we may classify them by aggregating similar theoretical frameworks (see Figure 1). Such a classification is intended to support us in anticipating and formulating the potential research trends of palliative care.

Most standardized protocols may be linked to existential therapy (Frankl, 1978) or, generally speaking, to a spiritual and meaning-centered perspective (e.g., CALM, MCT, DT). The main achievement of the existentialist approach is, surely, the progressive standardization of humanistic and frequently unstructured therapies. Although authors such as Frankl (1978) theoretically explored the human need for meaningfulness, they never defined standardized protocols that would be easy to supply and be trained on. Breitbart (2017) and colleagues demonstrate how standardization is urgently needed and does not conflict with an empathetic and personalized perspective. Similarly, CALM (Rodin et al. 2016) and DT (Chochinov, 2002) are fostering the process of scientific validation of this core part (i.e., the existential theory) of psycho-oncology. Moreover, the standardization process has been focused on relevant constraints of the palliative care setting (i.e., scarce temporal, cognitive, physical resources), developing interventions such as DT, for example, which is a very brief psychotherapy focused on just nine questions.

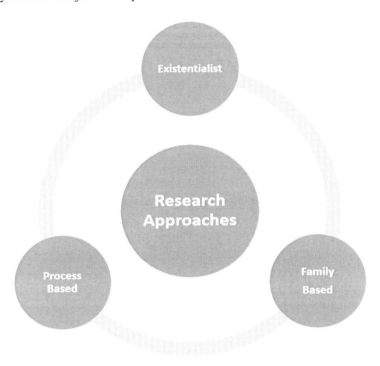

Figure 1. Psycho-oncology research approaches.

The issue of setting is relevant as well, though not easily handled. The most fertile contribution of FNT is probably that it constantly highlights the need for contextualized psychosocial interventions within the family, social and cultural narratives of the patient (Baider, 2008; Baider, Cooper, & Kaplan De-Nour, 2000). FNT may be considered a versatile tool that is theoretically rooted in a family therapy tradition (Jackson, 1968; Whitaker & Bumberry, 1988), and can include different techniques or strategies. The core assumption is that patients' experiences are defined and expressed through the narratives they live in. The work of Baider and colleagues is not simply circumscribed to family therapy, but is intended to be a systemic way of looking at the homeostasis processes of a family (i.e., maintenance and precipitating factors) and at the narrative frameworks (in terms of experiential constraints and possibilities) of a patient's social context (Baider, 2012). FNT urges palliative care teams to implement their strategies in terms of culturally sensitive and tailored approaches, so as to overcome a recurrent ecological bias when dealing with spirituality and suffering (Baider & Goldzweig, 2016).

Nowadays TW-CBT represents a popular psychotherapy framework, overtly focused on process-based and transdiagnostic approaches (Hayes & Hofmann, 2018). The process-based perspective has shaped and fostered the evolution of cognitive therapies. Recent advances are defining interventions that are based not on abstract psychopathological and diagnostic categories, but on cognitive, metacognitive and interpersonal processes recurring across such categories. This hermeneutic and integrative renaissance states that human suffering, beyond specific diagnoses, is due to dysfunctional patterns such as experiential avoidance, cognitive fusion, self-criticism, and so on. Existing therapeutic models try to face suffering by instead promoting healthy processes such as acceptance, mindfulness, compassion, decentering, etc. (Gilbert, 2009; Hayes, 2004; Tirch, Schoendorff, & Silberstein, 2014). In the last few years, many studies have tested and validated TW-CBT psycho-oncology approaches, specifically in palliative care, reporting promising results (Lotorraca et al., 2017). Even if the evidence's strengths with terminally ill patients are still limited, many observational studies highlight their usefulness. Indeed, the complex and differentiated target of palliative care patients may benefit from a transdiagnostic and process-based approach.

4. FUTURE RESEARCH AT A GLANCE

We are used to looking at theory and application, research and practice as separate fields. The more complexity we face, the more we tend to fall into this trap and reduce our ability to increase our knowledge (Braithwaite, Churruca, Long, Ellis, & Herkes, 2018). The question can be framed and overcome by remembering that both the researcher and the clinician are embedded inside the framework they are trying to change. Facing the unpredictability of complex systems requires accepting this unpredictability and intentionally promoting social change of the systems' rules. Practically speaking, if we want to promote psychosocial research in palliative care, we have to hypothesize, test and revise new perspectives, and define our field of interest.

In this chapter, I have attempted to summarize current evidence and future trends of standardized psychosocial interventions in palliative care. The premise of the present work is that the challenge of profiling a terminally ill patient's trajectory urges us to balance empathetic personalization with rigorous standardization. In short, I assume that modern healthcare cannot split these two constructs, but instead must find a more sustainable way to achieve both.

In conclusion, by reviewing methodological biases and challenges, I maintain that future research must outline, validate and share psychosocial interventions that are standardized, easy-to-apply, socially-grounded, and focused on transdiagnostic processes.

REFERENCES

Akechi, T., Okuyama, T., Onishi, J., Morita, T., & Furukawa, T.A. (2010). Psychotherapy for depression among incurable cancer patients. *Cochrane Database Systematic Reviews*, 16;(2):CD005537. doi: 10.1002/14651858.CD005537.pub2.

Baider, Lea (2008). Communicating about illness: A family narrative. *Supportive Care Cancer*, 16(6):607-11. doi: 10.1007/s00520-007-0370-4.

Baider, L. (2012). Cultural diversity: Family path through terminal illness. *Annals of Oncology*, 23(suppl 3): 62-5. doi: 10.1093/annonc/mds090.

Baider, L., Cooper, C.L., Kaplan De-Nour, A. (Eds.) (2000). *Cancer and the Family. Second Edition*. New York: Wiley.

Baider, L., & Goldzweig, G. (2016). The magic of dreams: conflicts and quandaries within multicultural societies in transition. In M. Silbermann (Ed.), *Cancer Care in Countries and Societies in Transition*, (pp. 47-64). New York: Springer.

Breitbart, W. (Ed.) (2017). *Meaning-Centered Psychotherapy in Cancer Setting: Finding Meaning and Hope in the Face of Suffering*. Oxford: Oxford University Press.

Breitbart, W., & Alici, Y. (Eds.) (2014). *Psychosocial Palliative Care*. Oxford: Oxford University Press.

Breitbart, W., & Poppito, S. (2014a). *Meaning-Centered Group Psychotherapy for Patients with Advanced Cancer*. Oxford: Oxford University Press.

Breitbart, W., & Poppito, S. (2014b). *Individual Meaning-Centered Psychotherapy for Patients with Advanced Cancer*. Oxford: Oxford University Press.

Braithwaite, J., Churruca, K., Long, J.C., Ellis, L.A., & Herkes, J. (2018). When complexity science meets implementation science: a theoretical and empirical analysis of systems change. *BMC Medicine*, 16, 63. doi: 10.1186/s12916-018-1057-z.

Campbell, C.L., & Campbell, L.C. (2012). A Systematic Review of Cognitive Behavioral Interventions in Advanced Cancer. *Patient Education and Counseling*, 89(1), 15–24. doi: 10.1016/j.pec.2012.06.019.

Chochinov, H.M. (2002). Dignity-conserving care-a new model for palliative care: helping the patient feel valued. *JAMA*, 287: 2253–2260. doi: 10.1001/jama.287.17.2253.

Chochinov, H.M., & Breitbart, W. (Eds.) (2000). *Handbook of Psychiatry in Palliative Medicine*. Oxford: Oxford University Press.

Connor, S.R. (2015). Hospice and home care. In J.C. Holland, W.S Breitbart, P.N. Butow, P.B Jacobsn, M.J. Loscalzo, & R. McCorkle (Eds.), *Psycho-Oncology. Third Edition* (pp. 249-242). Oxford: Oxford University Press.

Frankl, V.E. (1978). *The Unheard Cry for Meaning*. New York: Washington Square Press.

Fulton, J.J., Newins, A.R., Porter, L.S., & Ramos, K. (2018). Psychotherapy targeting depression and anxiety for use in palliative care: a meta-analysis. *Journal of Palliative Medicine*. doi: 10.1089/jpm.2017.0576.

Goelitz, A. (2003). Suicidal ideation at end-of-life: the palliative care team's role. *Palliative and Supportive Care*. 1(3):275-8. doi: 10.1017/S1478951503030244.

Gilbert, P. (2009). *The Compassionate Mind*. London: Robinson.

GRADE Working Group. (2004). Grading quality of evidence and strength of recommend-dations. *British Medical Journal*, 328(7454), 1490. doi: 10.1136/bmj. 328.7454.1490.

Greco, T., Zangrillo, A., Biondi-Zoccai, G., & Landoni, G. (2013). Meta-analysis: pitfalls and hints. *Heart, Lung and Vessels*, 5(4), 219–225.

Grossman, C.H., Brooker, J., Michael, N., & Kissane, D. (2017). Death anxiety interventions in patients with advanced cancer: a systematic review. *Palliative Medicine*, 32(1): 172 – 184. doi: 10.1177/0269216317722123.

Hayes SC. 2004. Acceptance and commitment therapy, relational frame theory, and the third wave of behavioral and cognitive therapies. *Behavior Therapy*, 35(4):639-665. doi: 10.1016/S0005-7894(04)80013-3.

Hayes, S.C., & Hofmann, S.C. (2018). *Process-Based CBT. The Science and Core Clinical Competencies of Cognitive Behavioral Therapy*. Oakland, CA: New Harbinger.

Jackson, D. (Ed.). (1968). *Communication, Family and Marriage*. Palo Alto, CA: Science & Behavior Books.

Jeffrey, D. (2003). What do we mean by psychosocial care in palliative care? In M. Lloyd-Williams (Ed.), *Psychosocial Issues in Palliative Care* (pp. 1-12). Oxford: Oxford University Press.

Lloyd-Williams (Ed.) (2003). *Psychosocial Issues in Palliative Care*. Oxford: Oxford University Press.

Lo, C., Hales, S., Chiu, A., Panday, T., Malfitano, C., Jung, J., Rydall, A., Li, M., Nissim, R., Zimmermann, C., & Rodin, G. (2016). Managing Cancer and Living Meaningfully (CALM): randomised feasibility trial in patients with advanced cancer. *BMJ Supportive & Palliative Care*. doi: 10.1136/bmjspcare-2015-000866.

Latorraca, C.O.C., Martimbianco, A.L.C., Pachito, D.V, Pacheco, R.L., & Riera, R. (2017). Mindfulness for palliative care patients. Systematic review. *International Journal of Clinical Practice*, 71(12). doi: 10.1111/ijcp.13034.

Lyman, G.H., & Kuderer, N.M. (2005). The strengths and limitations of meta-analyses based on aggregate data. *BMC Medical Research Methodology,* 55:14. doi: 10.1186/1471-2288-5-14.

Martínez, M., Arantzamendi, M., Belar, A., Carrasco, J., Carvajal, A., Rullán, M., & Centeno, C. (2017). 'Dignity therapy', a promising intervention in palliative care: A comprehensive systematic literature review. *Palliative Medicine*, 31(6): 492 – 509. doi: 10.1177/0269216316665562.

Okuyama, T., Akechi, T., Mackenzie, L., Furukawa, T. (2017). Psychotherapy for depression among advanced, incurable cancer patients: a systematic review and meta-analysis. *Cancer Treatment Reviews*, 56: 16-27. doi: 10.1016/j.ctrv.2017.03.012.

Poort, H., Peters, M., Bleijenberg, G., Gielissen, M.F., Goedendorp, M.M., Jacobsen, P., Verhagen, S., & Knoop, H. (2017). Psychosocial interventions for fatigue during cancer treatment with palliative intent. *Cochrane Database of Systematic Reviews* 2017, Issue 7. Art. No.: CD012030. doi: 10.1002/14651858.CD012030.pub2.

Prescott, Anna T.,Hull, Jay G.,Dionne-Odom, J. Nicholas,Tosteson, Tor D.,Lyons, Kathleen Doyle,Li, Zhigang,Li, Zhongze,Dragnev, Konstantin H.,Hegel, Mark T.,Steinhauser, Karen E.,Ahles, Tim A.,Bakitas, & Marie A. (2017). The role of a palliative care intervention in moderating the relationship between depression and survival among individuals with advanced cancer. *Health Psychology*, Vol 36(12): 1140-1146. doi: 10.1037/hea0000544.

Rodin, G., Lo, C., Rydall, A., Nissim, R., Malfitano, C., Shnall, Zimmermann, C., & Hales S. (2017). Managing cancer and living meaningfully (CALM): A randomized controlled trial of a psychological intervention for patients with advanced cancer. *Journal of Clinical Oncology*, 35(18). doi: 10.1200/JCO.2017.35.18_suppl.LBA10001.

Tirch, D.D., Schoendorff, B., & Silberstein, LR. (2014). *The ACT Practitioner's Guide to the Science of Compassion. Tools for Fostering Psychological Flexibility*. Oakland, CA: New Harbinger.

Whitaker, C.A. & Bumberry, W.A. (1988). *Dancing With the Family: A Symbolic-experiential Approach*. New York: Brunner/Mazel.

Wiener, L., Viola, A., Koretski, J., Perper, E.D., & Patenaude, A.F. (2015). Pediatric Psycho-oncology Care: Standards, Guidelines and Consensus Reports. *Psycho-Oncology*, 24(2), 204–211. http://doi.org/10.1002/pon.3589.

BIOGRAPHICAL SKETCH

Simone Cheli

Simone Cheli is adjunct professor in clinical psychology at the University of Florence, chief of research at the Psycho-oncology Unit, Central Tuscany Department of Oncology. He is visiting lecturer at many Italian and international courses in psycho-oncology and clinical mindfulness. He is currently involved in an open trial on a mindfulness-based and metacognitively oriented intervention for cancer patients and professionals, namely Metacognitive Awareness in Cancer Setting (MACS).

In: Palliative Care
Editor: Michael Silbermann

ISBN: 978-1-53616-199-1
© 2019 Nova Science Publishers, Inc.

Chapter 10

PALLIATIVE CARE SERVICE PROVISION AND OUTCOMES IN LOW AND MIDDLE INCOME COUNTRIES

Kennedy Nkhoma[1], Ping Guo[1,], Eve Namisango[1,2] and Richard Harding[1]*

[1]Cicely Saunders Institute of Palliative Care, Policy and Rehabilitation,
Florence Nightingale Faculty of Nursing, Midwifery and Palliative Care,
King's College London, London, UK
[2]African Palliative Care Association, Kampala, Uganda

ABSTRACT

As the world's population is aging, the need for palliative care is rapidly growing, particularly in low and middle income countries (LMICs). This chapter offers a much-needed summary of palliative care development and provision in LMICs. In the world's most populous nations, China and India, palliative care has advanced from localised service provision to some preliminary integration within the health care system. In Middle Eastern countries such as Jordan, the constant influx of a large number of refugees from neighbouring countries poses a challenge to the knowledge base and skills required by health care providers to respond to the needs of individuals with advanced illness and to address the broader humanitarian and political issues. In the African region, despite positive advances over the last decade including an increased number of service providers, the provision of palliative care on the continent remains inconsistent, still largely provided by isolated centres with restricted geographic and population coverage rather than being meaningfully and systematically integrated into healthcare structures. The chapter also draws attention to the role of advocacy organisations and current evidence base highlighting the importance of outcome measurement to inform the delivery of effective and appropriate palliative care. As well as looking at the ways in which the main barriers to the integration of palliative care in LMICs could be addressed, furthermore the chapter contains a discussion on palliative care interventions focusing on

---

* Corresponding Author's E-mail: ping.guo@kcl.ac.uk.

pain management in African context, and concludes with the crucial importance of capacity building across these regions.

Keywords: palliative care, service provision, outcomes, capacity building

INTRODUCTION

Palliative care is recognised as a human right by the World Health Organisation (WHO) [1], the United Nations Committee on Economic, Social and Cultural Rights and the International Covenant for Economic, Social and Cultural Rights [2-4]. The evolving demographics and epidemiology of life-threatening and life limiting diseases as well as chronic conditions across the globe have created an urgent and growing need for palliative care [5]. Although palliative care has been recognised as a human right and the integration of palliative care with basic health care has improved in recent years, in one third of the world, there is no access to palliative care for persons who need it [6]. In addition, there are huge disparities in the provision of and access to palliative care services for individuals with life-limiting illness across the globe [7]. Millions of people who die without palliative care in low and middle income countries (LMICs) often experience a high burden of health suffering [8]. This is largely due to factors such as the unavailability of opioids for moderate to severe pain management [9-11] and poor access to health care services [12]. LMICs are making some progress in palliative care development [13]. In this chapter, we will highlight some of these developments in palliative care services in low and middle income settings and implications for policy, clinical practice and education including capacity building. We will also discuss recent research evidence and outcome measurement to drive up quality of palliative care in these settings.

EPIDEMIOLOGY OF PALLIATIVE CARE

The need for palliative care is expanding due to the ageing population [14] and increase in the incidence and prevalence of both communicable and non-communicable diseases [6] such as HIV/AIDS and cancer [15]. Resource limited settings shoulder over 70% of the burden of such diseases. For example, in 2016, there were 36.7 million people living with HIV globally (including 1.8 million children). The majority of these live in LMICs - 25.5 million (70%) live in sub-Saharan Africa, of which 19.4 million live in East and Southern Africa [16]. More so, WHO estimates that more than 70% of deaths from cancer occur in developing countries [17]. In addition, tuberculosis is the second leading cause of death from infectious diseases, and its prevalence is higher in LMICs [6]. Patients with multi-drug-resistant tuberculosis have higher risk of death particularly if they are also HIV positive [6].

Of an estimated 40 million people globally in need of palliative care, just 14% receive it, most of whom are adults and children in high income countries [7]. The numbers of individuals who die without palliative care, largely in low income countries, is huge and so is the unmet need as only a few countries have implemented equitable access to palliative care programs through a public health approach. Moreover, in many countries, opioid analgesics are not available or accessible to the majority of patients suffering moderate or severe pain [11, 18], and the health systems in low resource settings are fragile [12].

The estimated global number of children in need of palliative care at the end of life is almost 1.2 million. The greatest number of children in need of palliative care died from congenital anomalies, followed by neonatal conditions, protein energy malnutrition, meningitis, HIV/AIDS and cardiovascular diseases [6]. Prognosis of the disease is more uncertain and treatment is often aggressive which makes palliative care important among children. The majority of children (98%) in need of palliative care at the end of life are from LMICs. Almost one-half (48.5%) concentrates in the lower middle income group and over one-third in the low income group. The African Region accounts for the majority of children in need of palliative care (49%), followed by the Southeast Asia (24%) and Eastern Mediterranean regions (12%) [6]. Children in need of progressive palliative care for non-malignant disease constitute by far the highest proportion of cases for all WHO regions (ranging from 78% in the African Region to 91% in the Eastern Mediterranean Region).

Measuring the scope of need for palliative care is difficult as most estimates are based on death rates, which do not include accurate numbers of person suffering earlier in the illness trajectory. Within LMICs, there has been comparatively little evidence in relation to the numbers of patients seen and the magnitude of need for palliative care [19]. The WHO estimates that 20 million people need palliative care at the end of life each year, 67% among older adults (60 years of age or older), and 6% among children. Cardiovascular disease-related deaths comprise over 38% of deaths, followed by cancer 34%, and chronic respiratory conditions 10.3% [20]. What is presented in terms of need for palliative care is thus largely underestimated.

Palliative care is driven by the universal health coverage, which covers two elements: 1) everyone should have access to full range of palliative care services, 2) services must be affordable, and patients should be protected from financial risk when they are accessing care [21]. The Lancet Commission report [8] acknowledges that palliative care services are not accessible and equitable globally. Patients in resource poor countries have no access to palliative care and pain relief, which leads to avoidable health suffering and the lancet commission argues that this has to be alleviated.

PALLIATIVE CARE DEVELOPMENT IN LOW AND MIDDLE INCOME COUNTRIES

Data describing the development and delivery of palliative care services in LMICs are limited. In the world's most populous nations, China and India, palliative care development has advanced from localised service provision to some preliminary integration within the health care system. However, large disparities in access to palliative medicine exist that are based on socioeconomic status. China faces its most pressing challenges from population ageing and the rising incidence of chronic conditions such as cardiovascular disease, which accounted for a third of all deaths in the country in 2012 [22]. Large geographical variations in health care make the quality of palliative care diverse [23]. Even though palliative care has increasingly received attention in China, uneven allocation of health resources, medical and cultural attitudes, and social and political factors make the speedier development of palliative care services in China highly challenging [23].

In India, the concept of palliative care was introduced in the 1980s. Hospice and palliative care services have been developed throughout the country, often in collaboration with international organisations [24]. The South Indian state of Kerala has been a leader in this field, with more widely available services provided by nongovernmental organisations, public and private hospitals, and hospices. Demand for palliative care services has increased substantially, with an increasing proportion of patients with cancer [24]. Improved access to palliative care is needed through the development of national health policies, a scale-up of existing services, and implementation of new health delivery systems. In addition, much of the research on refugees has focused on their movement from non-Western countries to Western countries where immigration policies have been developed, such as the US, Canada, and Australia [25].

In Middle Eastern countries such as Jordan they are also coping with the arrival of a large number of refugees from neighbouring countries and managing the ensuing protection efforts. The constant influx of Palestinian, Syrian and Iraqi refugees has strained the ability of local authorities to maintain service delivery and added a considerable burden on public expenditure [26]. This global refugee situation poses a challenge to the knowledge base and skills required by health care providers to respond to the needs of individuals with advanced illness and to address the broader humanitarian and political issues. Palliative care is still in the infancy stage in these Middle Eastern countries and many challenges have to be tackled to promote the development and delivery of palliative care at the national level.

In the African region, palliative care services started over 30 years ago with the founding of the Island Hospice and Bereavement Service in Harare, Zimbabwe [27, 28]. Driven by pioneering advocates, the discipline evolved outside mainstream government health systems, among faith- and secular-based agencies. Consequently, despite positive advances over the last decade including an increased number of service providers [29], the provision of palliative care on the continent remains inconsistent, still largely provided by isolated centres with restricted geographic and population coverage rather than being meaningfully and systematically integrated into healthcare structures. However, many countries continue to use a home-based model that is detached from mainstream care services, centred on trained health professionals, community-based volunteers, and family caregivers. The challenge with this model is that it does not address all components of the WHO's enhanced public health model for palliative care development [30]. Furthermore, international funding has arguably focussed on palliative care delivery opportunities [31] in response to the HIV epidemic, thereby limiting access with other chronic illnesses.

South Africa, Uganda, Rwanda and Kenya have the highest number of total hospice and palliative care services in Africa [13]. South Africa has been identified as achieving preliminary integration with existing health services, with some of the most advanced non-governmental organisation services on the continent. Palliative care is provided at three different levels: (1) through a 'palliative care approach' adopted by all healthcare professionals, provided that they are educated and skilled through appropriate training; (2) 'general palliative care' provided by primary care professionals and those treating patients with life-threatening diseases, with a good basic knowledge of palliative care; and (3) 'specialist palliative care' provided by specialised teams for patients with complex problems. A review of developments undertaken by the World Hospice and Palliative Care Alliance

(WHPCA) in 2011 revealed that sub-Saharan Africa has shown the most notable changes in service development [32]. A subsequent global mapping of palliative care developments in 2014 by the WHO and the WHPCA revealed additional positive developments in Africa [20].

Main barriers to the integration of palliative care in LMICs include (1) lack of national palliative care policies. As a result, the resources are allocated more on cure and acute care compared to palliative care; (2) lack of awareness by health professionals and the public, of what palliative care is and the benefits it can offer to patients and health systems; (3) cultural and social beliefs about death and dying, and misconceptions that palliative care is only for those in their last days of life, therefore referral of patients to the palliative care services is often delayed; and (4) the misconception that improving access to opioid analgesia could lead to increased substance abuse. Constraints on opioids prescribing and interruption in its availability still exist in some LMICs [18]. The most pressing challenges to overcome in LMICs are the need for healthcare provider training in palliative care, and patient access to palliative care services, and pain relief [8].

ROLE OF ADVOCACY ORGANISATIONS IN PALLIATIVE CARE DEVELOPMENT, POLICY, IMPLEMENTATION, AND RESEARCH

Advocacy organisations such as the African Palliative Care Association (APCA) are mechanisms that have helped to increase the provision of palliative care. APCA was formally founded in Tanzania in 2004 with a goal to reduce unnecessary pain and suffering from life-limiting illnesses across Africa. It works collaboratively with existing and potential palliative care services to help expand service provision. Furthermore, APCA works with governments and policymakers to ensure that the optimum policy and regulatory framework exists for the development of palliative care across Africa. So far, a number of nations in Africa have established National Palliative Care Associations which work hand in hand with APCA and their respective health ministries. APCA ascribes to the WHO's public health approach to palliative care development and has collaborative partnerships with Cicely Saunders Institute (CSI), WHPCA and many more. It also provides leadership and coordination in the development of palliative care Information, Education and Communication resources tailored to the needs of patients, families, policy makers and healthcare providers in the African region, which have impact across the globe. These materials cover awareness, policy, advocacy, education, research and service quality improvement in palliative care.

STATUS OF PALLIATIVE CARE RESEARCH IN LOW AND MIDDLE INCOME COUNTRIES

Palliative care as a scientific discipline thrives on research to inform policy and clinical practice - a recent study found a strong relationship between publications and the level of palliative care development [33]. A systematic review concluded that the evidence base for palliative care is expanding, however, LMICs continue to be underrepresented [33, 34]. The review further reported coverage for the overarching categories of research domains, which include evolution of services, evaluating benefits of services, access to care and needs, analysing legalisation and costs, end of life decision making, limited coverage for research related to patients and families, pain and symptom management, ethics and dignity, outcomes, spirituality, and cultural issues [33].

In a recent systematic review of the evidence for care models, interventions, and outcomes conducted by Singh and Harding [35], 16 articles were identified, reporting a small range of palliative care services in South Asia (14 from India, 1 from Nepal, and 1 from Pakistan). They found a dearth of evidence in terms of palliative care outcomes and the lack of data from beyond India, which highlight the urgent need for greater research investment and activities to guide the development of feasible, acceptable, appropriate, and effective palliative care services. High quality research to determine outcomes and costs of palliative care are urgently needed. Studies are also needed to better understand the cultural context of death and dying for patients and their families in South Asia, and to respond to the growing need for palliative and end-of-life care in the region.

Despite some notable research studies, the evidence base informing the delivery of effective and appropriate care in Africa remains in its infancy [36] and not well distributed and accessible [37]. In the last ten years, a number of palliative care research developments have taken place in Africa [38]. Research that addresses system level barriers to service access has a considerable impact on service development. A shining example of such research is the classical work on the development and validation of core outcome measures for palliative care [39, 40]. This work is based on high income – low income learning exchange model of implementation science [41]. This involved building on what works elsewhere, with a balance of fidelity and adaptation, to develop interventions that are suitable for LMICs. The goal of this initiative was to provide a platform for incorporating person-centered outcome measures into clinical care. Person-centered outcomes incorporate patients' subjective illness experiences and it is one of the robust strategies for involving patients and family caregivers in care and decision making [42]. The incorporation of patient-level data has been associated with improved communication between patients, families and care providers and outcomes of care [41].

Palliative care outcomes are the result of many complex factors inside and outside the health system. Poverty affects palliative outcomes not only through access to formal services, but shortage of essential drugs such as opioids for pain relief, and shortage of health care professionals. To better understand patients' symptoms and concerns, and to demonstrate objectively the difference palliative care makes for patients and their families, we need to have appropriate tools that are able to capture changes in symptoms and quality of life experienced by patients and families.

The Palliative care Outcomes Scale (POS) family of measures have been developed, refined, and adapted [39, 40] to capture physical symptoms, psychological, emotional and spiritual, and information and support needs of patients and families with chronic incurable illnesses or long-term conditions. These tools can help day-to-day clinical practice and care, as well as being valuable in research and education. They have been translated into different languages (e.g., Dutch, German, Portuguese, Spanish, Punjabi, Italian, Chinese, and so on), tested, and widely used by researchers and clinicians across the globe (www.pos-pal.org).

Drawing on existing psychometric studies of outcome measures in palliative care, the Outcome Assessment and Complexity Collaborative (OACC) project team at Cicely Saunders Institute has agreed standardised suite of measures (e.g., Phase of Illness, the Australia-modified Karnofsky Performance Status – AKPS, Integrated Palliative care Outcome Scale –

IPOS) to transform palliative care for patients and families [43]. In response to results from a Europe wide PRISMA project including an online survey on the use and experiences of professionals with outcome measurement in palliative care [44, 45], the OACC team also developed guidelines and training resources to facilitate the integration of these outcome measures into routine palliative care. The team worked with hospice, hospital, and community based palliative care teams in the UK to support the implementation and use of the measures routinely in practice through regular feedback of results at an individual and organisational level, webinars, and training workshops.

The African Palliative Care Association (APCA) African Palliative care Outcomes Scale (POS), hereafter referred known as APOS is one of the most commonly used patient and family-level outcome measure in Africa. It was developed to be administered by health professionals due to high levels of illiteracy in Africa. APOS was developed and validated in Africa to address the challenges of a lack of rigorously validated measures for research and clinical practice despite a high burden of life limiting illnesses [46]. It was validated in sub-Saharan Africa among 682 patients with HIV and cancer and 437 family caregivers. Validation was conducted across five African services and in 3 phases: face validity, construct validity, and internal consistency. The instrument showed sound psychometric properties, well understood and brief to use [41].

Following this implementation science breakthrough, several measures have been adapted for use in Africa. These include the Functional Assessment of Chronic Illness Therapy-Palliative care (FACIT-Pal) scale, the Spirit 8 and the Missoula Vitas quality of life Index [47-50]. This development addressed the lack of outcome measures for palliative care in Africa, which was a barrier for service development and ability to demonstrate the effectiveness of services. These measures are a critical resource in routine clinical care [51], and have been used in clinical trials to demonstrate the effectiveness of services [52, 53] and in clinical audits aimed at improving the quality of care [54].

Another implementation science model links to the regulatory barriers to accessibility of opioids for cancer pain in Africa and the Middle East [55]. The generation of this evidence, led to an increase in concerted efforts geared towards addressing barriers to the access of opioids for pain management in the two regions. There is some improvement in access to opioids, however, more work needs to be done to solve the barrier to opioids access [13, 56].

The regions are also making progress in promoting knowledge translation initiatives, as evidence is on a small scale being used to inform care guidelines [57] and policy development [58]. That said, the field continues to lag behind in terms of availing the evidence required to inform policy and guideline development in the regions [59]. This is a concern that needs urgent attention to reduce the overlay reliance on expert opinion for the development of policies and care guidelines [57].

For future direction, developing research in LMICs should address key challenges which include: the lack of a research culture, lack of research skills and knowledge among health care professionals, professional isolation, patient recruitment and attrition, lack of agreement on outcome measures, research funding, the dominance of the biomedical model rather than the biopsychosocial model, the absence of national strategies for palliative care research, and the absence of a strategic research vision [38]. Furthermore, there is extensive linguistic diversity in Africa with over 2,000 indigenous languages, making it important to ensure ethnic inclusiveness for overarching relevance of findings. The lack of resources also remains a main challenge that has promoted prioritisation of clinical care focusing on the biomedical model rather than person-centred care.

PAIN IN HIV: INTERVENTIONS IN AFRICAN CONTEXT IN PALLIATIVE CARE OUTCOMES

Research projects have been conducted in sub-Saharan Africa using robust design to evaluate the effectiveness of palliative care interventions. It had become common for care providers and public health specialists to argue that, with the advent of the lifesaving antiretroviral therapy (ART), pain and other symptoms were no longer a concern in this population. To explore the validity of this argument, a study was conducted to determine the prevalence, intensity, associated factors, and effect of pain among ambulatory HIV/AIDS patients [60]. The study revealed that 47% of the patients reported pain in the seven days prior to the survey and pain was a symptom at the time of diagnosis for 68%. Number of health comorbidities were significantly associated with pain intensity. Increasing pain intensity was associated with greater functional ability impairment and poorer quality of life. The authors concluded that pain is a common symptom among ambulatory HIV/AIDS patients and has a debilitating effect on quality of life and emphasised the problem of the significant unmet need for pain relief in the population. More evidence has been generated confirming that multi-dimensional symptoms and concerns persist from diagnosis to advanced disease even in the era of ART [61]. Following such evidence, pain and symptom management are increasingly being recognised as an important component of HIV care. This lead to further work in developing and evaluating complex interventions in palliative care and pain management in HIV/AIDS.

To assess the effectiveness of a nurse led palliative care intervention for patients with HIV/AIDS on ART, a randomised trial was conducted in Kenya and South Africa. The intervention was intensive training in palliative care for nurses delivering care to patients with HIV/AIDS, and the control group received care from nurses with no exposure to palliative care training. The intervention showed positive benefits on patients total palliative care outcomes [52]. Another intervention study was conducted in Malawi among HIV patients and family caregivers. The intervention consisted of an information leaflet, face-to-face discussion and a phone call. Both patients and family caregivers who received the intervention showed significant improvements in palliative care outcomes compared to those who received usual care [53]. These studies have made important contribution to knowledge in terms of the provision of palliative care for HIV/AIDS patients in clinical practice.

CONCLUSION

Capacity building in LMICs is important. A number of projects are currently conducted aimed at building research capacity and improving quality of palliative care to address the local challenges and needs. These project, led by researchers at Cicely Saunders Institute, include but not limited to 1) improving bereavement outcomes in Zimbabwe: a feasibility cluster trial of the 9-cell bereavement tool, 2) developing palliative care guidelines in burns management in Ghana, 3) exploring palliative care symptoms and concerns among Nigerian cohorts with kidney diseases, and 4) evaluating a nurse-led integrated palliative care in a randomised controlled trial for Multi-Drug resistant TB patients in Uganda. The findings will inform better policies and practices in LMICs.

In terms of policy, national palliative care guidelines are available in some countries. For example in Africa, to date, seven African countries have standalone national palliative care policies including Malawi, Mozambique, Rwanda, Swaziland, Tanzania, Botswana and Zimbabwe. Uganda has drafted a national policy that is in the process of being adopted. More so, several countries have cancer control strategies and other guidelines that give guidance on how palliative care related tasks should be handled [62]. LMICs continue to struggle with a lack of access to opioids and overlay restrictive policies which has been cited as a barrier to opioid availability. Revision of policies to remove stigmatising language such as "drug abuse" and the lack of balance between control and access [63]. Advocacy organisations have directed towards elimination of unduly restrictive laws on morphine prescription such as South Africa, Uganda [64] and Zambia [9, 65]. South Africa has the highest morphine consumption [9]. Morphine powder is constituted nationally in Kenya [66], Sierra Leona [67] and Uganda [9].

There are several training hubs in Africa, for example the Institute of Hospice and Palliative Care that offers diploma and degree courses in palliative care. The University of Cape Town is another leading training institution for upcoming palliative care professionals in the region [68]. In Uganda, Kenya, South Africa, Mauritius, Taiwan, Malawi, Tanzania, postgraduate diplomas in palliative care are available. Through international partnership capacity building initiatives, several scholars have had the opportunity to undergo training. For example, one scholarship is offered per year to outstanding students from developing countries to study at Cicely Saunders Institute and specialise in palliative care. Courses provided include MSc and PhD. All those who studied this course have made significant contribution in palliative care in their respective countries.

Palliative care in LMICs is making progress in areas of research, policy, practice, training, and capacity building. However, more work needs to be done in all areas to improve the patient outcomes and quality of palliative care services. Cicely Saunders Institute continues to provide mentorship and training for healthcare providers who will become future leaders in palliative care in LMICs.

REFERENCES

[1] WHO. *WHO definition of palliative care*. 1998.
[2] Brennan, F., D. B. Carr, and M. Cousins, Pain Management: A Fundamental Human Right. *Anesthesia & Analgesia*, 2007. **105**(1): p. 205-221.
[3] Gwyther, L., F. Brennan, and R. Harding, Advancing palliative care as a human right. *Journal of pain and symptom management*, 2009. **38**(5): p. 767-774.
[4] Brennan, F., Palliative Care as an International Human Right. *Journal of Pain and Symptom Management*, 2007. **33**(5): p. 494-499.
[5] World Health Organisation. *Strengthening of palliative care as a component of integrated treatment within the continuum of care*. 2014.

[6] World Health Organisation. *Global Atlas of Palliative Care at the End-of-Life 2014* [cited 2018 31/07/2018].

[7] Anderson, R. E. and L. Grant, What is the value of palliative care provision in low-resource settings? *BMJ Global Health*, 2017. **2**(1).

[8] Knaul, F. M., et al., Alleviating the access abyss in palliative care and pain relief-an imperative of universal health coverage: The Lancet Commission report. *Lancet*, 2018. **391**(10128): p. 1391-1454.

[9] Logie, D. E. and R. Harding, An evaluation of a morphine public health programme for cancer and AIDS pain relief in Sub-Saharan Africa. *BMC Public Health*, 2005. **5**: p. 82.

[10] Logie, D. and M. Leng, Africans die in pain because of fears of opiate addiction. *BMJ*, 2007. **335**(7622): p. 685-685.

[11] Seya, M. J., et al., A first comparison between the consumption of and the need for opioid analgesics at country, regional, and global levels. *J Pain Palliat Care Pharmacother*, 2011. **25**(1): p. 6-18.

[12] Kim, J. Y., P. Farmer, and M. E. Porter, Redefining global health-care delivery. *Lancet*, 2013. **382**(9897): p. 1060-9.

[13] Rhee JY, et al., *APCA Atlas of Palliative Care in Africa*. 2017, Houston TX: IAHPC Press.

[14] WHO. *Global Health and Aging*. 2011 [cited 2018 02/08/2018]; Available from: http://www.who.int/ageing/publications/global_health.pdf.

[15] Reville, B. and A. M. Foxwell, The global state of palliative care-progress and challenges in cancer care. *Ann Palliat Med*, 2014. **3**(3): p. 129-38.

[16] UNAIDS. *Ending AIDS: progress towards the 90–90–90 targets*. 2017; Available from: http://www.unaids.org/en/resources/documents/2017/20170720_Global_AIDS_update_2017.

[17] WHO. *Cancer* 2018; Available from: http://www.who.int/en/news-room/fact-sheets/detail/cancer.

[18] Hartwig, K., et al., *Where there is no morphine: The challenge and hope of palliative care delivery in Tanzania*. 2014, 2014. **6**(1).

[19] Harding, R., et al., How Can We Improve Palliative Care Patient Outcomes in Low- and Middle-Income Countries? Successful Outcomes Research in Sub-Saharan Africa. *Journal of Pain and Symptom Management*, 2010. **40**(1): p. 23-26.

[20] World Health Organization and World Hospice Palliative Care Alliance. Global Atlas of Palliative Care at End of Life. . 2014 [cited 2018 12/07/2018].

[21] World Hospice Palliative Care Alliance. *Universal Health Coverage and Palliative Care 2014*; Available from: file:///C:/Users/k1632994/Downloads/Global_Atlas_of_Palliative_Care.pdf.

[22] Guo, P., R. Harding, and I. J. Higginson, Palliative care needs of heart failure patients in China: putting people first. *Current Opinion in Supportive and Palliative Care*, 2018. **12**(1): p. 10-15.

[23] Liu, W. and P. Guo, Exploring the challenges of implementing palliative care in China. *European Journal of Palliative Care*, 2017. **24**(1): p. 12-17.

[24] Krishnan, A., et al., Palliative Care Program Development in a Low- to Middle-Income Country: Delivery of Care by a Nongovernmental Organization in India. *Journal of Global Oncology*, 2018(4): p. 1-8.

[25] Lacroix, M. and T. Al-Qdah, Iraqi refugees in Jordan: lessons for practice with refugees internationally. *European Journal of Social Work*, 2012. **15**(2): p. 223-239.

[26] Stevens, M. R., The collapse of social networks among Syrian refugees in urban Jordan. *Contemporary Levant*, 2016. **1**(1): p. 51-63.

[27] Mwangi-Powell, F. N., et al., Palliative care in Africa. In *Textbook of Palliative Nursing*, B. R. Ferrell and N. Coyle, Editors. 2015, Oxford University Press: New York. p. 1118-1129.

[28] Wright, M. and D. Clark, *Hospice and Palliative Care in Africa: A review of developments and challenges*. 2006, Oxford: Oxford University Press.

[29] Grant, L., et al., Palliative care making a difference in rural Uganda, Kenya and Malawi: three rapid evaluation field studies. *BMC Palliative Care*, 2011. **10**(1): p. 8.

[30] Stjernsward, J., Uganda: initiating a government public health approach to pain relief and palliative care. *Journal of Pain & Symptom Management*, 2002. **24**: p. 257 - 264.

[31] Kates, J., A. Wexler, and E. Lief, Financing the Response to HIV in Low-and Middle-Income Countries. 2016.

[32] Lynch, T., S. Connor, and D. Clark, Mapping levels of palliative care development: a global update. *J Pain Symptom Manage*, 2013. **45**(6): p. 1094-106.

[33] Pastrana, T., et al., Disparities in the contribution of low- and middle-income countries to palliative care research. *J Pain Symptom Manage*, 2010. **39**(1): p. 54-68.

[34] Lodge, M. and M. Corbex, Establishing an evidence-base for breast cancer control in developing countries. *Breast*, 2011. **20 Suppl 2**: p. S65-9.

[35] Singh, T. and R. Harding, Palliative care in South Asia: a systematic review of the evidence for care models, interventions, and outcomes. *BMC Res Notes*, 2015. **8**: p. 172.

[36] Harding, R., et al., Generating an African palliative care evidence base: The context, need, challenges and strategies. *J Pain Symp Manage*, 2008. **36**: p. 304 - 309.

[37] Jang, J. and M. Lazenby, Current state of palliative and end-of-life care in home versus inpatient facilities and urban versus rural settings in Africa. *Palliat Support Care*, 2013. **11**(5): p. 425-42.

[38] Powell, R., et al., Advancing palliative care research in sub-Saharan Africa: from the Venice declaration, to Nairobi and beyond. *Palliat Med*, 2008. **22**: p. 885 - 887.

[39] Hearn, J. and I. J. Higginson, Outcome measures in palliative care for advanced cancer patients: A review. *Journal of Public Health Medicine*, 1997. **19**(2): p. 193-199.

[40] Hearn, J., I. J. Higginson, and P. Palliative Care Core Audit, Development and validation of a core outcome measure for palliative care: the palliative care outcome scale. *Quality in Health Care*, 1999. **8**(4): p. 219-227.

[41] Harding, R., et al., Validation of a core outcome measure for palliative care in Africa: the APCA African Palliative Outcome Scale. *Health Qual Life Outcomes*, 2010. **8**(10).

[42] Fayers P. M. and D. Machin, *Quality of Life* second edition ed. The assessment, analysis and interpretation of patient reported outcomes 2000.

[43] Pinto, C., et al., Perspectives of patients, family caregivers and health professionals on the use of outcome measures in palliative care and lessons for implementation: a multi-method qualitative study. *Annals of Palliative Medicine*, 2018.

[44] Harding, R., et al., The PRISMA Symposium 1: outcome tool use. Disharmony in European outcomes research for palliative and advanced disease care: too many tools in practice. *J Pain Symptom Manage*, 2011. **42**: p. 493 - 500.

[45] Harding, R. and I. J. Higginson, PRISMA: share best practice in end-of-life cancer care research and measurement. *European Journal of Palliative Care*, 2010. **17**(4): p. 182-184.
[46] Harding, R. and I. J. Higginson, Palliative care in sub-Saharan Africa. *Lancet*, 2005. **365**.
[47] Harding, R., et al., Validation of a core outcome measure for palliative care in Africa: the APCA African Palliative Outcome Scale. *Health Qual Life Outcomes*, 2010. **8**: p. 10.
[48] Namisango, E., et al., Validation of the Missoula-Vitas Quality-of-Life Index among patients with advanced AIDS in urban Kampala, Uganda. *J Pain Symptom Manage*, 2007. **33**(2): p. 189-202.
[49] Selman, L., et al., The "Spirit 8" successfully captured spiritual well-being in African palliative care: factor and Rasch analysis. *J Clin Epidemiol*, 2012. **65**(4): p. 434-43.
[50] Selman, L., et al., 'Peace' and 'life worthwhile' as measures of spiritual well-being in African palliative care: a mixed-methods study. *Health Qual Life Outcomes*, 2013. **11**: p. 94.
[51] Defilippi K and Downing J, Feedback from African palliative care practioners on the use of the APCA POS *International Journal of Palliative Nursing*, 2013 **19**(12): p. 577-581.
[52] Lowther, K., et al., Nurse-led palliative care for HIV-positive patients taking antiretroviral therapy in Kenya: a randomised controlled trial. *The Lancet HIV*, 2015. **2**(8): p. e328-e334.
[53] Nkhoma, K., J. Seymour, and A. Arthur, An Educational Intervention to Reduce Pain and Improve Pain Management for Malawian People Living With HIV/AIDS and Their Family Carers: A Randomized Controlled Trial. *Journal of Pain & Symptom Management*, 2015. **50**(1): p. 80-90.e4 1p.
[54] Selman, L. and R. Harding, How can we improve outcomes for patients and families under palliative care? Implementing clinical audit for quality improvement in resource limited settings. *Indian J Palliat Care*, 2010. **16**(1): p. 8-15.
[55] Cleary, J., et al., Formulary availability and regulatory barriers to accessibility of opioids for cancer pain in Africa: a report from the Global Opioid Policy Initiative (GOPI). *Ann Oncol*, 2013. **24 Suppl 11**: p. xi14-23.
[56] Clark, B. A., H. Siden, and L. Straatman, An integrative approach to music therapy in pediatric palliative care. *Journal of Palliative Care*, 2014. **30**(3): p. 179-187.
[57] Distelhorst, S. R., et al., Optimisation of the continuum of supportive and palliative care for patients with breast cancer in low-income and middle-income countries: executive summary of the Breast Health Global Initiative, 2014. *Lancet Oncol*, 2015. **16**(3): p. e137-47.
[58] Nabudere, H., E. Obuku, and M. Lamorde, Advancing palliative care in the Uganda health system: an evidence-based policy brief. *Int J Technol Assess Health Care*, 2014. **30**(6): p. 621-5.
[59] Mutatina, B., et al., Identifying and characterising health policy and system-relevant documents in Uganda: a scoping review to develop a framework for the development of a one-stop shop. *Health Res Policy Syst*, 2017. **15**(1): p. 7.

[60] Namisango, E., et al., Pain among ambulatory HIV/AIDS patients: Multicenter study of prevalence, intensity, associated factors, and effect. *The Journal of Pain*, 2012. **13**(7): p. 704-713.

[61] Simms, V., et al., Multidimensional patient-reported problems within two weeks of HIV diagnosis in East Africa: a multicentre observational study. *PLoS One*, 2013. **8**(2): p. e57203.

[62] Luyirika, E. B. K., et al., Best practices in developing a national palliative care policy in resource limited settings: lessons from five African countries. *ecancermedicalscience*, 2016. **10**: p. 652.

[63] Namisango, E., et al., Investigation of the Practices, Legislation, Supply Chain, and Regulation of Opioids for Clinical Pain Management in Southern Africa: A Multi-sectoral, Cross-National, Mixed Methods Study. *J Pain Symptom Manage*, 2018. **55**(3): p. 851-863.

[64] Clark, D., et al., Hospice and Palliative Care Development in Africa: A Multi-Method Review of Services and Experiences. *J Pain Symp Manage*, 2007. **33**: p. 698 - 710.

[65] Logie, D. E., An evaluation of a public health advocacy strategy to enhance palliative care provision in Zambia. BMJ Supportive & amp; *Palliative Care*, 2012. **2**(3): p. 264-269.

[66] Scholten, W. K. and B. Milani, Providing paediatric palliative care in Kenya. *Lancet*, 2010. **376**(9757): p. 1988.

[67] Bosnjak, S., et al., Improving the availability and accessibility of opioids for the treatment of pain: The International Pain Policy Fellowship. *Supportive Care in Cancer*, 2011. **19**(8): p. 1239-1247.

[68] Rawlinson, F., et al., The current situation in education and training of health-care professionals across Africa to optimise the delivery of palliative care for cancer patients. *ecancermedicalscience*, 2014. **8**: p. 492.

BIOGRAPHICAL SKETCHES

Kennedy Bashan Nkhoma

Affiliation: Cicely Saunders Institute

Business Address: King's College London
Cicely Saunders Institute of Palliative Care, Policy & Rehabilitation
Florence Nightingale Faculty of Nursing, Midwifery & Palliative Care
Bessemer Road, London SE5 9PJ, UK
Email: kennedy.nkhoma@kcl.ac.uk

Education:
PhD in Nursing Studies, University of Nottingham
MSc in Palliative Care, University of Nottingham
BSc Nursing, University of Malawi

Research and Professional Experience:

Dr Kennedy Bashan Nkhoma is a researcher interested in pain and symptom management in chronic illnesses including HIV/AIDS, Cancer and COPD. He has research skills in quantitative and qualitative methods including randomised controlled trials, systematic reviews and epidemiological studies. Kennedy has worked both clinically and in the academia delivering teaching and research in both low and middle-income countries and the UK. He has also experience in designing, and developing complex interventions using the MRC framework. Currently, he is delivering a clustered randomised trial in Cape Town for COPD patients and families, an NIHR (national institute for health research) funded project aimed at strengthening the health system in sub-Saharan Africa (https://www.kcl.ac.uk/kghi/projects/asset.aspx).

Appointments:

March 2018 to present: Research Associate in Global Health Palliative Care, King's College London, Florence Nightingale Faculty of Nursing, Midwifery and Palliative care

August 2016-March 2018: Research Fellow, King's College London, Florence Nightingale Faculty of Nursing, Midwifery and Palliative care.

September 2013 to December 2014: Postgraduate Research Student Teacher, University of Nottingham, Faculty of Health Sciences.

Publications from the Last Three Years:

Nkhoma, K.; Norton, C.; Sabin, C.; Winston, A.; Merlin, J.; Harding, R. Self-management Interventions for Pain and Physical Symptoms Among People Living With HIV: A Systematic Review of the Evidence. *JAIDS Journal of Acquired Immune Deficiency Syndromes.* 2018; 79: 206–225.

Nkhoma, K., Ahmed, A., Ali, Z., Gikaara, N., Sherr, L., and Harding, R. Does being on TB treatment predict a higher burden of problems and concerns among HIV outpatients in Kenya? A cross-sectional self-report study. *AIDS care.* 2018; 30: 28-32.

Nkhoma, K., J. Seymour, and A. Arthur, An Educational Intervention to Reduce Pain and Improve Pain Management for Malawian People Living with HIV/AIDS and Their Family Carers: A Randomized Controlled Trial. *Journal of Pain and Symptom Management.* 2015; 50: 80-90.

Ping Guo

Affiliation: King's College London, UK

Education: PhD in Nursing Studies, University of Nottingham, UK
MSc in Advanced Nursing, University of Nottingham, UK
BSc in Nursing part time, Changzhi Medical College, China
Diploma in Nursing, Henan University, China

Business Address: Cicely Saunders Institute of Palliative Care,
Policy & Rehabilitation,
Florence Nightingale Faculty of Nursing, Midwifery & Palliative Care,
King's College London,
Bessemer Road, London, SE5 9PJ

Research and Professional Experience:
Dr Ping Guo has experience of leading and managing different projects in clinical trials and observational studies, undertaking documentary reviews and qualitative interviews. Her research and teaching has focused on casemix classification in palliative care, global health, outcome measurement, psychosocial and education interventions for both patients and family caregivers, and self-management. Currently, she is working on building research capacity and partnerships, and improving person-centred quality of palliative care across Middle East and North Africa (MENA). It is under the Research for Health in Conflict (R4HC-MENA) project (https://r4hc-mena.org/), funded by ESRC Economic and Social Research Council (Global Challenges Research Fund).

Professional Appointments:
Research Associate, Cicely Saunders Institute of Palliative Care, Policy and Rehabilitation, King's College London, UK

Nurse Specialist, the First Affiliated Hospital of Henan University of Science and Technology, China

Honors: Palliative Care Research Society (PCRS) membership (2014-present, No. 1372)

Publications from the Last Three Years:
Pinto C, Bristowe K, Witt J, Davies JM, de Wolf-Linder S, Dawkins M, Guo P, Higginson IJ, Daveson B and Murtagh FEM. Perspectives of patients, family caregivers and health professionals on the use of outcome measures in palliative care and lessons for implementation: a multi-method qualitative study. *Annals of Palliative Medicine*, 2018. doi: 10.21037/apm.2018.09.02 (accepted for publication 21st Aug 2018).

Huang SJ, Huang CY, Woung LC, Lee OKS, Chu DC, Huang TC, Wang YW, Guo P, Harding R, Kellehear A, & Curtis JR (2018) The 2017 Taipei Declaration for Health-Promoting Palliative Care. *Journal of Palliative Medicine*, 21, 581-582. (Letter to the Editor).

Guo P, Dzingina M, Firth AM, Davies JM, Douiri A, O'Brien SM, Pinto C, Pask S, Higginson IJ, Eagar K & Murtagh FEM (2018) Development and validation of a casemix classification to predict costs of specialist palliative care provision across inpatient hospice, hospital and community settings in the UK: a study protocol. *BMJ Open*, 8: e020071.

Pask S, Pinto C, Bristowe K, van Vliet L, Nicholson C, Evans CJ, George R, Bailey K, Davies JM, Guo P, Daveson BA, Higginson IJ & Murtagh FEM (2018) A framework for complexity in palliative care: A qualitative study with patients, family carers and professionals. *Palliative Medicine*, 32, 1078-1090.

Guo P, Gao W, Higginson IJ & Harding R (2018) Implementing outcome measures in palliative care. *Journal of Palliative Medicine*, 21, 414. (Letter to the Editor).

Guo P, Harding R & Higginson IJ (2018) Palliative care needs of heart failure patients in China: putting people first. *Current Opinion in Supportive and Palliative Care*, 12, 10-15.

Mather H, Guo P, Firth A, Davies JM, Sykes N, Landon A & Murtagh FEM (2018) Phase of Illness in Palliative Care: Cross-sectional analysis of clinical data from community, hospital, and hospice patients. *Palliative Medicine*, 32, 404-412.

Liu W & Guo P (2017) Exploring the challenges of implementing palliative care in China. *European Journal of Palliative Care*, 24, 12-17.

Guo P (2017) *Palliative care in Mainland China: Past, present and future.* EAPC Blog. Posted on 29th March 2017: https://eapcnet.wordpress.com/2017/03/29/palliative-care-in-mainland-china-past-present-and-future/

Guo P, Harris R (2016) The effectiveness and experience of self-management following acute coronary syndrome: A review of the literature. *International Journal of Nursing Studies*, 61, 29-51.

Schildmann EK, Groeneveld EI, Denzel J, Brown A, Bernhardt F, Bailey K, Guo P, Ramsenthaler C, Lovell N, Higginson IJ, Bausewein C & Murtagh FEM (2016) Discovering the hidden benefits of cognitive interviewing in two languages: The first phase of a validation study of the Integrated Palliative care Outcome Scale. *Palliative Medicine,* 30, 599-610.

Eve Namisango

Affiliation: Cicely Saunders Institute,
King's College London and African Palliative Care Association

Business Address: African Palliative Care Association
PO Box 72518, Plot 95, Dr Gibbons Road, Kampala, Uganda
eve.namisango@africanpalliativecare.org/eve.namisango@kcl.ac.uk

Research and Professional Experience:

Eve Namisango's specialty is in Clinical Epidemiology, Biostatistics, Palliative Care, Policy and Rehabilitation. For the last 15 years, she has led research palliative care related research HIV, Cancer, and Tuberculosis. She has also undertaken in research in the following fields; medicines and technology, psychometrics, systematic reviews, mhealth, end of life care, policy and mapping levels of palliative care in development. She engages in teaching, student supervision, knowledge synthesis & translation and building capacity for the use of person-centered outcome measures in clinical care.

Professional Appointments:
Research and Development Manager at the African Palliative Care Association and PhD Training Fellow, Cicely Saunders Institute King's College London

Publications from the Last Three Years:

Namisango E, Bristowe K, Allsop M, Murtagh FEM, Melanie Abas Irene J Higginson, Julia Downing, Richard Harding. Symptoms and concerns among children and young people with life-limiting and life-threatening conditions: A systematic review highlighting meaningful health outcomes *The Patient: Patient-Centered Outcomes Research-* 2018.

Downing J, Namisango E, Harding R. Outcome measurement in paediatric palliative care: lessons from the past and future developments. *Ann Palliat Med* 2018.

Fraser, BA; Powell RA; Faith N. Mwangi-Powell, FN; Namisango E, Hannon B; Zimmermann C. Palliative Care Development in Africa: Lessons From Uganda and Kenya. *Journal of Global Oncology* 2018.

John Y Rhee, Eduardo Garralda, Carlos Torrado, Santiago Blanco, Ibone Ayala, Eve Namisango, Emmanuel Luyirika, Liliana de Lima, Richard A Powell, Carlos Centeno. Palliative care in Africa: a scoping review from 2005–16. *Lancet Oncol* 2017; 18: e522–31

Rhee JY, Garralda E Torrado C4, Blanco S, Ayala I, Namisango E, Luyirika E, de Lima L, Powell RA, López-Fidalgo J, Centeno C. Publications on Palliative Care Development Can Be Used as an Indicator of Palliative Care Development in Africa. *J Palliat Med.* 2017 Jun 29.

Rhee JY Garralda E, Namisango E, Luyirika E, de Lima L, Powell RA López-Fidalgo J Centeno C. An Analysis of Palliative Care Development in Africa: A Ranking Based on Region-Specific Macro-indicators. *J Pain Symptom Manage.* 2018 Aug; 56(2): 230-238. doi: 10.1016/j.jpainsymman.2018.05.005

Namisango E, Ntege C, Luyirika EB, Kiyange F, Allsop MJ. Strengthening pharmaceutical systems for palliative care services in resource-limited settings: piloting a mHealth application across a rural and urban setting in Uganda. *BMC Palliat Care.* 2016 Feb 19; 15:20. doi: 10.1186/s12904-016-0092-9.

Namisango E, Kiyange F, Luyirika EB. Possible directions for palliative care research in Africa. *Palliat Med.* 2016 Jun; 30(6): 517-9. doi: 10.1177/0269216316647879.

Namisango E, Harding R, Katabira ET, Siegert RJ, Powell RA, Atuhaire L, Moens K, Taylor S.A novel symptom cluster analysis among ambulatory HIV/AIDS patients in Uganda. *AIDS Care.* 2015; 27(8): 954-63. doi: 10.1080/09540121.2015.1020749. Epub 2015 Mar 18.

Moens K, Siegert RJ, Taylor S, Namisango E, Harding R. Symptom Clusters in People Living with HIV Attending Five Palliative Care Facilities in Two Sub-Saharan African Countries: A Hierarchical Cluster Analysis.; *PLoS One.* 2015 May 12; 10(5): e0126554. doi: 10.1371/journal.pone.0126554. Collection 2015. ENCOMPASS; EURO IMPACT.

Allsop, M. J, Powell, R. A, Namisango, E. The state of mHealth development and use by palliative care services in sub-Saharan Africa: a systematic review of the literature, Jun 2016. *Supportive and Palliative Care.*

Professor Richard Harding

Affiliation: Cicely Saunders Institute, King's College London, UK

Education:
Professor Richard Harding did his first degree in Social Anthropology and Sociology (including a EC ERASMUS scholarship), followed by a Masters degree in Social Policy and Social Work studies with a Diploma in Social Work (UK Home Office Award), and a PhD in Public Health (competitive studentship awarded). He worked as an HIV/palliative care Care Manager before taking up his PhD studentship.

Business Address: King's College London
Cicely Saunders Institute of Palliative Care, Policy & Rehabilitation
Florence Nightingale Faculty of Nursing, Midwifery & Palliative Care
Bessemer Road, London SE5 9PJ, UK
Tel: +44 (0) 20 7848 5518
Email: richard.harding@kcl.ac.uk

Research and Professional Experience:
Professor Harding is Director of the Centre for Global health Palliative Care, a post-Graduate Degrees co-ordinator, and a member of the King's Global Health Institute. His research focuses on outcome measurement and tool validation, HIV/AIDS, heart failure, family caregivers, sub-Saharan Africa, Global Health, audit and quality improvement, mixed methods, intervention development and testing, paediatrics. He is a Board member of the International Association for Hospice Palliative Care, a member of the World Health Organisation Palliative Care Technical Working Group, and Leader of the WHO Collaborating Centre.

Professional Appointments:

2017-present	Professor of Palliative Care
Herbert Dunhill chair, King's College London, Cicely Saunders institute, Department of Palliative Care, Policy and Rehabilitation.
2017-present	Director of the Centre for Global Health Palliative Care
King's College London, Cicely Saunders Institute, Department of Palliative Care, Policy and Rehabilitation.
2011-present	Visiting Professor
School of Public Health and Family Medicine, Faculty of Health Sciences, University of Cape Town.
2011-	present Director of African Programmes
Cicely Saunders International.
2010-2017	Reader (equivalent associate professor)
King's College London, Cicely Saunders institute, Department of Palliative Care, Policy and Rehabilitation.
2007-2010	Senior Lecturer

	King's College London, Cicely Saunders Institute, Department of Palliative Care, Policy and Rehabilitation.
2006-2010	Adjunct Professor
	Department of Community Health Science, Faculty of Medicine, University of Manitoba.
2004-2007	Lecturer
	King's College London, Cicely Saunders Institute, department of palliative care, policy and rehabilitation.

Honors:
European Research Council Consolidator Award. Euros 1,799,820. 2018-2022.

Children's Palliative care Outcome scale.Harding R, Higginson IJ, Murtagh F, WEIGAO, Bluebond-Langner M, Farsides B, Curtis H.
WHO. £39,497. 2017-2017.

Commissioned call for rapid review of service delivery models for older people at the end-of-life that maximise quality of life.Harding R, Evans C, Maddocks M, Higginson I, Ellis-Smith C, Namisango E, Bajwah S, Yi D, Gao W.
NIHR. £164,964. 2018-2019.

Improving communication between clinicians and LGBT patients with serious illness: a national qualitative study to develop and deliver evidence-based guidance. Harding R, Rose R, Bristowe K, Johnson K, Sleeman K.
NIHR. £6,997,730. 2017-2021.

careSSA. Prince M (PI), Harding R *(Co-applicant) from a cross-national group of co-applicants, HARDING responsible for leading platform on palliative care and health systems strengthening cross-cutting theme on person-centred care*
ESRC. £5,989,759. 2017-2021.

Developing capability, partnerships and research in the Middle and Near East (RH4C-MENA). Sullivan R, Patel P, Kienzler H, Bowen W, HARDING R *(Co-applicant, responsible for leading palliative care work package)*, Moran M, Chalkidou K, Darzi A, King L, Coutts A, Ruggeri K.
Marie Curie. £185,673. 2017-2019.

Bereavement outcomes for LGB (lesbian, gay and bisexual) and heterosexual partners: a population-based cross sectional mixed methods study. Harding R (PI), Bristowe K, Gaowei, Yi D, King M, Johnson K, Almack K, Gazzard B.
The Dunhill Medical Trust. £134,798. 2015-17.

Improving palliative rehabilitation in palliative care using goal attainment. Maddocks M, Higginson IJ, Turner-Stoke L, Siegert R, Ashford S, Harding R, Gao W, Murtagh FE.
Open Society Foundations. £196,490. 2015-2018.

BUILDcare Africa.Harding R (PI).
Marie Curie. £116,000. 2014-2016.

ACCESSCare: Advanced Cancer Care Equality Strategy for Sexual minorities. Harding R (PI), Daveson B, Johnson K, Almack K, Koffman J.
EC FP7. Primary health Care Support Programme. €1,155,518.74. 2011-2015.

Health care users experience, as a focus for unlocking opportunities to access quality health. Harding R, (Co-applicant). *Work Package lead for KCL. (Local PI)*

Publications from the Last Three Years:
BMC Infectious Disease. 2018; 18 (1):55
Place of death for people with HIV: a population-level comparison of eleven countries across three continents using death certificate data.
Harding R, Marchetti S, Onwuteaka-Philipsen BD, Wilson DM, Ruiz-Ramos M, Cardenas-Turanzas M, Rhee Y, Morin L, Hunt K, Teno J, Hakanson C, Houttekier D, Deliens L, Cohen J.

BMC Infectious Disease. 2018; 18 (27).
Active ingredients of a person-centred intervention for people on HIV treatment: analysis of mixed methods trial data.
Lowther K, Harding R, Simms V, Ahmed A, Ali Z, Gikaara N, Sherr L, Kariuki H, Higginson RJ, Selman L.

Journal of Palliative Medicine. 2018; 21:581-582
The 2017 Taipei declaration for health-promoting palliative care.
Huang S.J, Huang C.Y, Woung L.C, Lee K.S, Chu D.C, Huang T.C., Wang Y.W, Guo P, Harding R, Kellehear A, Curtis J.R.

Journal of Palliative Medicine. 2018; 21:414.
Implementing outcome measures in palliative care.
Guo P, Gao W, Higginson IJ, Harding R.

Journal of Pain and Symptom Management (E-Publication)
Investigation of the practices, legislation, supply chain and regulation of opioids for clinical pain management in Southern Africa: A multi-sectoral, cross-national, mixed methods study.
Namisango E, Allsop MJ, Powell RA, Friedrichsdorf SJ, Luyirika EB, Kiyange F, Mukooza E, Ntege C, Garanganga E, Ginindza-Mdluli MN, Mwangi-Powell F, Mondlane LJ, Harding R.

Current Opinion in Supportive & Palliative Care. 2018; 12: 10-15.
Palliative care needs of heart failure patients in China: putting people first.

Guo P, Harding R, Higginson IJ.

Health and Quality of Life Outcomes. 2017. DOI: 10.1186/s12955-017-0778-6.
Measuring quality of life among people living with HIV: a systematic review of reviews.
Cooper V, Clatworth J, Harding R, Whetham J, Emerge Consortium.

BMC Palliative Care. 2017; 13(1):8.
The impact of antiretroviral therapy on symptom burden among HIV outpatients with low CD4 count in rural Uganda: nested longitudinal cohort study.
Wakeham K, Harding R, Levin J, Parkes-Ratanshi R, Kamali A, Lalloo DG.

BMJ Supportive & Palliative Care. 2017; 7(2): 158-163.
Transition: the experiences of support workers caring for people with learning disabilities towards the end of life.
O'Sullivan G, Harding R.

BMJ Supportive & Palliative Care. 2017; 7(2):128-132.
Out of the shadows: non-communicable diseases and palliative care in Africa.
Powell RA, Ali Z, Luyirika E, Harding R, Radbruch L, Mwangi-Powell FN.

Palliative Medicine. [Epub ahead of print]. DOI: 10.1177/0269216317705102.
Recommendations to reduce inequalities for LGBT people facing advanced illness: ACCESSCare national qualitative interview study.
Bristowe K, Hodson M, Wee B, Almack K, Johnson K, Daveson BA, Koffman J, McEnhill L, Harding R.

BMJ Global Health. 2017 DOI: 10.1136/bmjgh-2016-000168.
'They will be afraid to touch you'. LGBTI people and sex workers' experiences of accessing healthcare in Zimbabwe: an in-depth qualitative study.
Hunt J, Bristowe K, Chidyamatare S, Harding R.

Journal of Palliative Medicine. 2017; 20(4):313.
Outcome Measurement for Children and Young People.
Harding R, Wolfe J, Baker JN.

Intensive Care Medicine. 2017; 43(3):463-464.
Do we have adequate tools and skills to manage uncertainty among patients and families in ICU?
Harding R, Hopkins P, Metaxa V, Higginson IJ.

Journal of Pain and Symptom Management. 2017; 53(2):e3-e4.
How to Establish Successful Research Partnerships in Global Health Palliative Care.
Harding R, Namisango E, Radbruch L, Katabira ET.

Journal of Cancer Policy. 2016; (10):16-20.
Palliative Care: When and how, and what are the implications for global cancer policy?
Harding R, Luyirika E, Sleeman K.

Cochrane Database of Systematic Reviews. 2016; 20:10:CD007354.
Benzodiazepines for the relief of breathlessness in advanced malignant and non-malignant diseases in adults.
Simon ST, Higginson IJ, Booth S, Harding R, Bausewein C.

South African Medical Journal.2016;106 (9):940-4.
What are the communication skills and needs of doctors when communicating a poor prognosis to patients and their families? A qualitative study from South Africa.
Ganca LL, Gwyther L, Harding R, Meiring M.

Palliative Medicine. 2016; 30(9):862-8.
What palliative care-related problems do patients with drug-resistant or drug-susceptible tuberculosis experience on admission to hospital? A cross-sectional self-report study.
Harding R, Defilippi K, Cameron D.

AIDS Care. 2016; 28(12):1495-1505.
Evaluation of a physiotherapy-led group rehabilitation intervention for adults living with HIV: referrals, adherence and outcome.
Harding R, Claffey A, Brown, D.

AIDS Care. 2016; 28 (1):1-2.
"We are our choice" - AIDS impact special issue Amsterdam 2015.
Davidovich U, Jonas K, Catalan J, Cluver L, Harding R, Hedge B, Prince B, Rietmeijer, K Spire B, van den Boom F, Sherr L.

Palliative Medicine. 2016; 30 (8):730-44.
The bereavement experiences of lesbian, gay, bisexual and/or trans* people who have lost a partner: A systematic review, thematic synthesis and modelling of the literature.
Bristowe K, Marshall S, Harding R.

AIDS Care. 2016; 28(1):60-3.
Conducting experimental research in marginalised populations: clinical and methodological implications from a mixed-methods randomised controlled trial in Kenya.
Lowther K, Harding R, Ahmed A, Gikaara N, Ali Z, Kariuki H, Sherr L, Simms V, Selman L.

BMC Palliative Care. 2016; 15(1):9.
The needs, models of care, interventions and outcomes of palliative care in the Caribbean: a systematic review of the evidence.
Harding R, Maharaj S.

Archives of Disease in Childhood. 2016; 101(1):85-90.
Children's palliative care in low- and middle-income countries.
Downing J, Powell RA, Marston J, Huwa C, Chandra L, Garchakova A, Harding R.

Palliative Medicine. 2016; 30(1):6-22.
EAPC White Paper on outcome measurement in palliative care: Improving practice, attaining outcomes and delivering quality services - Recommendations from the European Association for Palliative Care (EAPC) Task Force on Outcome Measurement.
Bausewein C, Daveson BA, Currow DC, Downing J, Deliens L, Radbruch L, Defilippi K, Lopes Ferreira P, Costantini M, Harding R, Higginson IJ.

Palliative Medicine. 2016; 30(1):64-74.
Home care by general practitioners for cancer patients in the last 3 months of life: An epidemiological study of quality and associated factors.
Pivodic L, Harding R, Calanzani N, McCrone P, Hall S, Deliens L, Higginson IJ, Gomes B; on behalf of EURO Impact.

Journal of Epidemiology & Community Health. 2016; 70(1):9.
Response to 'Place of death in the population dying from diseases indicative of palliative care need: a cross-national population-level study in 14 countries'.
Harding R.

BMJ Supportive & Palliative Care. 2016; 6(1):60-5.
'My body's falling apart.' Understanding the experiences of patients with advanced multimorbidity to improve care: serial interviews with patients and carers.
Mason B, Nanton V, Epiphaniou E, Murray SA, Donaldson A, Shipman C, Daveson BA, Harding R, Higginson IJ, Munday D, Barclay S, Dale J, Kendall M, Worth A, Boyd K.

Journal of Cardiovascular Nursing. 2016; 31(4):313-22.
The Prevalence and Associated Distress of Physical and Psychological Symptoms in Patients With Advanced Heart Failure Attending a South African Medical Center.
Lokker ME, Gwyther L, Riley JP, van Zuylen L, van der Heide A, Harding R.

Journal of Epidemiology & Community Health. 2016; 70(1):17-24.
Place of death in the population dying from diseases indicative of palliative care need: a cross-national population-level study in 14 countries.

Pivodic L, Pardon K, Morin L, Addington-Hal J, Miccinesi G, Cardenas-Turanzas M, Onwuteaka-Philipsen B, Naylor W, Ruiz Ramos M, Van den Block L, Wilson DM, Loucka M, Csikos A, Rhee YJ, Teno J, Deliens L, Houttekier D, Cohen J; on behalf of EUROImpact.

In: Palliative Care
Editor: Michael Silbermann

ISBN: 978-1-53616-199-1
© 2019 Nova Science Publishers, Inc.

Chapter 11

GLOBAL PALLIATIVE CARE DEVELOPMENT RESEARCH

Stephen R. Connor[*]*, PhD*
Worldwide Hospice Palliative Care Alliance, London, UK

ABSTRACT

Understanding the growth and development of palliative care worldwide poses significant challenges. In this chapter we explore the overall definition and concept of global palliative care development, the assessment of need for palliative care, national levels of palliative care development, progress in achieving the public health model of palliative care including policy development, educational development, access to essential medicines, implementation of palliative care and need for research. Also discussed are clinical measurement, cost and utilization outcomes of palliative care.

Keywords: palliative care, hospice, need assessment, measurement, public health

INTRODUCTION

The measurement of palliative care development globally poses numerous challenges and continues to be a work in progress. Though the modern field of palliative care is now over fifty years old it is still a new and emerging specialization with a shifting definitional nature. The official World Health Organization (WHO) definition of palliative care [1] has been modified twice and may be moving toward a third iteration. Measuring a field such as palliative care is difficult without a clearly defined and operational definition. However, progress is being made as we come to a better understanding of the nature and measurement of suffering. A recent Lancet Commission Report has introduced the concept of "serious health related suffering" to help us better understand who needs palliative care [2].

---

[*] Corresponding Author's E-mail: sconnor@thewhpca.org.

Palliative care should be about more than the absence of suffering though relief from serious health related suffering is essential before healing and growth can occur. In the whole person model of palliative care, illness is experienced in several domains, physical, psychological, social, and spiritual and we do not just treat persons we prevent bad outcomes and promote growth. Measuring all these concepts and understanding what constitutes quality palliative care is a considerable challenge.

Taking all this to the national level is another degree of difficulty. National level measurement of the progress and development of palliative care in a country poses additional challenges including meaningfulness, accuracy of data sources and methods, and the ability to monitor long term trends.

In this chapter we will explore some of the challenges and concepts being used to help measure the global development of palliative care. This will include measurement of the need for palliative care; levels of palliative care development; progress in policy adoption; access to medicines; educational outcomes; program implementation; clinical outcome measurement; cost impact of palliative care; and national level development.

NEED FOR PALLIATIVE CARE

The first attempts to measure the need for palliative care focused on the use of mortality data. Limiting measurement to mortality tends to underestimate the need for palliative care because it does not include those needing palliative care prior to the year they die. This is especially true for children who may need care for one day or for a decade or more. Connor [3] estimated the need for hospice care in the United States using death certificate data and national mortality follow back survey data (NMFBS) [4]. Three groups were identified including 1) those that, due to the trajectory of illness would not be expected to be able to access hospice or palliative care; 2) those that would be relatively easy to identify as qualified for the Medicare Hospice Benefit, and 3) those that would need hospice care but would be difficult to identify due to uncertain prognosis. Sixty-seven percent of all deaths fell into the second and third group. The remaining 33% were not considered candidates for palliative care as they died suddenly of accidents, acute cardiac events, stroke, or other acute conditions. This was consistent with the findings from the NMFBS where 30% of decedents were not known to have had any limitations on their activities of daily living the day prior to their death.

Gomez-Batiste [5] used a population approach to estimate the need in the Catalan Region of Spain and estimated that 1.5% of the population was in need of palliative care including a large number of the frail elderly. This finding may be useful in high income countries with a large elderly population.

These efforts were based in high income countries with quite elderly populations. Mortality in low-and-middle-income countries with much younger populations has a much different profile. There is a lot more death from communicable diseases and injury. The first attempt to measure the need for palliative care worldwide was undertaken by the Worldwide Hospice Palliative Care Alliance (WHPCA) in cooperation with the WHO. The *Global Atlas of Palliative Care at the End-of-Life.* [6] The Atlas primarily used WHO mortality data to estimate the need for the 18 major diagnostic groups needing palliative care. The result was an estimate of over 20 million at the end of life, which was doubled to account for those prior to the end of life, giving an overall estimate of over 40 million patients per year. This estimate was conservative as the WHO did not want to overestimate the need, however it was the first attempt to quantify the need and acknowledged that palliative care was indeed much more than care for oncology and AIDS patients.

The Atlas methodology used mortality and pain prevalence as a marker for the need for palliative care, which was inherently limited since palliative care patients have a host of different symptoms in addition to pain. To help address this limitation another report was developed as part of a Lancet Commission Report on palliative care and pain relief [2].

This report also used WHO mortality data but included a method for identifying and quantifying days of suffering from 18 common symptoms and 20 diagnostic groups. The results were that two groups were identified that needed palliative care; decedents and non-decedents. Over 25 million decedent patients were identified along with over 35 million non-decedents. Together the need for palliative care was estimated at approximately 61 million annually.

LEVELS OF PALLIATIVE CARE DEVELOPMENT

Efforts to measure the development of palliative care globally began in 2008 when the WHPCA commissioned the development of a schema that divided countries into four categories: 1) countries where no palliative care was available and no champions were known to be working on its development, 2) countries where there were champions that wanted to develop palliative care but no service delivery had yet begun, 3) countries where some services existed but were not integrated in to the country's health care system, and 4) countries where services were available and integration was occurring [7]

A second initiative to measure palliative care development globally was published in 2012 and the schema was expanded to six levels by bifurcating levels three and four. Level three was divided into 3a for countries where some palliative care was in operation but care was not widely available and 3b for countries where there were many services, but they were not yet integrated into the country healthcare system. Similarly, level four was divided into 4a where integration was beginning and 4b where it was well integrated. At that time only 20 countries had palliative care well integrated, notably in North America, Western Europe, and Australia/New Zealand [8].

MEASUREMENT OF POLICY

Progress in inclusion of palliative care in national policies is based on the WHO public health model for palliative care development [9]. There are a number of key milestones that can be measured to determine if progress is being made, though these vary from country to country depending on local norms. They include:

- National Needs Assessment – an estimate of the need for palliative care by diagnosis for all ages, including barriers, qualitative data, and ideally an analysis of the gap

between need and capacity to deliver palliative care. Includes qualitative data from patients, families, and providers.
- A concept note or policy paper describing palliative care in the country
- Legislation defining palliative care and its place in the national health care system
- National standards for the provision of palliative care
- Clinical guidelines for the treatment of palliative care patients
- Recognition of palliative care as an area of specialization in health care
- A national strategy for the implementation of palliative care
- Inclusion of palliative care in major national strategies for areas such as:
  - National cancer control plan
  - National Non-communicable disease plan
  - National HIV and TB plans

All these policy documents should be officially endorsed or approved by the national government.

ACCESS TO MEDICINES

The WHO model list of essential medicines includes a section for palliative care and pain relief. There are twenty-two medications on this list and ideally every country should have all of them registered, available and accessible. Most of these medicines are controlled substances and come in a variety of forms. The most important of these medicines are opioids, which are needed for pain control and for treatment of shortness of breath. In 75% of the world there is a severe shortage of availability of opioids [10]. This is due to concerns about potential for misuse, however there is no reason to limit access to these medicines for palliative care patients and most current guidelines note that there should be no limitations in access for palliative and end-of-life patients.

In addition, while morphine may technically be available it is essential that it be available in both oral, and parenteral forms and that unduly restrictive barriers to prescribing are removed. The process of ensuring access to these medicines is complex and involves a number of steps.

These include:

- Approval/permission by MoH to register the medicine
- Finding a manufacturer/Importer
- Contracting, pricing, estimating
- Registration of the medicine
- Import/Export licensing
- Storage, distribution, & stocking
- Education of prescribers
- Community education

Educational Outcomes

Education is one of the pillars of the public health model for palliative care. As such it is important to be able to monitor progress in training and preparing the workforce that will be needed to provide services to the over 60 million people that need palliative care globally. There are several aspects to this that can be considered that I've broken down into six areas.

First it is necessary to have curricula in the language of the country where training is to occur. Curricula is needed for at least the following disciplines: medicine, nursing, social work, psychology, chaplaincy, and pharmacy. Second you must have faculty that are qualified to teach these curricula. Third you must include curricula in all the professional schools that train these disciplines including medical school, nursing colleges, religious schools, and universities that train social workers, psychologists, and pharmacists.

Fourth you need to include palliative care in post graduate training including for residents and interns, as well as for major specialties including family medicine and internal medicine. Fifth you need to have palliative care courses included for continuing medical education and sixth there needs to eventually be a process whereby physicians and nurses can achieve specialization in palliative care. Usually this is done as a sub-specialty.

As far as actual measurement of course the number of persons trained can be quantified. As are numbers of people that complete training and receive diplomas or certificates. Palliative care can't simply be taught in a classroom though. Basic principles can but in order to understand the real work of palliative care bedside teaching and mentoring are needed. Measuring changes in knowledge acquisition, competence, and changes in both attitudes and practice behavior are also needed and can be more challenging. Pre-post testing of knowledge is easiest. Competence in doing procedures, assessment and so forth can be observed. There are measures of attitudes toward palliative care that can be taken both before and after training. Seeing real changes in practice may be hardest to measure.

Program Implementation

The easiest part of measuring program implementation is to quantify the number of specialized palliative care programs delivering palliative care and the number of patients being admitted along with information on the services delivered including mean and median length of service. However, as we aim to integrate palliative care into existing health care systems, we should take note of how we are implementing palliative care into mainstream health care and primary care.

Palliative care can be thought of in at least three levels; 1) the palliative care approach that can be integrated into any trained professional's routine practice, 2) the delivery of primary palliative care mainly by primary clinical practices and clinics, usually by family and internal medicine including oncology, and 3) specialized palliative care services that are organized to deliver palliative care services primarily.

CLINICAL OUTCOMES

Clinical outcomes in palliative care are very important to ensuring that the services are effective, and that patients and families are not suffering. There are many validated instruments used in palliative care and they could be grouped in the following categories:

- Measures of symptom severity
- Measures of functional status
- Measures of quality of life
- Measures of consumer evaluation of care
- Measures of healthcare utilization and cost

While quality of life is frequently referred to as the goal of palliative care it can be difficult to use as an accountability measure as there are many things that affect one's perception of QOL that may not have anything to do with the palliative care services delivered. Still there are QOL measures that have been developed specifically for palliative care populations.

UTILIZATION AND COST OUTCOMES

Policy makers are very interested in measures of the cost of care and cost effectiveness. Many studies, primarily in high income countries, have demonstrated the cost effectiveness of palliative care (refs) and a few have shown the same in low-and-middle income countries [11, 12, 13, 14, 15, 16]. The basic premise of palliative care's impact on health care costs is to avoid unnecessary expenditures. Home based palliative care, when instituted early enough, reduces the need for expensive hospitalizations that are unnecessary. They are unnecessary because the interdisciplinary palliative care team prepares the patient and family for anticipated symptom problems and prevents crises that cause families to return the patient from home to the emergency wards and acute care hospitals. Also, palliative care prevents unnecessary lab and diagnostic testing, and with complete evidence-based information patients and families are less likely to opt for futile and often expensive treatments, therefore lessening the likelihood of financial impoverishment. Despite wide variation in study type, characteristic and study quality, there are consistent patterns in the results. Palliative care is most frequently found to be less costly relative to comparator groups, and in most cases, the difference in cost is statistically significant [17].

To achieve these outcomes, the palliative care service should be available 24 hours a day 7 days a week so that the family can report any significant changes in the patient's condition and respond appropriately to solve the problem or if necessary, make a visit to the home. This capacity usually results in the patient being kept stable and comfortable up until the time of death.

Measurement of the actual cost of palliative care delivery at the country level is also important. Metrics such as cost per visit, cost per day, cost per month, cost per admission are important indicators that can be based on local costs for human resources, medications, equipment and supplies, transport, indirect costs, and so forth. One study that has developed a matrix that local authorities can use to compute these costs is available [18].

Palliative care advocates need to be careful not to posit their services as saving money but as better value for money. While in some circumstances there may be savings, but these are offset by additional costs for training, delivering home care services, post death family bereavement support and so forth. Much more evidence is needed to understand the complex impact that palliative care has on health care systems.

NATIONAL LEVEL DEVELOPMENT

Reporting that can be used to measure progress in palliative care development at the national level is challenging. There is currently only one national measure approved by the United Nations though there are several that are under consideration. When the shift occurred from communicable to non-communicable disease focus one measure for palliative care was included as one of 24 WHO approved measures. That measure is the ratio of morphine equivalent opioid consumption minus methadone (used globally primarily for treatment of opioid use disorder) against cancer mortality.

There are some problems with this indicator in that both cancer mortality data and opioid use data can be unreliable for many countries. Cancer mortality data is often underreported and opioid use data to the International Narcotics Control Board is sometimes erratic. Death from cancer is still stigmatized in many parts of the world and death certificates may instead say cardiac arrest. Some countries do not report opioid consumption for particular years. Inaccuracy may be ameliorated by doing a multi-year average for both mortality and opioid use.

Other measures, particularly for universal health coverage, have been proposed including number of palliative care services per million population and per capita consumption of opioids but these have not been agreed by WHO because they don't' exactly correspond with insurance coverage and cost.

WHO's general program of work under the leadership of the new director general may also include some required country level reporting on palliative care. Under consideration are new ways of looking at opioid access including numbers of facilities and pharmacies that stock and fulfill prescriptions for opioids.

CONCLUSION

The global measurement of palliative care has begun and is improving but still has a long way to go. Progress has been made in measurement of the need for palliative care. Measurement of changes in levels of palliative care development for all countries has been accomplished and is now undergoing its third round of measurement. Overall progress is being made though some countries have slipped behind. Key milestones in the development of palliative care using the public health model are noted including essential policy actions needed, education and training needed, medications that must be available, and implementation actions that must be undertaken. Measurement of clinical outcomes should be standardized and based on current evidence. Cost measurement should be undertaken along with utilization outcomes. Finally, we need more valid and reliable national level measures to compare countries progress in palliative care development. Accurate global measurement of palliative care is essential to advocate for closing the access abyss in access to palliative care.

REFERENCES

[1] World Health Organization. *Definition of palliative* care. Accessed 14 October 2018 at: https://www.who.int/cancer/palliative/definition/en/

[2] Knaul F, Farmer P, Krakauer E, de Lima L, Bhadelia A, Xiaoxiao JK, Arreola-Ornelas H, Dantes OG, Rodriquez NM, Alleyne G, Connor, S, Hunter D, Lohman D, Radbruch L, Saenz R, Atun R, Foley K, Frenk J, Jamison D, & Rajagopal MR. (2017). Alleviating the Access Abyss in Palliative Care and Pain Relief: an imperative of universal health coverage: Report of the Lancet Commission on Global Access to Palliative Care and Pain Control. *Lancet* http://www.thelancet.com/commissions/palliative-care.

[3] Connor, S. (1999). New initiatives transforming hospice care, *The Hospice Journal*, 14(3/4), p. 193-203.

[4] United States Department of Health and Human Services. Center for Disease Control and Prevention. National Center for Health Statistics. *National Mortality Follow-Back Survey Data*, 1993 (ISPCSR 2900). Available at: https://www.icpsr.umich.edu/icpsrweb/ICPSR/studies/2900.

[5] Gomez-Batiste X, Blay C, Martínez-Muñoz M, Lasmarías C, Vila L, Espinosa J, Costa X, Sánchez-Ferrin P, Bullich I, Constante C, Kelley E, The Catalonia WHO Demonstration Project of Palliative Care: Results at 25 years (1990-2015), *Journal of Pain and Symptom Management* (2016), doi: 10.1016/j.jpainsymman.2015.11.029.

[6] Connor, S & Sepulveda, C (Eds.). (2014) *Global Atlas of Palliative Care at the End-of-Life* London UK, Geneva CH: Worldwide Palliative Care Alliance and World Health Organization. http://www.who.int/cancer/publications/palliative-care-atlas/en/.

[7] Wright M, et al. Mapping Levels of Palliative Care Development: A Global View. Wright, Michael et al. *Journal of Pain and Symptom Management*. 2007, Volume 35, Issue 5, 469 – 485.

[8] Lynch T, Connor S, Clark D. (2013). Mapping levels of palliative care development: A global update. *Journal of Pain & Symptom Management;* 45(6):1094-1106.

[9] Stjernsward J, Foley K, Ferris F. The public health strategy for palliative care. *J Pain &Sympt Mgmt*, 2007; 33(5)486-493.

[10] World Health Organization. *Ensuring balance in national policies on controlled substances Guidance for availability and accessibility of controlled medicines*. 2011. Available at: http://www.who.int/medicines/areas/quality_safety/guide_nocp_sanend/en/.

[11] Morrison RS, Penrod JD, Litke A, Meier DE, Cassel JB, Caust-Ellenbogen M, Spragens L. Cost savings associated with US hospital palliative care consultation programs. *Archives of Internal Medicine* 2008; 168(16):1783–1790.

[12] Morrison RS, Meier DE, Dietrich J, Ladwig S, Quill T, Sacco J, Tangeman J. The care span: Palliative care consultation teams cut hospital costs for Medicaid beneficiaries. *Health Affairs* 2011; 30(3):454–463.
[13] Penrod JD, Deb P, Luhrs C, Dellenbaugh C, Zhu CW, Hochman T, Morrison RS. Cost and utilisation outcomes of patients receiving hospital-based palliative care consultation. *Journal of Palliative Medicine* 2006; 9(4):855–860.
[14] Serra-Prat M, Gallo P, Picaza JM. Home palliative care as a cost-saving alternative: Evidence from Catalonia. *Palliative Medicine* 2001; 15(4):271–278.
[15] Brumley R, Enguidanos S, Jamison P, Seitz R, Morgenstern N, Saito S, Gonzalez J. Increased satisfaction with care and lower costs: Results of a randomised trial of in-home palliative care. *JAGS*, 2007; 55(7):993–1000.
[16] Wright AA, Trice E, Zhang B, Ray A, Balboni T, Block SD, Maciejewski PK. Associations between end of life discussions, patient mental health, medical care near death, and caregiver bereavement adjustment. *JAMA*, 2008; 300(14):1665-1673.
[17] Smith, Brick, O'hara, Normand. Evidence on the cost and cost-effectiveness of palliative care: A literature review. *Palliative Medicine*. 2014, 28(2):130-150.
[18] Mosoiu D, Dumitrescu M, & Connor SR. (2014). Developing a costing framework for palliative care services. *J Pain Symptom Mgmt;* 48(4): 719-729.

BIOGRAPHICAL SKETCH

Stephen R. Connor, PhD

Stephen R. Connor, PhD is Executive Director of the UK charity, Worldwide Hospice Palliative Care Alliance (WHPCA), a global alliance of 320 national and regional hospice and palliative care organizations in 100 countries & territories advocating for hospice palliative care development worldwide and in official relations with WHO. WHPCA, advocates, communicates, and helps develop palliative care worldwide with a focus on low-and-middle income countries.

Dr. Connor has worked in palliative care continuously for the past 44 years as a researcher, licensed clinical health psychologist, consultant, author, educator, advocate, & executive. For the last 18 years Dr. Connor has worked on global palliative care development in over 25 countries in Eastern Europe, sub-Saharan Africa, and Asia. He a trustee of the International Children's Palliative Care Network, a board member of the Elizabeth Kubler-Ross Foundation, on the scientific advisory board of the (US) National Palliative Care Research Center and is a member of the editorial board of the *Journal of Pain & Symptom Management*.

Connor has published over 125 peer reviewed journal articles, reviews, and book chapters on issues related to palliative care for patients and their families and is the author of *Hospice: Practice, Pitfalls, and Promise (1998)*, *Hospice and Palliative Care: The Essential Guide* (2009 & 2017) and co-editor of the WHPCA/WHO *Global Atlas of Palliative Care at the End-of-Life* (2014) and *Building Integrated Palliative Care Programs and Services* (2017).

In: Palliative Care
Editor: Michael Silbermann

ISBN: 978-1-53616-199-1
© 2019 Nova Science Publishers, Inc.

Chapter 12

RESEARCH METHODS IN PALLIATIVE CARE

Paz Fernández Ortega[1]*, PhD
and Julio C. de la Torre-Montero[2], PhD

[1]Institut Català d'Oncologia, University of Barcelona, Faculty of Health Sciences,
Barcelona, Spain
[2]San Juan de Dios School of Nursing and Physical Therapy,
Comillas Pontifical University, Madrid, Spain

ABSTRACT

This chapter briefly reviews palliative care research. The first section argues for its importance and describes current trends in the field. Specifically, qualitative approaches have proven beneficial, and evidence-based data and mixed methods are having an impact on modern practice. We describe selected European and international reviews that explain palliative care teams' research strategies and experiences, the barriers they have encountered, and (in the second section), some implications for knowledge translation. The third section presents general symptoms and supportive management approaches in palliative care, while the final section presents studies focused on specific symptoms, namely pain, nutrition, elimination, sleep, relationships/sexuality, and spirituality.

Keywords: research, palliative care, qualitative, quantitative, evidence-based, symptoms management, supportive care

1. RESEARCH METHODS FOR THE END OF LIFE. GENERAL OVERVIEW

It is undeniable that health sciences research contributes to better diagnostic, therapeutic and organizational decisions. Research is an essential element to evidence-based decisions and provides the only path for increasing quality and excellence. This chapter outlines the

---

* Corresponding author's e-mail: mpax2001@gmail.com

processes related to end-of-life research, as they relate to both patients and the teams who are caring for them.

While many professionals are motivated to perform research, the number of publications relating to palliative care is quite low compared to research in drugs and treatments. A greater awareness of the importance of publishing and disseminating results, and in translating knowledge to practice, is therefore necessary. In a 2016 survey of palliative care teams in Spain (Doblado et al. 2016), 45% of respondents recognized that research was an essential part of their activity and that they needed specific research skills.

Another question is the use of different research paradigms for approaching complexity in people at the end of their life. For many years, only quantitative research—derived from positivist, objectivist thinking—was recognized as a valid way to quantify the distribution and frecuencies of variables influencing health. Nowadays, the development of qualitative methods has improved research approaches to understanding patients' and their families' realities (Lim et al. 2017). These approaches permit an in-depth exploration of the phenomena affecting people's understanding and perceptions, allowing them to have a "voice" in research about their lives, experiences and health.

A good example of qualitative research contributing to evidence-based knowledge comes from Scotland (Finucane et al. 2018), where a systematic palliative care scoping review identifed all palliative care research in the country from 2006 to 2015. Authors were able to map the most relevant topics in clinical practice, concluding that numerous and valuable descriptive research had been undertaken and that now it was more urgent to perform intervention studies.

Randomized, double-blinded studies are not always possible, especially for complex interventions. Thus, researchers should be flexible, evaluating the benefits and harms of innovative methods and the integration of both quantitative and qualitative research paradigms. This may be an adequate and holistic approach to complex research questions; mixed-methods research is a good contemporary example that is having an impact on the research panorama today.

End-of-life research is also associated with different barriers, including the short time available for follow-up in this population, paternalistic attitudes in families and professionals, and ageism toward older patients. In a systematic literature review including 21 original studies from the UK, the United States, and several northern European countries (Blum et al. 2015), recruitment, attrition, and gatekeeping frequently represented hindrances to research, patients had misgivings around the possibility of complications and adverse events as well as the complexity of the intervention, but they were willing to take part for altruistic reasons. Additionally, patients may be excluded from some studies if they are near death or if family members are considered vulnerable; Bruera and Hui (2013) describe their experience with these concerns based on over 25 years of experience in the field of palliative care.

Bearing in mind the specific characteristics of patients at the end of life, the tools used to screen and assess advanced patients (Limonero and Gil-Moncayo 2014) should be characterized by their simplicity in language and format, adaptability to patients, and ease of implementation. Simple tools that do not require training are easier to adopt in practice. For example, symptoms checklists and abridged versions of some scales have been developed for conditions and specific symptoms associated with the end of life (such as pain, dypsnoea, constipation, fatigue, and anorexia). By contrast, long questionnaires with many items are difficult to complete and may be daunting for patients. Qualitative research methods that use in-depth interviews and participative techniques, on the other hand, can provide excellent data (Digiulio 2013).

Palliative care team members are often poorly prepared to evaluate studies or to coordinate multicenter research. Some authors have described important difficulties arising from a lack of research training and education, calling for institutions and policies to increase opportunities in post-graduate education, both at universities and through continuous training inside the teams (Bruera and Hui 2013). These educational initiatives require additional investments in different health system contexts, with a high commitment from the governments to achieve better coverage for citizens at the end of their life.

2. SCIENTIFIC PRACTICE AND KNOWLEDGE TRANSLATION IN PALLIATIVE CARE

Research in palliative care presents numerous challenges that must be overcome to achieve expected goals. Patients referred to specialized palliative care units come from areas where precision in symptom management is not always the goal, so a special focus on this kind of specific care is needed.

One of the hallmarks of palliative care is multidisciplinary teamwork, as the combination of knowledge, skills, and experience can provide patients with support and care in all aspects of their lives, not only those related to their illness. Teams comprise nurses, physicians, psychologists, physical therapists, and social workers, with strong support from pain specialist professionals (anesthesia), priests (spiritual companions and advisors), and economic support managers. Cooperation among specialists to ensure expert assistance is essential for care and research goals. Clinical research is not possible where health care is inadequate.

Evidence-based clinical practice goes hand-in-hand with research questions oriented toward improving patients' quality of life. However, scientific practice is not always easy in palliative care: previous negative experiences and clinical inertia are some examples. Clinical research needs to overcome many barriers to succeed.

The driving goal of palliative care is to provide the most complete care, preserving the highest possible quality of life at every stage of illness and dying. This process involves a series of development and care-building projects in which all parties involved have specific tasks regarding patients and their families. We cannot forget that in palliative care, family care and primary caregiving is a key aspect of our work as well as a research topic.

After establishing our conceptual framework, we can develop the basics of palliative care research. This is a two-way street: feedback from clinical practice improves research programs and vice versa.

3. RESEARCH ON GENERAL SYMPTOMS AND SUPPORTIVE MANAGEMENT

General care research, quality of life (Tabano, Condosta and Coons 2002, 223-230), and longer maintenance of stabilized performance status scores are significant components of the patient experience. In addition, patients, caregivers and professionals all need general knowledge about how to face stressful, painful and difficult situations. Because specialists delivering palliative care have diverse attitudes (Smallwood et al. 2018, 115), deepening their knowledge is essential to improving services. Despite cultural considerations that affect palliative care (Busolo and Woodgate 2015, 99-111), Palliative care should not only be in line with modern clinical evidence, it should also be culturally sensitive (Busolo and Woodgate 2015, 99-111).

4. Research on Specific Symptoms: Pain, Nutrition and Elimination, Sleep Disturbances, Human Relations and Sexuality and Spirituality

If we had to write an index or directory of all patient needs, the checklist would probably be quite long. This section focuses on the the most important patient needs that come up in clinical practice.

4.1. Pain

Pain is probably one of the most researched symptoms, but many studies face limitations that are inherent to this special patient population, especially the short-term follow-up relative to studies of chronic diseases. Pain control and management is a challenge, wherein adequate monitoring and treatment could be extremely useful. For example, research in pain scales could be applicable not only to severe cases, but also in patients with moderate and low levels of pain.

A useful scale would measure intensity, depth, chronology, irradiation, focus, types, and so on. It would also be important to study patients' adaptation to illness in relation to pain (Chabowski et al. 2017, 1447-1452).

Pain is a totally personal and subjective sensation, so it can be difficult to measure and treat. Research in end-of-life patients has been hindered by difficulties related to experimentation (there are more randomized clinical trials of treatments for diseases than of associated symptoms), and in many cases, published evidence is based only on observational studies. However, these difficulties should serve as an incentive to carry out more research, not less.

Pain has a certain cultural importance, described both in classical and modern literature (James 2011) as well as in music (Gore 2005), with a focus on sensations that can be expressed.

The researcher must take these cultural factors into account, both to avoid bias and to adjust evaluations based on the patient's origin, culture, religion and spiritual beliefs.

Regarding pain treatments, and despite the existence of consensus documents for pain control and integrated care (Bhatnagar and Gupta 2016, 196-208; Kaasa et al. 2018), patients have no real access to these treatments in many places in the world. Again, culture and religion can be powerful influences, sometimes keeping dying patients from finding relief for their symptoms, and even making them wish for death.

4.2. Nutrition

Nutrition and food are common concerns for patients and their families. In view of that concern and its direct relationship with patients' quality of life, professionals should systematically address nutritional questions. Like pain, food (and therefore nutrition) has strong cultural roots, with different connotations in Western, Eastern, and African cultures. Nutritional advice from specialists is especially important, with ethics playing a very important role (Rucker and Rucker 2016, 1183-1192). In relation to patients' food intake, elimination is also a major concern in patients receiving palliative care: opioid-based treatments can cause both constipation and diarrhea (Stapleton et al. 2016, 3863-3871).

4.3. Sleep Disturbances

In addition to other painful symptoms, lack of sleep can result from high levels of anxiety, depressive symptoms, and different aspects of disease and treatment (due to the action and side effects of some drugs) (Grote 2018, 161-168). Many non-pharmaceutical therapies, such as acupuncture and yoga treatments, could help to control and reduce symptoms associated with cancer (Lopez et al. 2018, 3613-3619).

4.4. Relationships and Sexuality

Communication and sexual expression continue to be important for palliative care patients, even those of advanced age (Leung, Goldfarb, and Dizon 2016, 11). For LGBTQ minorities with advanced disease, heteronormative behaviours and stereotypical attitudes remain a common barrier (Griebling 2016, 95-101).

Disease—especially when it is terminal—influences the experience of interpersonal relationships and sexuality. A healthy expression of affection, friendship and sexuality has considerable benefits for quality of life. These topics must be fully investigated to promote wider knowledge, and the application of such research can undoubtedly help patients and their relatives to accept experiences in both the past and present. Humanistic movements around intensive care units (White et al. 2018, 2365-2375) are the expression of a new, non-technical view of care. In some ways, this approach recalls the 16th century care revolution in Granada, Spain, led by St. John of God, who not only tended to disease, but considered the holistic needs of the sick person and developed some of the earliest scales of humanized care (Galán González-Serna, Ferreras-Mencia, and Arribas-Marín 2017, e2919).

4.5. Spiritual Needs

In palliative care, the need for spiritual expression is accentuated. Spirituality is conceived not only as a religious expression of one's relationship with God, but as their relationship with transcendence and communication with the beyond. The adequacy of existing spiritual programs aimed at meeting palliative care patients' needs is an important research topic. It is central to have a wise vision of the different perspectives of many religions, and to break the silence surrounding disease. Although many integrative views have been expressed, many more should be addressed in our research on spiritual matters (Steinhauser et al. 2017, 428-440, Evangelista et al. 2016, 591-601, Delgado-Guay 2014, 308-313).

REFERENCES

Bhatnagar, Sushma and Mayank Gupta. 2016. "Integrated Pain and Palliative Medicine Model". *Annals of Palliative Medicine,* 5 (3): 196 - 208. doi:10.21037/apm.2016.05.02.

Blum, David, Roman Inauen, Jacqueline Binswanger and Florian Strasser. 2015. "Barriers to Research in Palliative Care: A Systematic Literature Review". *Progress in Palliative Care,* 23 (2): 75 - 84. https://doi.org/10.1179/1743291X14Y.0000000100.

Bruera, Eduardo and David Hui. 2013. "Palliative Care Research: Lessons Learned by Our Team over the Last 25 Years". *Palliative Medicine,* 27 (10): 939 - 51. https://doi.org/10.1177/0269216313477177.

Busolo, David and Roberta Woodgate. 2015. "Palliative Care Experiences of Adult Cancer Patients from Ethnocultural Groups: A Qualitative Systematic Review Protocol". *JBI Database of Systematic Reviews and Implementation Reports,* 13 (1): 99 - 111. doi:10.11124/jbisrir-2015-1809.

Chabowski, Mariusz, Michał Junke, Jan Juzwiszyn, Magdalena Milan, Maciej Malinowski and Dariusz Janczak. 2017. "Adaptation to Illness in Relation to Pain Perceived by Patients After Surgery". *Journal of Pain Research,* 10: 1447 - 1452. doi:10.2147/JPR.S129936.

Delgado-Guay, Marvin O. 2014. "Spirituality and Religiosity in Supportive and Palliative Care". *Current Opinion in Supportive and Palliative Care,* 8 (3): 308 - 313. doi:10.1097/SPC.0000000000000079.

Digiulio, Sarah. 2013. *Ethical Dilemmas in Cancer Care New Research on Why Conflicts Arise and How to Help Nurses Speak Up.* Vol. 35.

Doblado, Rafael, Emilio Herrera, Silvia Librada, Miguel Ángel Lucas, Ingrid Muñoz and Zacarías Rodríguez. 2016. "Análisis y Evaluación de Los Recursos de Cuidados Paliativos de España [Analysis and Evaluation of Palliative Care Resources in Spain]". *Monografias Secpal,* 9 (5): 139. www.siosigrafico.com.

Evangelista, Carla Braz, Maria Emilia Limeira Lopes, Costa, Solange Fatima Geraldo da, Batista, Patricia Serpa de Souza, Jaqueline Brito Vidal Batista and Oliveira, Amanda Maritsa de Magalhães. 2016. "Palliative Care and Spirituality: An Integrative Literature Review". *Revista Brasileira De Enfermagem,* 69 (3): 591 - 601. doi:10.1590/0034-7167.2016690324i.

Finucane, Anne M., Emma Carduff, Jean Lugton, Stephen Fenning, Bridget Johnston, Marie Fallon, David Clark, Juliet A. Spiller and Scott A. Murray. 2018. "Palliative and End-of-Life Care Research in Scotland 2006-2015: A Systematic Scoping Review". *BMC Palliative Care,* 17 (1): 1 - 14. https://doi.org/10.1186/s12904-017-0266-0.

Galán González-Serna, José María, Soledad Ferreras-Mencia and Juan Manuel Arribas-Marín. 2017. "Development and Validation of the Hospitality Axiological Scale for

Humanization of Nursing Care". *Revista Latino-Americana De Enfermagem,* 25: e2919. doi:10.1590/1518-8345.1767.2919.

Gore, Martin. 2005. *A Pain that I'M used to.* Depeche Mode. Sony/ATV Music Publishing LLC.

Griebling, Tomas L. 2016. "Sexuality and Aging: A Focus on Lesbian, Gay, Bisexual, and Transgender (LGBT) Needs in Palliative and End of Life Care". *Current Opinion in Supportive and Palliative Care,* 10 (1): 95 - 101. doi:10.1097/SPC.0000000000000196.

Grote, Ludger. 2018. "Drug-Induced Sleep-Disordered Breathing and Ventilatory Impairment". *Sleep Medicine Clinics,* 13 (2): 161 - 168. doi:10.1016/j.jsmc.2018.03.003.

James, Erika Leonard. 2011. *Fifty Shades of Grey.* London, UK: Arrow Books.

Kaasa, Stein, Jon H. Loge, Matti Aapro, Tit Albreht, Rebecca Anderson, Eduardo Bruera, Cinzia Brunelli et al. 2018. "Integration of Oncology and Palliative Care: A Lancet Oncology Commission". *The Lancet. Oncology,* doi:10.1016/S1470-2045(18)30415-7.

Leung, Margaret W., Shari Goldfarb and Don S. Dizon. 2016. "Communication about Sexuality in Advanced Illness Aligns with a Palliative Care Approach to Patient-Centered Care". *Current Oncology Reports,* 18 (2): 11. doi:10.1007/s11912-015-0497-2.

Lim, Christopher T., Avia Tadmor, Daisuke Fujisawa, James J. MacDonald, Emily R. Gallagher, Justin Eusebio, Vicki A. Jackson et al. 2017. "Qualitative Research in Palliative Care: Applications to Clinical Trials Work". *Journal of Palliative Medicine,* 20 (8): 857 - 61. https://doi.org/10.1089/jpm.2017.0061.

Limonero, Joaquín T. and Francisco Gil-Moncayo. 2014. "Palliative Medicine and Hospice Care Importance of Psychological Research in Palliative Care: Barriers in Its Development". *Palliat. Med. Hosp. Care Open J.,* 1 (1): 1 - 3. http://dx.doi.org/PMHCOJ/PMHCOJ-1-101.

Lopez, Gabriel, M. Kay Garcia, Wenli Liu, Michael Spano, Susan Underwood, Seyedeh S. Dibaj, Yisheng Li et al. 2018. "Outpatient Acupuncture Effects on Patient Self-Reported Symptoms in Oncology Care: A Retrospective Analysis". *Journal of Cancer,* 9 (19): 3613 - 3619. doi:10.7150/jca.26527.

Rucker, Robert B. and Michael R. Rucker. 2016. "Nutrition: Ethical Issues and Challenges". *Nutrition Research, (New York, N.Y.)* 36 (11): 1183 - 1192. doi:10.1016/ j.nutres.2016.10.006.

Smallwood, Natasha, David Currow, Sara Booth, Anna Spathis, Louis Irving and Jennifer Philip. 2018. "Attitudes to Specialist Palliative Care and Advance Care Planning in People with COPD: A Multi-National Survey of Palliative and Respiratory Medicine Specialists". *BMC Palliative Care,* 17 (1): 115. doi:10.1186/s12904-018-0371-8.

Stapleton, Stephen J., Janean Holden, Joel Epstein and Diana J. Wilkie. 2016. "Symptom Clusters in Patients with Cancer in the Hospice/Palliative Care Setting". *Supportive Care in Cancer: Official Journal of the Multinational Association of Supportive Care in Cancer,* 24 (9): 3863 - 3871. doi:10.1007/s00520-016-3210-6.

Steinhauser, Karen E., George Fitchett, George F. Handzo, Kimberly S. Johnson, Harold G. Koenig, Kenneth I. Pargament, Christina M. Puchalski, Shane Sinclair, Elizabeth J. Taylor and Tracy A. Balboni. 2017. "State of the Science of Spirituality and Palliative Care Research Part I: Definitions, Measurement, and Outcomes". *Journal of Pain and Symptom Management,* 54 (3): 428 - 440. doi:10.1016/j.jpainsymman.2017.07.028.

Tabano, Maggi, Deborah Condosta and Mary Coons. 2002. "Symptoms Affecting Quality of Life in Women with Gynecologic Cancer". *Seminars in Oncology Nursing,* 18 (3): 223 -

230. doi:10.1053/sonu.2002.34084. http://www.sciencedirect.com/science/article/pii/S0749208102800080.

White, Douglas B., Derek C. Angus, Anne-Marie Shields, Praewpannarai Buddadhumaruk, Caroline Pidro, Cynthia Paner, Elizabeth Chaitin et al. 2018. "A Randomized Trial of a Family-Support Intervention in Intensive Care Units". *New England Journal of Medicine*, 378 (25): 2365 - 2375. doi:10.1056/NEJMoa1802637. https://doi.org/10.1056/NEJMoa1802637.

Chapter 13

EARLY INTERVENTION OF PALLIATIVE CARE: AN INNOVATIVE, EFFECTIVE AND EFFICIENT MODEL OF CARE TO MEET THE CHALLENGE OF THE PHENOMENA OF DISEASE CHRONICATION AND DEMOGRAPHIC TRANSITION IN THE 21ST CENTURY: WHAT IS THE SITUATION IN FRANCE?

Rana Istambouly[*]
Palliamed, Paris, France
Université Paris-Est, Champs-Sur-Marne, France
IAE Gustave Eiffel, Graduate School of OMI (Organizations, Markets, Institutions), Créteil, France

*We have been mistaken in our work in medicine,
believing that our job is to ensure "health" and survival. However,
the matter is rather to allow everyone "to be", and well-being is the reason
for wishing to be alive.*

I owe loads to my family members who keep me in their thoughts and prayers.
I address my heartiest affection to my mother, my motivation and power.
Her sacrifices for my education have been my daily beacon overseas.
She taught me perseverance
and autonomy. I thank her for her perpetual encouragement and support.
She believed in me, making my achievements a harvest of her love and endeavor.
A heavenly thought to dad, who shadows my steps in excelsis;
I hope I am making you proud.
To you I dedicate this chapter.

---

[*] Corresponding author's e-mail: rana.313@hotmail.com

Abstract

In parallel with the epidemiological (from infectious to chronic disease (CD) or non-transmissible diseases) and demographical transitions (aging of populations, namely in developed countries), the traditional concept of palliative care (PC), i.e., accompanying the last days of a hopeless dying patient, is inclined to switch to a modern model: Early Palliative Care (EPCM). This new model of care takes healthcare to a new level where *living with* illness is symbiotic with *battling against* it.

Modern Palliative medicine is concerned about the use of certain treatments that can limit or prolong signs of life. Questions about the appropriateness of an action challenge insight about the benefits and adversity of curative treatments. They not only stimulate thinking about which criteria to include in the decision-making process, but incite considering the patients as persons, their wishes, objectives, plans, experience with illness, their symptoms of discomfort and their suffering. Modern PC offers greater autonomy: patients contribute to advanced care planning that communicates their wishes at different disease stages according to their goals and values. There is strong evidence that EPC, when combined with curative treatments, leads to better results for patients and their family caregivers and for healthcare system. Studies firmly demonstrate that EPC is efficacious and efficient in managing CDs. International associations recommend the model of early and primary PC in management of CDs as soon as diagnosed. Several international studies have shown that EPCM presents better results in CD management.

France, though having been one the first countries to develop the concept of PC as a pioneer in this domain since 1874, it mostly conserved the traditional model of terminal PC and seldom developed EPCM.

Keywords: Early Palliative Care, advanced care planning, Chronic Diseases (CDs), Non-Transmissible Diseases (NTDs), Quality Of Life (QOL), epidemiological transition, demographic transition, healthcare system

"Palliative Medicine of the Future"

In this chapter I will highlight a new model of care for innovative health and social policies in the management of chronic diseases (CDs) which is both reflective and prospective. Palliative medicine is a medically effective practice, socially useful and personally indispensable for patients, their carers and their families. Palliative care (PC) means patient-and family-centered care that optimizes quality of life (QOL) by anticipating, preventing and treating suffering. PC throughout the continuum of illness involves addressing physical, emotional, spiritual and social needs and facilitating patient autonomy, access to information and choice [1]. I will show briefly how this care model creates a new link to science and chronic and incurable diseases by

1. *Evolution of the doctor–patient relationship to a patient–interdisciplinary healthcare team relationship:*
   Palliative care has accentuated the development of interprofessional collaboration by bringing together different disciplines and domains to respond to the multiple and complex needs of patients. The patients' needs are often subject to complex situations and difficulties in therapeutic decisions. The singular colloquium

and singularity of treatment myth have been reevaluated, since no single health professional can provide all the competences necessary for the diverse needs of patients with chronic illnesses. Indeed, all professionals are now largely dependent on each other in their care actions.

2. *Evolution of the patient's representation; from management of a disease to that of patients in their globality:*

   Palliative medicine goes beyond the traditional medical model centered on the disease. It consists of holistic care that includes physical, psychosocial, spiritual and existential care centered on patients in their entirety.

3. *Evolution of the paternalistic model to a model of autonomous decision-making patient:*

   At first, palliative medicine articulated a "sickness" perception with the treatment of the disease and day-to-day decisions based on necessary adaptations. It has redefined the patient's position in the healthcare system, particularly the handling of therapeutic projects, from disease control to the fight against discomfort and enhancement of the patient's quality of life (QOL). We caregivers must consider that patients are able to determine what is right for them. They want to be autonomous, not passive, participate in their healthcare and be masters of their fates. Having unlimited confidence in the practitioner is no longer a central preoccupation, as we have moved from a paternalistic model to a dual relationship where the patient's word often counts with legal validity.

   Palliative medicine has exacted a renewed caregiver–cared for relationship. The doctor must consider patient preferences and respect their dignity during the disease. This trend towards health democracy is characterized by a coupling of pragmatism and ethics.

4. *Transcendence toward the integration of an ethical reflection*

   Current medicine appears obsessed with prolonging life through extreme measures. The progress of medical science has permitted a relentless pursuit of signs of life. Nonetheless, healthcare professionals perceive the complexity of situations engendered by this progress. This situation raises several questions:

   - Should the doctor prolong patients' existence at all costs, despite their physical deterioration, or take actions which might precipitate their demise??
   - What limits do we set on our competences and therapeutic capabilities?
   - How far should the doctor go in an intervention that scientific breakthroughs permit?
   - Can we and should we do everything against death? What benchmarks and limits should be set?
   - How do we avoid therapeutic relentlessness and early cessation of therapy? What is the alternative?

Palliative medicine is concerned about the use of certain treatments that can limit or prolong signs of life. Questions about the appropriateness of an action are thought-provoking about the benefits and adversity of curative treatments. They not only stimulate thinking about which criteria to include in the decision-making process, but consider the patient as a person, their wishes, objectives, plans, experience with illness, their symptoms of discomfort and their suffering [2].

Palliative medicine is not just an antonym of curative medicine. At stake is the articulation between curative and palliative care that facilitates living with the disease. With this perspective, a proposal for a model of palliative medicine can be fruitful, and with techno-scientific medicine, could take healthcare to a new level where living with illness is symbiotic with battling against it.

FROM INFECTIOUS EPIDEMIC TO EPIDEMIC OF CHRONIC DISEASE AND DEMOGRAPHIC TRANSITION: FROM TERMINAL PC TOWARD EARLY PC

For millennia, populations suffered devastating epidemics of plagues, cholera, and influenza. In the 19th century, such epidemics were generated by population changes due to industrial development, and most deaths were caused by infectious diseases [3]. In the 20th century, end-of-life patients would die abandoned in really poor conditions, as medicine was centered on healing, curation and technique. Since the post-war therapeutic revolution with its cohort of miracle drugs, the notion of battling the disease has dominated medical logic. Medicine focused solely on treatments and on technicalities. At that time, it was urgent to improve end-of-life conditions. Here the idea of PC began to take over incurable cases to improve end-of-life quality. PC was practiced by a multidisciplinary team after the cessation of all curative treatment, aiming to relieve the patient and accompanying the family to ensure a good death [4].

Historically, palliative and end-of-life care were designed to help mostly cancer patients manage symptoms and satisfy psychosocial needs during their final months. A person suffering from cancer would generally receive curative interventions until there were no more modifying treatments left. At this stage care was no longer focused on healing but on comfort. PC was only provided when treatment stopped. To be eligible for palliative programs, patients had to be on the verge of death and, like their family, agree to give up active treatment. At that time, the sick person benefited from services such as pain and symptom management, psychosocial and spiritual support to improve QOL, whereas the family was accompanied till death and could receive a bereavement follow-up if requested [5].

FROM CHRONIC DISEASE EPIDEMIC AND DEMOGRAPHIC TRANSITION TOWARD MODERNIZATION OF PALLIATIVE MEDICINE

A century ago, death was generally quite sudden, and the main causes were infections, accidents and complications of childbirth [6]. Today, sudden death is less common. In fact, the improvement of medicine has enabled

- *Prolonging the life of severely ill* patients with cancer, or renal, cardiac, respiratory or other chronic physical dysfunctions. For example, new targeted therapies or chemotherapies allow the disease to be stabilized for longer than

before. New technologies may, however, have adverse and even permanent effects which encumber patients and significantly diminish their QOL.
- *Extending the life expectancy* of patients spectacularly. The average age at time of death was 65 in 2000 and increased to 74 years in 2012. The ageing of world population continues because of advances in medicine. There are today in the world 600 million people 60 years of age or older. This total will double by 2025 and reach 2 billion in 2050. More and more people will live beyond 80 or 90 years. Those aged 80 years or above, for example, will quadruple to 395 million between 2000 and 2050 [7].

This prolongation of life has also produced the phenomenon of chronication. People are living longer with CDs that are getting worse, weigh heavily on them and affect their QOL [8,9]. Towards the end of their lives, most will suffer from serious progressive illness, such as cardiovascular disease, cancer, kidney or respiratory disorders, which will increasingly damage their normal activities until end of life [10]. Techno-scientific medicine is certainly efficacious, but in turn, has generated a new phenomenon, namely an increase in life expectancy of CDs with disability.

Nowadays, two out of three deaths result from CDs [11]– also called non-transmissible diseases (NTDs) – killing 41 million people each year, representing 71% of deaths worldwide. The future global projection shows that CD deaths are expected to reach 80% by 2030 [12]. As the World Health Organization (WHO) states, CDs affect the entire planet: "In both developed and developing countries, chronic NTDs are the main causes of mortality, morbidity and disability in elders". The 73rd session of the United Nations (UN) General Assembly report in September 2018 stressed that NTDs constitute a major issue of global public health and socio-economic impact, and the UN called for actions, urgent measures and Rethinking Health Policies [13].

CDs or NTDs tend to be of long duration and derive from an association of genetic, physiological, environmental and behavioral factors. The CDs by their durable and evolutive character engender loss of autonomy and physical, emotional and spiritual suffering that degrades QOL for patients, carers and family members. Most often, the CD develops suddenly, and its discovery is experienced as a time of crisis. It distressing the patients and disrupting their lifestyle, their projects and the landmarks of their life. It provokes shock, disbelief, anguish, fear of losing one's mental faculties, or seeing physical functions degrade. The patient may face existential fears and questions: how to continue finding meaning in life, how to continue projects, how to live as they wish and believe in the value of continuation when there is no hope of healing. The disease will accompany them until death. But how to alleviate suffering? How to maintain dignity until and as they die? How to prevent unnecessary aggravation and complications and to give meaning to the processes of dying? How to become resilient in the face of incurability and when facing death?

These changes affect every decision of daily life and are made in a climate of suspense and uncertainty. The uncertainty which accompanies the evolution of the disease is difficult to staunch as it represents an onset of fragility. All these upheavals have physical and also psychic, spiritual, familial, relational and socio-professional repercussions. These ramifications affect patients from diagnosis until end of life. Moments of profound despair and of hope may alternate, while our techno-scientific medicine is assumed to have all the answers.

FROM THE EPIDEMIC OF CHRONIC DISEASE TO THE EVOLUTION OF EARLY PALLIATIVE CARE

WHO notices that health systems are based on old-fashioned, acute disease centered organizations and are merely adapted to chronic disease monitoring. WHO assigns a global public health priority to the improvement of QOL of persons with CDs (or NTDs) [14, 15]. How to reform healthcare systems, and which strategy should address chronicity and its serious impact on QOL of affected persons and the economic repercussions?

To meet the considerable challenges posed by the management of CDs, including the impact on QOL, also linked to WHO precognizance, management models of chronic pathologies have been developed (among others, disease and case management, chronic care models and early PC) [16].

One of them, particularly promising, is inspired by PC models. Referred to as "Early Palliative Care Model" (EPCM), it consists of integrating PC intervention models since the diagnosis of a chronic disease [17, 18, 19, 20].

PC integrated into medical care in CD situations will help to better manage symptoms. It will fulfill all needs and reinforce personal autonomy, enabling patients to participate more actively in their own care. It respects their right to make informed decisions about their care and life plans [21]. In fact, the patient will have better access to key elements at the appropriate time, in the context of choice of care. It will thus be feasible to discuss the range of possible treatments and their benefits/risks and prognosis. It will define their objectives, planning beforehand and readjusting the strategies of care throughout the trajectory of the disease. Frank discussions about the prognosis and trajectory of the disease do not destroy hope; instead, they can reduce anguish, obviate ineffectual therapies, and improve QOL and the death process [22].

This medicine which we will call "palliative" is a particularly sophisticated modern medicine. It allows persons with chronic incurable illness to experience the least uncomfortable or less deconstructing sensations. The intent of administering PC is to maintain a more peaceful relationship with their body and their care. It is important to limit the symptoms related to the evolution of the disease. PC is administered with consciousness of its deficiencies, and the side effects of the treatment on daily life which are both physical, cognitive, social, psychological and spiritual.

There is strong evidence that early palliative medicine, when combined with curative treatments, leads to better results for patients and their family caregivers and for healthcare system. Studies firmly demonstrate that the modern model of primary early PC is efficacious in managing CDs. International associations recommend the model of early and primary PC in management of CDs as soon as diagnosed [23, 24].

Several international studies have shown that EPCM presents better results in CD management [25, 26, 27, 28, 29]:

- *For patients:* it offers better QOL and ability to live with the disease, greater autonomy (patients contribute to advanced care planning that communicates their wishes at different disease stages according to their goals and values), a greater respect for their will and less distress during their care.
- *For families and caregivers:* it facilitates their accompaniment of the patients and lightens the burden of the illness and care.
- *For health professionals:* it allows better therapeutic decisions in complex situations by planning and anticipating care goals and advance care planning with the patient throughout the disease; unreasonable prolongations of certain therapies may be limited as well as emergency decisions; it ensures better coordination between health professionals and limits stress.
- *For Health System Management:* through a more adequate referral to hospitals, recourse to more appropriate specialists, a reduction in emergency cases, and limitation of costly and ineffective intensive interventions at end of life, health costs can be managed efficiently.

The WHO assembly recognized that palliative medicine is a fundamental of integrated, person-centered health services, not a supplement or an option, and considers it a human right. For this reason, the WHO executive Board called on all countries to reinforce PC and include it in CD management. Its June 2018 report states: "It is crucial to invest in a better management of non-transmissible diseases also called chronic diseases, comprising detection, screening, treatment, as well as access to primary palliative care for those who need it" [30]. WHO published new guides for integrating primary PC into healthcare in October 2018. Similarly, ESMO (European Society for Medical Oncology), ASCO (American Society of Clinical Oncology) and NCCN (National Comprehensive Cancer Network) have drawn up a guide for the integration of early PC upon diagnosis of a cancer [31, 32]. Several international research efforts have finally begun to develop primary PC in CD management. A reference group on primary care was recently established by the European Hospice Palliative Care Association (EAPC) to develop early PC in CD management [33].

WHAT IS THE SITUATION IN FRANCE REGARDING THE INTEGRATION OF EARLY PALLIATIVE CARE?

France is also affected by the CD epidemic: 20 million out of 57 million insured persons of the general regime, comprising one third of the population, resorted to the care system for a CD in 2015. In 2020, 584,000 additional people are expected to suffer from at least one CD. CDs also have weighty economic repercussions because they are very costly and consume two-thirds of health insurance expenditure, for instance, 90 billion euros in 2011 and 125 billion euros in 2016 [34]. In the future, the share of people with long duration affections (LDA) may jump from 15.4% of the population in 2011 to 19.7% in 2020. In addition to economic effects, CDs, by their sustainable and evolving nature over many years, or throughout life, degrade the QOL of patients and their entourage. It is a public health problem in France [35].

The LDA health system, which was created for the management of chronic diseases, is poorly adapted, according to several findings. Some great difficulties are those of accompaniment, the protocolization of the pathways of care, and the coordination of professionals [36]. Despite the strengths of the current system, it remains severely partitioned and its dysfunctions generate high costs compared to services rendered. The segmentation of care, with the lack of coordination and access to medical information, leads hospital professionals to repeat acts or benefits, to prescribe unnecessary treatments, and perform unjustified emergency interventions. The direct impact of such disorganization is a lack of overall vision and of global conception of CD management [37]. Thus, hospital-centrism, with the doctor as a pivot, is no longer suitable for CDs; the healthcare system must be reorganized around patients at home to meet their needs [38].

Recently, scholarly societies have reported the existence of programs "juxtaposed" to each chronic pathology, while noting the absence of a CD management program and of homogeneous management practices by stage of disease evolution. Several findings from a review of the scientific and grey literature, supplemented by expert opinions, have stated that the LDA system does not provide a basis for improving practices [39, 40]. Nor is it able to respect the control of health expenses or to ensure equity in access to care for patients with CD [41]. Currently, managing these pathologies is not optimal from either a clinical, organizational, functional or structural aspect. This engenders a loss of efficiency [42, 43, 44].

The 21st century has heralded a greater use of technological innovations, interoperability, and interconnectivity which challenge medicine and health systems. The foundation of the medicine of future, such as digital technology, (e-health, big data), 5 Ps of medicine (Preventive, Predictive, Participatory, Personalized, Pertinent), nanotechnologies, artificial intelligence, and genomic medicine, have enabled us to advance treatments far beyond 10 or 20 years ago. These innovations have not yet overhauled our health system, which remains unfit to adequately manage treatment of CDs on both organizational and financial levels.

The vast majority (two out of three deaths) of the 603,000 French who die each year is due to CDs. Only 17% have access to palliative care, and most only receive these services in the last days or weeks of life[45]. For example, a CNSPFV (Centre National de Soins Palliatifs et de Fin de Vie) report on the year 2016 indicates that less than half of patients hospitalized in France received the classification of "palliative care." These patients must wait until the end of their lives to benefit from holistic PC care to improve QOL. The moment of death is sometimes sudden and always difficult to predict; being diagnosed as "close to death" can no longer be a PC trigger, because too many people with incurable and progressive diseases who die "unexpectedly with suffering" will not receive care that could improve QOL and end of life. Lack of access to early PC represents a widening gap in care deficit and a growing public health concern [46, 47].

France has retained the traditional model of terminal PC, whereas some other countries have managed to adapt it to respond to the challenge of CD and its grave consequences on QOL by turning it into a specialty [46]. However, France was among the first countries to develop this concept and pioneered in this field with Maison Jeanne Garnier in Paris (1874) created by les Dames du Calvaire, la Maison Médicale Notre Dame du Lac in Rueil-Malmaison (1946) and la Maison Médicale Jean XXIII) in the north at Frelinghien near Lille, founded in 1966 by les Oblates de l'Eucharistie. Many health professionals have also contributed, and the circular of Geneviève Laroque on August 26, 1986 led to the development of the French PC model, with the creation in 1989 of la Société Française d'Accompagnement et de Soins Palliatifs (SFAP) and le CNSPFV in 2016 [47]. It was necessary to respond urgently to all those patients who were dying in desperate circumstances. The movement then developed in different French regions but still restricted itself to the end-of-life. That is why in 2018 the word "palliative" is linked solely to death and is still avoided by some professionals.

In short, PC development in France was laid somewhat piecemeal, in response to social movements, lacking global strategy or long-term vision. Professional palliative caregivers are now realizing that people with serious illnesses can benefit from numerous aspects of early PC. To address shortcomings in QOL management of end-of-life patients, the barriers and limits of development of early PC, some have resolved to legalize euthanasia or clinician assisted dying.

Will a new law on euthanasia or clinician assisted suicide

- resolve deficits and lacunas in the QOL management of patients with CDs?
- correct the disorganization of patients with CDs in the health sector?
- remedy health system failures?
- optimize and ensure the comfort of end-of-life patients?
- compensate for the development of early PC?

In other words, is it logical to limit our perceptions and role to the eradication of suffering by law? When in difficulty, an automatic reflex is to assume the absence of adequate legislation and propose new laws that are mainly ignored and not enforced. This was the case with the 1999 Law on the Protection of the Right to PC access, the Kouchner Act (2002) on the rights of the sick and the quality of the health system, the Leonetti Act (2005) on the rights of patients and end-of-life persons, and the Claeys-Leonetti law (2016) [47]. Regardless of future legislation, the development of early PC requires a solution.

EARLY INTERVENTION OF PALLIATIVE CARE: AN INNOVATIVE, EFFECTIVE AND EFFICIENT MODEL OF CARE THAT WILL MEET THE CHALLENGE OF THE INCREASE IN CHRONIC DISEASE IN AN AGING POPULATION IN THE 21ST CENTURY

Those who seek euthanasia or assisted suicide do not really want to end their life, but just to end the pain, distress and suffering accrued for months or even years by evolving diseases. Such patients want to maintain dignity and autonomy. In fact, they are mainly treated according to the single purpose of healing. A grievance such as "I can no longer bear it, I want to die" is understandable when the assessment of their QOL and the management of their symptoms is inappropriate and lacking since diagnosis.

Our challenge today is not to create healthcare systems but rather caring systems of health to improve QOL and alleviate suffering. We have mistakenly believed that our job is to ensure health and survival. However, the matter is rather to allow everyone "to be", and well-being is the reason for wishing to be alive. It is time for in-depth reflection on the pertinence of care and the QOL generated, for rethinking the link between biomedical and human approaches, to identify weaknesses, and reform health systems within new perspectives, progressing in the continuum of care for CDs.

What is at stake today otherwise is the overall quality of continuing life for our loved ones affected by CD: our children and grandchildren, our parents and grandparents. It would be better, therefore, for early PC to become part of the great modern organizational innovations of all healthcare systems. Let us strive to implement this new QOL policy in France for the sake of our population!

REFERENCES

[1] Weems K. & Leavitt MO. (2008). Medicare and Medicaid Programs: Hospice Conditions of Participation; Final Rule. *Federal Register*, **73(109):** 32088–3220.

[2] Ricœur P. (2001). La prise de décision dans l'acte médical et dans l'acte judiciaire [Decision-making in the medical act and in the judicial act]. *Le Juste*, **2:** 245–255.

[3] Saunders C. (1964). The symptomatic treatment of incurable malignant disease. *Prescribers J*, **4:** 68–73.

[4] Thoresen L. (2003). A reflection on Cicely Saunders? Views on a good death through the philosophy of Charles Taylor. *International journal of palliative nursing*, **9(1):** 19–23.

[5] Saunders C. (1969). The moment of truth: care of the dying person. In Pearson L's "Death and Dying: Current Issues in the Treatment of the Dying Person." *The press of Case Western University*, 49–78.

[6] Nakatani H. (2016). Global Strategies for the Prevention and Control of Infectious Diseases and Non-Communicable Diseases. *Journal of Epidemiology*, **26(4):** 171–178.

[7] Organisation Mondiale pour la Santé. (2015). *Résumé: rapport mondial sur le vieillissement et la santé [Summary: World Report on Aging and Health]*. who.int/iris/bitstream/handle/10665/186469/WHO_FWC_ALC_15.01_fre.pdf.

[8] Beaglehole R, Bonita R, Horton R, Adams C, Alleyne G, Asaria P, Baugh V, Bekedam H, Billo N, Casswell S, Cecchini M, Colagiuri R, Colagiuri S, Collins T, Ebrahim S, Engelgau M, Galea G, Gaziano T, Geneau R, Haines A, Hospedales J, Jha P, Keeling A, Leeder S, Lincoln P, McKee M, Mackay J, Magnusson R, Moodie R, Mwatsama M, Nishtar S, Norrving B, Patterson D, Piot P, Ralston J, Rani M, Reddy KS, Sassi F, Sheron N, Stuckler D, Suh I, Torode J, Varghese C, Watt J. (2011). Priority actions for the non-communicable disease crisis. *Lancet*, **377(9775):** 1438–1447.

[9] Mercer AJ. (2018). Updating the epidemiological transition model. *Epidemiology and Infection*, **146:** 680–687.

[10] Murray SA Kendall M, Boyd K, Sheikh A. (2005). Illness trajectories and palliative care. *BMJ*, **330:** 1007–1011.

[11] Organisation Mondiale pour la Santé. (2014). *Strengthening of palliative care as a component of comprehensive care throughout the life course*. Resolution WHA67.19.

[12] *Organisation Mondiale pour la Santé*. (2018). http://www.who.int/fr/news-room/fact sheets/detail/noncommunicable-diseases.

[13] *Organisation des Nations Unis*, (2018). https://www.un.org/press/fr/2018/ag12069.doc.htm.

[14] Karanikolos M., Adany R., McKee M. (2017). *European Journal of Public Health*, **27(S4):** 4–8.

[15] Bigdeli M., Shroff ZC., Godin I, Ghaffar A. (2018). Health systems research on access to medicines: unpacking challenges in implementing policies in the face of the epidemiological transition. *BMJ Global Health*, **2:** e000941. doi:10.1136/bmjgh-2018-000941.

[16] Brunn M. (2013). Care for patients with chronic illness – concepts, assessment and foreign experiences. *Santé Publique*, **25(1):** 87–94.

[17] Fins, J.J. & Calahan D. (1992). Palliation in the Age of Chronic Disease. *Hastings Center Report*, **22(1):** 41–42.

[18] Murray S, Kendall M, Mitchell G, Moine S, Amblàs-Novellas J, Boyd K. (2017). Palliative care from diagnosis to death. *BMJ*, **356:** j878.

[19] Jackson K., Head B., Twaddle M., Grant W. (2011). Complex Chronic Illness in Palliative Care: Adult Case Study Involving the Interdisciplinary Team. *Journal of Pain and Symptom Management*, **41(1):** 166–167.

[20] Baines M. (2011). From pioneer days to implementation: lessons to be learnt, *European Journal of Palliative Care*, **18(5):** 223–227.

[21] Klick JC., Ballantine A. (2007). Providing Care in Chronic Disease: The Ever-Changing Balance of Integrating Palliative and Restorative Medicine. *Pediatric Clinics of North America*, **54(5):** 99–812.

[22] Baxter S., Buchanan S., Hirst L., Mohan H., O'Brien LA., Randall-Wood D. (2013). A Model to Guide Hospice Palliative Care: Based on National Principles and Norms of Practice. *Canadian Hospice Palliative Care Association (CHPCA)*.

[23] Hawley PH. (2014). The Bow Tie Model of 21st Century Palliative Care. *Journal of Pain and Symptom Management*, **47(1):** 2–5.

[24] Temel JS., Greer JA., Muzikansky A., Gallagher ER., Admane S., Jackson VA., Dahlin CM., Blinderman CD., Jacobsen J., Pirl WF., Billings JA., Lynch TJ. (2010). Early palliative care for patients with metastatic non-small-cell lung cancer. *New England Journal of Medicine*. **363:** 733–742.

[25] May P., Garrido MM., Del Fabbro E., Noreika D., Normand C., Skoro N., Cassel JB. (2018). Does modality matter? Palliative care units associated with more cost-avoidance than consultations. *Journal of Pain and Symptom Management*, **55(3):** 2018, 766–774.

[26] Bridget M. (2017). Economics of palliative care: Measuring the full value of an intervention. *Journal of Palliative Medicine*, **20(3):** 222–226.

[27] Luckett T., Phillips J., Agar M., Virdun C., Green A., Davidson PM. (2014). Elements of effective palliative care models: a rapid review. *BMC Health Services Research*, **14:** 136.

[28] Gomes B. Calanzani N., Curiale V., McCrone P., Higginson IJ. (2013). Effectiveness and cost-effectiveness of home palliative care services for adults with advanced illness and their caregivers. *The Cochrane Database of Systematic Reviews*, **6:** CD007760.

[29] Hodgson C. (2013). *Coût–efficacité des soins palliatifs: Analyse de la documentation* [*Cost-Effectiveness of Palliative Care: Literature Review*]. Association canadienne des soins palliatifs, http://www.hpcintegration.ca/media/24546/TWF-Economics-report-FR-final-.pdf.

[30] Ferrell BR. Temel JS., Temin S., Smith TJ. (2017). Integration of Palliative Care Into Standard Oncology Care: ASCO Clinical Practice Guideline Update Summary. *Journal of oncolgy practice*, **13(2):** 119–121.

[31] Dans M., Smith T., Back A., Baker JN., Bauman JR., Beck AC., Block S., Campbell T., Case AA., Dalal S., Edwards H., Fitch TR., Kapo J., Kutner JS., Kvale E., Miller C., Misra S., Mitchell W., Portman DG., Spiegel D., Sutton L., Szmuilowicz E., Temel J., Tickoo R., Urba SG., Weinstein E., Zachariah F., Bergman MA., Scavone JL. (2017). NCCN Guidelines Insights Palliative Care, Version 2.2017. *Journal of the National Comprehensive Cancer Network*, **15(8):** 989–997.

[32] EAPC. (2017). https://www.eapcnet.eu/eapc-groups/reference/primary-care.

[33] Schrijvers D. & Cherny NI., on behalf of the ESMO Guidelines Working Group. (2014). ESMO Clinical Practice Guidelines on palliative care: advanced care planning. *Annals of Oncology*, **25(S3):** 138–142.

[34] Blanpain N & Chardon O. (2010). Projections de population à l'horizon [Projections of population on the horizon]. *Paris: Insee Première*, **(1320):** 1–4.

[35] Vernay M., Bonaldi C., Grémy I. (2015). Les maladies chroniques: tendances récentes, enjeux et perspectives d'évolution [Chronic Diseases: Recent Trends, Challenges and Prospects for Evolution]. *Santé Publique*, *s1,(HS)*, 189–197. doi:10.3917/spub.150.0189.

[36] De Chambine S., Morin A. (2010). Protocolisation et qualité du parcours de soins dans le dispositif des affections de longue durée [Protocol and quality of the care pathway in the long-term condition]. *Actualité et dossier en santé publique*, **72:** 25–29.

[37] Delval D. & Bildstein V. Conseil de l'Ordre des Médecins. (2017). Améliorer l'observance: traiter mieux et moins cher [Improve adherence: treat better and cheaper]. *Webzine Santé*, ImsHealth/Crip 2014.

[38] Baumann C., Briançon S. (2010). Maladie chronique et qualité de vie: enjeux, définition et mesure [Chronic Illness and Quality of Life: Issues, Definition and Measurement]. *Actualité et dossier en santé publique*, **72:** 19–21.

[39] Martin D. (2010). Les différentes composantes du dispositif de prise en charge des malades chroniques [The different components of the management system for chronic patients]. *Actualité et dossier en santé publique*, **72:** 30–32.

[40] Leo M. (2010). Le dispositif ALD: point de vue des patients [The ALD device: patients' point of view]. *Actualité et dossier en santé publique*, **72:** 48–49.

[41] Vinquant J-P., Mayo-Simbsler S. (2010). Vieillissement et prise en charge des maladies chroniques [Aging and managing chronic diseases]. *Actualité et dossier en santé publique*, **72:** 33–36.

[42] Haute Autorité de Santé, Organisation des Parcours. (2016). Note méthodologique et de synthèse documentaire; mise au point sur la démarche palliative [Methodological note and documentary synthesis; focus on the palliative approach]. https://www.has-sante.fr/portail/ upload/ docs/ application/ pdf/ 2016-12/ mc_ 247_ note_ methodo_ demarche_ palliative_web.pdf.

[43] Institut Montaigne. (2016). Réanimer le système de santé; propositions pour 2017 [Revitalize the health system; proposals for 2017]. https://www.institutmontaigne.org/ressources/pdfs/publications/reanimer_systeme_de_sante.pdf.

[44] Ministère de la Santé, de la Jeunesse, des Sports et de la Vie Associative. (2007). Plan 2007 - 2011: pour l'amélioration de la qualité de vie des personnes atteintes de

maladies chroniques [2007 - 2011 plan: improving the quality of life of people with chronic diseases]. https://solidarites-sante.gouv.fr/IMG/pdf/plan2007_2011.pdf.

[45] Centre national des soins palliatifs et de la fin de vie. (2017). Rapport d'activité 2016 [Activity Report 2016]. https://www.parlons-fin-de-vie.fr/wp-content/uploads/2018/09/CNSPFVRapport Activite2016.pdf.

[46] Haute Autorité de la Santé. (2016). Note méthodologique et de synthèse documentaire, Mise au point sur la démarche palliative [Methodological note and documentary synthesis, Update on the palliative approach.].

[47] Ravanello A., Rotelli-Bihet L. (2018). *Atlas des soins palliatifs et de la fin de vie en France, Première édition* [*Atlas of Palliative and End-of-Life Care in France, First Edition*]. Centre national des soins palliatifs et de la fin de vie (CNSPFV).

Part III. Eastern Europe

In: Palliative Care
Editor: Michael Silbermann

ISBN: 978-1-53616-199-1
© 2019 Nova Science Publishers, Inc.

Chapter 14

MEDICAL RESEARCH IN PALLIATIVE MEDICINE IN POLAND: THE BOTTOM-UP VERSUS THE TOP-DOWN APPROACH

Zbigniew (Ben) Zylicz MD, PhD[1,*] and Aleksandra Kotlińska-Lemieszek MD, PhD[2]

[1]Institute of Experimental and Clinical Medicine, University of Rzeszów, Poland
[2]Palliative Medicine Chair and Department, Karol Marcinkowski University of Medical Sciences, Poznan, Poland

ABSTRACT

Palliative medicine started to develop in Poland in the early 1980s but only after the significant political changes in the country did it emerge as a new discipline in medicine. The first research institutes appeared in Poznań, Kraków, Bydgoszcz and Gdańsk. In the first phase of development, many Western researchers helped to establish new research lines. Today, palliative care research is much more autonomous in the country but universities remain short of the money needed to finance new developments. Most of the research is done in a "bottom-up" way, in response to what doctors' experience at the bedside. This kind of research has resulted in a couple of interesting innovations, now used worldwide. However, research should also be planned "top-down", to solve problems in the organization and quality assurance of palliative care. There is a great need for a new fund, partially financed by the government and partially by private donors. Palliative care in Poland needs a boost to attract young people and provide them with attractive careers. Changing societies need different, more dynamic approaches.

Keywords: palliative care medicine, Poland, history, hospice, research institutes, bottom-up research, top-down research

---

* Corresponding Author's E-mail: z.zylicz@ur.edu.pl.

INTRODUCTION

In principle, there are two different approaches to medical research. The first is the top-down type of research: a national science foundation formulates a research vision and designates the resources needed. Scientists submit projects befitting this vision and some are granted money. This approach is suited to large institutions such as universities accustomed to the immense amount of paperwork involved. However, it also causes disappointment because only the best win, the competition is usually strong, and institutions with a multitude of publications enjoy priority. Another problem is that palliative medicine is rarely represented in national or special programmes.

The other approach is to employ bottom-up research. This is dependent on you and your invention. The following is a story that fascinated one of our team (ZZ) and inspired further research.

An 88-year-old ship's captain was admitted to our hospice because of severe pruritus that complicated widespread bronchial cancer [1]. He was scratching so intensely that his wounds were bleeding. The evening following admission, he tried to commit suicide by cutting his wrists. After his bleeding had been stopped, he was given paroxetine against his supposed depression.

To our surprise, the patient slept well that night and, the next day, he awoke in good spirits and declared that his itch had diminished. Within two weeks, the intensity of his itch was approaching zero, and his skin healed without leaving scars. He left the hospice and died two months later, without the itch.

This was a kind of miracle. You can consider it a unique phenomenon and leave it at that, but you can also become interested in the subject, digging through masses of articles and books. This is what we did but, to our disappointment, we found nothing. At least we could now be sure that nobody else had described this phenomenon before.

We started to treat a couple of cancer patients with paroxetine who had recalcitrant itch [1]. In this uncontrolled series, they both, as expected, responded very well to the drug. I cannot remember any adverse effects. We were now sure this was an interesting issue. Together with Małgorzata Krajnik, who was at this time looking for a subject of her doctorate, we decided to conduct a formal clinical trial; no easy task in a hospice environment. We wrote a protocol and found a hospital pharmacist who would prepare identical capsules, one with a placebo and one with paroxetine, and code them for randomization. The Ethics Commitee agreed to the study. We devised it as a double-blind, placebo-controlled trial with a crossover design. The problem was that the interim period between the treatments, which for our patients could not be very long, needed a substantial washout period. If the trial lasted many weeks, most patients would be unable to complete it, as their prognosis was usually short. So, we decided to do it all in two weeks. This was based on the observation that our patients responded to paroxetine almost instantly. We could, however, expect a considerable carryover effect.

We started the trial without any financial support or knowledge of how it would end. As accrual was slow, we looked for suitable patients in a number of hospitals. Finally, we completed a trial with 26 patients. Two patients experienced severe nausea and vomiting and were excluded [2]. The trial found that approximately 30% of the patients with intractable itch who took part benefited from paroxetine and adverse effects were usually mild and acceptable.

Now, 20 years later, we can proudly state that by treating the first index patient with paroxetine, we started a new era in the understanding of pruritus, and not only in cancer [3, 4]. This whole process can be described by a beautiful English word: "serendipity". Although miracles often happen in our practice of palliative care (PC), we need to be attuned to them. You must get inspired and be fascinated. Now that a couple of controlled trials have been performed elsewhere with paroxetine and other related drugs, [5, 6] we are sure this therapy is efficacious. It is now heralded as the first choice by many national and international guidelines on itch.

Nonetheless, for many years, we did not know how selective serotonin reuptake inhibitors (SSRIs) worked. Several hypotheses were proposed, but none were proved experimentally. Now we know that paroxetine is a strong inhibitor of P2X4 [7-9] and probably of Toll-like receptor [7, 10, 11] receptors and, in this way, totally independent of serotonin metabolism, it inhibits the propagation of itch impulses.

Moreover, we can expect that the pharmaceutical industry will, in the near future, be interested in the synthesis of new drugs, not necessarily antidepressants, that act on these receptors and could be tried against itch.

Palliative medicine is a young specialty, not only in Poland. It evolved from the idealistic hospice movement started by Dame Cicely Saunders in the late 1960s in London. From the beginning, British hospices were carefully observed by Polish doctors and nurses. Saunders, who always had a soft spot for Poles, visited Poland in 1976 and gave important impetus to the development of several hospices [12]. The first hospices appeared under communist rule, before it's fall in 1989. British hospice leaders and researchers contributed immensely by supporting and stimulating these developments [12]. This support was supplemented by researchers from all over Europe, such as Robert Twycross, Pål Klepstad, Stein Kaasa, Ilora Finlay, Kris Vissers, Yvonne Engels, Sam Ahmedzai, Lukas Radbruch and many others. They frequently visited Poland to give lectures and courses and invited us to participate in European research projects by writing and publishing with them. They even invited some of us to their universities, first to attend courses for free, but later to teach on them. There were also a couple of Polish expats living and working in PC outside Poland. Important roles were played here by Piotr Sobański (Switzerland) and Zbigniew (Ben) Zylicz (the Netherlands and the UK). They provided a bridge between Poland, the rest of Europe and the world, finding institutes and the right people willing to help in Polish research. Soon, in addition to a network of hospices and PC units, a number of centres started specific research in PC medicine. However, governments, especially in post-Communist Poland, had no money for PC research. Thus, most studies were of a clinical, bottom-up nature, with little or no outside financial support. Studies were performed enthusiastically and even resulted in a number of doctorates. Research was needed to develop, gain experience, modernize our practice, connect with colleagues from the West, and finally to attract young people to the specialty. Most important, however, was learning to work according to the rules of evidence-based medicine.

After three decades of such efforts, we can cite established research centres in Poland. First is the centre in Poznan, founded by Professor Jacek Łuczak, now succeeded by his students: Prof. Wojciech Leppert, Aleksandra Kotlińska-Lemieszek and Maciej Sopata. All three developed their own research lines, one of which will be discussed shortly. Another centre emerged in Kraków at St Lazarus Hospice and the Jagiellonian University, the oldest university in the country. This university has a long tradition of pain research within molecular biology and anaesthesiology. In recent decades, interest has extended to other problems and to PC [13]. For example, Tomasz Grądalski et al. have specialized in the treatment of lymphatic oedema [14-24].

After gaining experience in the Netherlands, **Małgorzata** Krajnik started another research centre in Bydgoszcz. Her first area of expertise, after itch studies, was the use of nebulized morphine to treat breathlessness. Previous data, obtained elsewhere in a single controlled clinical trial, suggested that morphine, although efficacious, was equal in potency to the saline used as a placebo control [25]. However, these data were obtained without knowledge of where the receptors are in the airways or how to reach them with nebulized morphine. First, Krajnik conducted immune-histopathological studies in Berlin on lung tissues resected from patients with tumours. These studies revealed that opioid receptors are mainly localized in medium-sized bronchi on the pulmonary neuroendocrine cells (PNEC) [26, 27]. Later, nebulization that specifically targets receptors was developed and tested [28]. The optimal method [28] was applied in a controlled trial with COPD patients experiencing breathlessness [29]. The study revealed a significant difference between the placebo and morphine and patients nebulizing morphine reported a marked improvement in breathlessness. Further, more complete studies were planned but failed to receive financial support. It is significant, however, that nebulized morphine is effective in treating breathlessness and this cutting-edge research gives hope to many suffering patients.

Another centre emerged in Gdańsk, where, during the time of the "Solidarność" movement, its medical university founded a facility for research and education in PC that was related to the nephrology clinic (Prof. Monika Lichodziejewska-Niemierko) and the lung disease clinic (Prof. Ewa Jassem). This centre researches problems around the syndromes of fatigue, [30-32] breathlessness and cough [29, 33, 34]. The two most active clinicians and researchers are Tomasz Buss and Aleksandra Modlińska.

No less interesting were studies performed in Poznań by Aleksandra Kotlińska-Lemieszek. She and Prof. J. Łuczak were the first to describe their experience with subanaesthetic doses of ketamine adjuvant to opioids [35]. For many years, we were all excited by this subject, which gained many supporters as well as opponents. Unfortunately, a systematic review of the controlled trials available neither confirmed nor denied the role of ketamine as an adjuvant in the control of cancer pain [36]. Nor did a more recent study concerning the use of oral ketamine confirm its efficacy in cancer-related neuropathic pain [37]. The authors suggested there may be a group of disorders with central sensitization that responds to ketamine. As the study did not specifically address this group, however, its results were inconclusive. Future studies that examine ketamine in chronic neuropathic pain should focus on patients with central sensitization, which can be established by a bedside test. This approach would be congruent with preclinical knowledge and addresses an important question.

Kotlińska-Lemieszek only recently became known as an expert in the field of the rational use and pharmacology of drugs used in PC [13]. Polypharmacy and drug interactions relevant to the field drew her particular attention [38, 39]. Other studies by her with a group of international experts were essential for the development of rational guidelines involved the prescription of drugs used for symptom control in patients with renal impairment [40-43].

In the first phase of PC development in Poland, we simply translated articles and, sometimes, whole books on the subject. We copied models of Western hospices and PC units and sometimes literally copied their guidelines. In the next phase, however, we achieved integration between the young discipline of PC and pain and pharmacology research. We started to write our own guidelines and publish our own studies. A couple of good books were published thanks to many integrated efforts. In 1999, palliative medicine and, a couple of years later, PC nursing were officially recognized in Poland as medical specialties. Since then, young colleagues have been able to pursue careers in this field.

Unfortunately, experience is not enough to solve all the problems of the third phase. Societies, including ours, are continuously changing. First comes ageing and a shortage of young people to care for the elderly and terminally ill. Another problem is the use of new technologies and PC drugs, as we lack sufficient technologies of our own. Even if somebody devises something new and exciting here, there is only a small chance this technology will be recognized and developed. The best inventions often migrate abroad, without serving our society or solving our problems. Nor do we have the mechanisms to adapt and adopt foreign technologies and assess them independently, without the support of the industry that produces them. This makes our services not sufficiently cost-efficient.

In Poland, we have two journals devoted solely to PC and a third to pain. Sadly, none of them are listed on MEDLINE and they are not cited very often, as they are published in Polish. Only one journal, Palliative Medicine in Practice, publishes papers in English and Polish. Most researchers publish their papers abroad in widely cited journals. On the other hand, these English papers are read by minority of Polish doctors and nurses. Improving the quality of the papers published, getting published in English and Polish, and being listed on MEDLINE should now be the top priorities for at least one of these journals.

The government has new ideas regarding how to reform healthcare but do we have a proper voice in this discussion? Do we have arguments supported by evidence that our solutions are better and cheaper? We owe this to our patients! Almost nobody in our country is conducting studies on new care models, better adapted to the changing circumstances in which we work.

That is why conducting only reactive or bottom-up research will never be enough. We need to proceed to the third phase. We need designated funding from the government or public donations that will be distributed in the right way to the right people. Where to obtain this money? PC is always presented as a specialty that costs money but will never be profitable. Nobody here conducts studies to show how important well-organized PC could be for the well-being of our society, for other specialties and for hospital budgets. Certainly, we need more studies on patients' acceptance and appreciation of PC. For example, how does PC, which is a typical Western concept, fit in with our culture? Why do so many patients fear admission to hospices and PC units? We sometimes calculate the direct costs of procedures or technologies, but this is just the tip of the iceberg. We should also invent mechanisms and algorithms to estimate the indirect costs of such care.

The number of patients under our care will increase, that is certain. Will we be able to cope with this increase and maintain a proper quality of patient care?

REFERENCES

[1] Zylicz Z, Smits C, Krajnik M. Paroxetine for pruritus in advanced cancer. *Journal of pain and symptom management* 1998;16:121-4.
[2] Zylicz Z, Krajnik M, Sorge AA, Costantini M. Paroxetine in the treatment of severe non-dermatological pruritus: a randomized, controlled trial. *Journal of pain and symptom management* 2003;26:1105-12.
[3] Twycross R, Greaves, MW, Handwerker H, Jones EA, Libretto SE, Szepietowski JC, Zylicz Z. Itch: scratching more than the surface. *QJM* 2003;96:7-26.
[4] Weisshaar E, Weiss M, Mettang T, Yosipovitch G, Zylicz Z. Special Interest Group of the International Forum on the Study of I. Paraneoplastic itch: an expert position statement from the Special Interest Group (SIG) of the International Forum on the Study of Itch (IFSI). *Acta Dermato-Venereologica* 2015;95:261-5.
[5] Mayo MJ, Handem I, Saldana S, Jacobe H, Getachew Y, Rush AJ. Sertraline as a first-line treatment for cholestatic pruritus. *Hepatology* 2007;45:666-74.
[6] Stander S, Bockenholt B, Schurmeyer-Horst F, et al. Treatment of chronic pruritus with the selective serotonin re-uptake inhibitors paroxetine and fluvoxamine: results of an open-labelled, two-arm proof-of-concept study. *Acta Dermato-Venereologica* 2009;89:45-51.
[7] Nagata K, Imai T, Yamashita T, Tsuda M, Tozaki-Saitoh H, Inoue K. Antidepressants inhibit P2X4 receptor function: a possible involvement in neuropathic pain relief. *Mol. Pain* 2009;5:20.
[8] Abdelrahman A, Namasivayam V, Hinz S, et al. Characterization of P2X4 receptor agonists and antagonists by calcium influx and radioligand binding studies. *Biochemical Pharmacology* 2017;125:41-54.
[9] Zarei M, Sabetkasaei M, Moini Zanjani T. Paroxetine attenuates the development and existing pain in a rat model of neurophatic pain. *Iran Biomed. J.* 2014;18:94-100.
[10] Taves S, Ji RR. Itch control by Toll-like receptors. *Handb. Exp. Pharmacol.* 2015;226:135-50.
[11] Liu T, Gao YJ, Ji RR. Emerging role of Toll-like receptors in the control of pain and itch. *Neurosci. Bull.* 2012;28:131-44.
[12] Bogusz H, Pekacka-Falkowska K, Magowska A. Under the British Roof: The British Contribution to the Development of Hospice and Palliative Care in Poland. *Journal of palliative care* 2018;33:115-9.
[13] Wordliczek J, Kotlinska-Lemieszek A, Leppert W, et al. Pharmacotherapy of pain in cancer patients - recommendations of the Polish Association for the Study of Pain, Polish Society of Palliative Medicine, Polish Society of Oncology, Polish Society of Family Medicine, Polish Society of Anaesthesiology and Intensive Therapy and Association of Polish Surgeons. *Pol. Przegl. Chir.* 2018;90:55-84.
[14] Ochalek K, Gradalski T. Manual lymph drainage may not be a necessary component in lymphedema treatment. *Journal of pain and symptom management* 2010;39:e1-2.
[15] Olszewski WL, Jain P, Ambujam G, Zaleska M, Cakala M, Gradalski T. Tissue fluid pressure and flow during pneumatic compression in lymphedema of lower limbs. *Lymphat Res. Biol.* 2011;9:77-83.

[16] Olszewski WL, Cwikla J, Zaleska M, Domaszewska-Szostek A, Gradalski T, Szopinska S. Pathways of lymph and tissue fluid flow during intermittent pneumatic massage of lower limbs with obstructive lymphedema. *Lymphology* 2011;44:54-64.

[17] Ochalek K, Gradalski T, Szygula Z. Five-year assessment of maintenance combined physical therapy in postmastectomy lymphedema. *Lymphat. Res. Biol.* 2015;13:54-8.

[18] Gradalski T, Ochalek K, Kurpiewska J. Complex Decongestive Lymphatic Therapy With or Without Vodder II Manual Lymph Drainage in More Severe Chronic Postmastectomy Upper Limb Lymphedema: A Randomized Noninferiority Prospective Study. *Journal of Pain and Symptom Management* 2015;50:750-7.

[19] Gradalski T, Kurpiewska J, Ochalek K, Bialon-Janusz A. The application of negative pressure wound therapy combined with compression bandaging for the decubitus ulcer of an advanced primary lower limb lymphedema. *International Journal of Dermatology* 2017;56:e144-e7.

[20] Ochalek K, Gradalski T, Partsch H. Preventing Early Postoperative Arm Swelling and Lymphedema Manifestation by Compression Sleeves After Axillary Lymph Node Interventions in Breast Cancer Patients: A Randomized Controlled Trial. *Journal of Pain and Symptom Management* 2017;54:346-54.

[21] Ochalek K, Gradalski T, Szygula Z, Partsch H. Physical Activity With and Without Arm Sleeves: Compliance and Quality of Life After Breast Cancer Surgery-A Randomized Controlled Trial. *Lymphat. Res. Biol.* 2018;16:294-9.

[22] Gradalski T. Diuretics Combined With Compression in Resistant Limb Edema of Advanced Disease-A Case Series Report. *Journal of Pain and Symptom Management.* 2018;55:1179-83.

[23] Gradalski T, Ochalek K, Rybak D. Lymphedema or Rather End-of-Life Edema? *J. Palliat. Med.* 2018;21:585.

[24] Ochalek K, Partsch H, Gradalski T, Szygula Z. Do Compression Sleeves Reduce the Incidence of Arm Lymphedema and Improve Quality of Life? Two-Year Results from a Prospective Randomized Trial in Breast Cancer Survivors. *Lymphat. Res. Biol.* 2018.

[25] Noseda A, Carpiaux JP, Markstein C, Meyvaert A, de Maertelaer V. Disabling dyspnoea in patients with advanced disease: lack of effect of nebulized morphine. *The European Respiratory Journal* 1997;10:1079-83.

[26] Krajnik M, Schafer M, Sobanski P, et al. Enkephalin, its precursor, processing enzymes, and receptor as part of a local opioid network throughout the respiratory system of lung cancer patients. *Hum. Pathol.* 2010;41:632-42.

[27] Krajnik M, Schafer M, Sobanski P, et al. Local pulmonary opioid network in patients with lung cancer: a putative modulator of respiratory function. *Pharmacol. Rep.* 2010;62:139-49.

[28] Krajnik M, Podolec Z, Siekierka M, et al. Morphine Inhalation by Cancer Patients: A Comparison of Different Nebulization Techniques Using Pharmacokinetic, Spirometric, and Gasometric Parameters. *Journal of Pain and Symptom Management* 2009;38:747-57.

[29] Janowiak P, Krajnik M, Podolec Z, et al. Dosimetrically administered nebulized morphine for breathlessness in very severe chronic obstructive pulmonary disease: a randomized, controlled trial. *BMC Pulm. Med.* 2017;17:186.

[30] Buss T, Modlinska A, Chelminska M, Niedoszytko M. [Cancer related fatigue. I. Prevalence and attempt to define the problem]. *Pol. Merkur. Lekarski.* 2004;16:70-2.

[31] Buss T, Kruk A, Wisniewski P, Modlinska A, Janiszewska J, Lichodziejewska-Niemierko M. Psychometric properties of the Polish version of the Multidimensional Fatigue Inventory-20 in cancer patients. *Journal of Pain and Symptom Management* 2014;48:730-7.

[32] Modlinska A, Kowalik B, Buss T, Janiszewska J, Lichodziejewska-Niemierko M. Strategy of coping with end-stage disease and cancer-related fatigue in terminally ill patients. *Am. J. Hosp. Palliat. Care* 2014;31:771-6.

[33] Krajnik M, Damps-Konstanska I, Gorska L, Jassem E. A portable automatic cough analyser in the ambulatory assessment of cough. *Biomedical Engineering Online* 2010;9:17.

[34] Krajnik M, Podolec Z, Zylicz Z, Jassem E. Air humidity may influence the aerosol distribution of normal saline administered by closed or vented nebulizers operated continuously or dosimetrically. *J. Aerosol. Med. Pulm. Drug. Deliv.* 2009;22:29-34.

[35] Kotlinska-Lemieszek A, Luczak J. Subanesthetic ketamine: an essential adjuvant for intractable cancer pain. *Journal of Pain and Symptom Management* 2004;28:100-2.

[36] Bell RF, Eccleston C, Kalso E. Ketamine as adjuvant to opioids for cancer pain. A qualitative systematic review. *Journal of Pain and Symptom Management* 2003;26:867-75.

[37] Fallon MT, Wilcock A, Kelly CA, et al. Oral Ketamine vs Placebo in Patients With Cancer-Related Neuropathic Pain: A Randomized Clinical Trial. *JAMA Oncol.* 2018;4:870-2.

[38] Kotlinska-Lemieszek A, Klepstad P, Haugen DF. Clinically significant drug-drug interactions involving opioid analgesics used for pain treatment in patients with cancer: a systematic review. *Drug Des. Devel. Ther.* 2015;9:5255-67.

[39] Kotlinska-Lemieszek A, Paulsen O, Kaasa S, Klepstad P. Polypharmacy in patients with advanced cancer and pain: a European cross-sectional study of 2282 patients. *Journal of Pain and Symptom Management* 2014;48:1145-59.

[40] Wilcock A, Charlesworth S, Twycross R, et al. Prescribing Non-Opioid Drugs in End-Stage Kidney Disease. *Journal of Pain and Symptom Management* 2017;54:776-87.

[41] Deskur-Smielecka E, Kotlinska-Lemieszek A, Chudek J, Wieczorowska-Tobis K. Assessment of renal function in geriatric palliative care patients - comparison of creatinine-based estimation equations. *Clin. Interv. Aging.* 2017;12:977-83.

[42] Twycross R, Ross J, Kotlinska-Lemieszek A, Charlesworth S, Mihalyo M, Wilcock A. Variability in response to drugs. *Journal of Pain and Symptom Management* 2015;49:293-306.

[43] Deskur-Smielecka E, Kotlinska-Lemieszek A, Niemir ZI, Wieczorowska-Tobis K. Prevalence of Renal Impairment in Palliative Care Inpatients: A Retrospective Analysis. *J. Palliat. Med.* 2015;18:613-7.

Part IV. Middle East

In: Palliative Care
Editor: Michael Silbermann

ISBN: 978-1-53616-199-1
© 2019 Nova Science Publishers, Inc.

Chapter 15

EARLY PALLIATIVE CARE (EPC) TRIALS FOR PATIENTS WITH ADVANCED INCURABLE CANCER: WHAT HAVE WE LEARNED AND HOW CAN WE IMPROVE FUTURE TRIALS AND PATIENTS' CARE

Haris Charalambous[1],*, MD and Angelos P. Kassianos[2], PhD

[1]Consultant Clinical Oncologist, BOC Oncology Centre, Nicosia, Cyprus
[2]Researcher, Department of Applied Health Research, UCL, London, UK

ABSTRACT

In the recent past, trials of Early Palliative Care (EPC) have been undertaken to address symptoms and improve quality of life of patients with advanced, incurable cancer, and improve on the practice of late referral to palliative care towards the end of life. In this chapter, we review trials of EPC to examine the benefits of this approach in relation to Health-Related Quality of Life (HRQoL), symptom improvement, End of Life (EOL) communication, aggressiveness of EOL care and survival. We also discuss their main differences especially in relation to the model of EPC used and the intensity of the EPC intervention. Finally, we refer to methodological issues, potential weaknesses and lessons learned from these trials, and as to issues that need to be addressed in future EPC studies in order to improve care of patients with advanced incurable cancer.

Keywords: trials, early palliative care, specialized palliative care, advanced cancer

INTRODUCTION

According to the World Health Organization (WHO), Palliative Care (PC) has a focus of providing "active, holistic care of patients with advanced, progressive illness, including management of pain and other symptoms and provision of psychological, social and spiritual

---

* Corresponding Author's E-mail: haris.charalambous@bococ.org.cy.

support is paramount. The goal of PC is achievement of the best quality of life for patients and their families" [1]. Furthermore, it is recognized that "many aspects of PC are also applicable earlier in the course of the illness in conjunction with other treatments" (WHO 1990).

Specialist palliative care (SPC) is provided by the PC team, i.e., health care professionals with expertise in PC, and who are exclusively occupied in providing PC, dealing with management of refractory pain and other symptoms, complex depression, anxiety, grief, and existential distress, and assistance with conflict resolution and in addressing futility issues [2]. Basic PC is provided by oncologists or primary care physicians addressing basic pain and symptom management, basic management of depression and anxiety, and basic discussion about goals, prognosis, and suffering [2].

The concept of Early Palliative Care (EPC) originated out of the realization that patients with advanced, incurable cancer were referred late or not at all to SPC services [3, 4, 5]. Equally data from the US would suggest that there was an excessive aggressiveness of care towards the end of life (EOL) [6], with patients continuing to receive chemotherapy [7, 8], resulting in high hospital and Intensive Care Unit (ICU) mortality, and care being fully focused on disease-directed therapy with little attention to quality of life and symptom control [9].

Following the emergence of studies showing benefit from the introduction of EPC in patients with advanced / progressive illness or metastatic / incurable cancer [10, 11], the American Society of Clinical Oncology (ASCO) issued in 2012 a provisional clinical opinion (PCO) recognizing the importance and benefits of PC in terms of improvement of patients' symptoms, quality of life and satisfaction, whilst reducing caregiver's burden, and has made a firm suggestion that PC should be considered early in the course of illness of all patients with metastatic cancer [12]. Subsequently in 2017 ASCO in a Clinical Oncology Clinical Practice Guideline Update, recommended that "inpatients and outpatients with advanced cancer should receive dedicated palliative care services, early in the disease course, concurrent with active treatment" [13].

In this review of trials of EPC we summarize the main findings of these studies in relation to Health-Related Quality of Life (HRQoL), symptom improvement, EOL communication, aggressiveness of EOL care and survival. We also discuss their main differences especially in relation to the model of EPC used and the intensity of the EPC intervention. Finally, we refer to methodological issues, potential weaknesses and lessons learned from these trials, and as to issues that need to be addressed in future EPC studies in order to improve care of patients with advanced incurable cancer.

METHODS

Even if this is not a systematic review, we used a systematic method in searching and screening studies to ensure that relevant EPC trials were not missed. The PICO [14] method was used for inclusion/exclusion criteria of studies identified for the review (Box 1).

Box 1. Developing the inclusion/exclusion criteria for EPC trials

P	I	C	O
Population	**Intervention**	**Comparison**	**Outcome**
Patients diagnosed with any type of cancer	Specialized Palliative Care (SPC) as defined by Qill and Abernethy [2].	The trials should be (a) comparing SPC with any type of control, and (b) implementing the SPC earlier than the late stages of the disease (EPC)	Health-Related Quality of Life (HRQoL), symptom improvement, end-of-life (EOL) discussions / patient communication, aggressiveness of EOL care, survival

Eligibility Criteria

Studies published in peer-reviewed journals were eligible to be reviewed provided they include patients > 18 years old diagnosed with any primary and metastatic cancer. Eligible studies should be evaluating interventions aiming to provide EPC to cancer patients by a Specialized Palliative Care (SPC) Team/within 12 weeks of a diagnosis of an advanced, incurable cancer diagnosis. Study authors in the abstract should mention 'Early' integration of SPC in order to be included for review. We note that we may have missed studies that may have used EPC but did not report this as 'early' integration in the abstract even though we assume that very few studies did so.

SPC service was defined as care provided from professionals / teams, with training / expertise in PC, who coordinate or provide comprehensive care for cancer patients. Studies that provided supportive care or any other psychosocial intervention or care that was not coordinated/provided by a specialized PC team were excluded.

Studies that included cancer patients together with other patient groups, and where there was no separate analysis for the cancer patients, were excluded.

Non-Randomized Controlled Trials (RCTs) including prospective and retrospective studies with pre- and post- assessment as well as cross-sectional, qualitative, feasibility and pilot studies were excluded. No publication date restriction was used and only studies published in English were included for pragmatic reasons.

Search Strategy and Study Selection

The keywords for search aimed to cover the following areas: the type of care, the type of patients and the timing of the referral to SPC. The search was in line with the PRESS checklist to ensure a more systematic approach and that we don't miss any relevant publications [15]. A search strategy was designed and developed targeting relevant databases (MEDLINE, EMBASE, PsycINFO, Global Health Archive, and PubMed). The combinations of keywords used were *[palliative care]; *[terminal care]; *[hospice care]; *[cancer* or neoplasm* or tumor* or carcinoma*]; *[quality of life* or qol* or *hrqol]; *[early]. One MSc student conducted the search and screened the papers together with the chapter authors.

RESULTS

Study Selection

There were 1274 papers identified in initial search in all databases and after title, abstract and full text screening a set of 10 different clinical trials, were included as eligible. The initial search was conducted in 2016. Initial title screening identified 921 studies that were excluded as non-peer reviewed (n = 460), non-RCTs (n = 23), including no cancer patients (n = 5) and published in languages other than English (n= 112) and with duplicates removed (n = 321). The remaining 353 abstracts were screened and another 327 papers were removed because they used a non-RCT research design (n = 138), did not differentiate cancer population outcomes (n = 14), were pilot/feasibility studies (n = 16), measured other outcomes (n = 46), did not use EPC (n = 57), or had no full text available (e.g., conference abstracts, n = 56). Finally, 26 full text articles were reviewed and 17 were removed because they did not evaluate the impact of EPC. Following an update in 2018 another three papers were identified resulting in the final 12 papers. Three papers [10, 16, 17] reported results from the same trial and therefore the final number of identified trials was 10.

Study Characteristics

Ten (10) trials were included in the review with a total of 2447 patients with advanced cancer.

It is important to recognize that we are only reporting on studies undertaken with cancer patients, and studies with both cancer patients and patients with progressive, incurable illnesses have not been included, as those did not provide a separate analysis for cancer patients.

Intervention and Control Procedures

In Table 1, there is a summary of the intervention (model of SPC provision) and control procedures used in each study.

All studies reported on the team or health professionals delivering SPC. The main difference was that five studies used a predominantly advanced/SPC nurse intervention (Bakitas 2009 [11], Bakitas 2015 [18], Tattersall [19], McCorkle [20] and Vanbutsele [21]), whilst the other five studies used a PC physician led/PC team-based intervention (Temel 2010 [10], Zimmermann [22], Maltoni [23], Temel 2017 [24], Groenveld [25]).

The control groups' procedures were reported in most RCTs as 'usual care', and referral to PC was usually initiated either by the patient or treating oncologist request. In only one study, by Bakitas 2015, EPC was offered to the control group after a three (3) month delay, whilst results regarding the primary endpoint were reported prior to the integration of EPC in the control arm.

Table 1. Description of intervention and control procedures of EPC trial studies

Study	Description of EPC	Team: Who is delivering the EPC	Control group procedures
Bakitas et al 2009 USA	Palliative care is based on the chronic care model, using a case management, educational approach to encourage patient activation, self-management, and empowerment. Education and advice provided predominantly via telephone consultations.	Delivered by two advanced practice nurses with palliative care training, a palliative care physician and a nurse practitioner.	Received usual care by a medical oncologist and consisting of symptom control and supportive care. Allowed to use all oncology and supportive services, without restrictions including referral to the institutions' interdisciplinary palliative care service.
Bakitas et al 2015 USA	Palliative care is based on the chronic care model, using a case management, educational approach to encourage patient activation, self-management, and empowerment. Education and advice provided predominantly via telephone consultations.	Delivered by two advanced practice nurses with palliative care training, a palliative care physician and a nurse practitioner.	Received usual care by a medical oncologist and consisting of symptom control and supportive care. Allowed to use all oncology and supportive services, without restrictions including referral to the institutions' interdisciplinary palliative care service.
Groenvold et al 2017 Denmark	Using the guidelines and expertise based on the European Association for Palliative Care White Paper, the WHO guidelines and national/local guidelines. Patients had both 1 face-to-face contact with the SPC team with additional telephone contacts	SPC team (different for each site included doctors, nurses, physiotherapists, psychologists, social workers, chaplains, secretaries, volunteers and pharmacists.	Received standard care provided by oncology GPs or home care services. Some patients had >1 face-to-face contact with the SPC team.
Maltoni et al. 2016 Italy	A checklist used to determine conversation with PC specialist. General PC guidelines used for appointments and interventions. PC specialist referred patients for further support (medical, physical, psychological, spiritual).	PC specialist who referred to other specialists according to patients' needs.	Only provided with an appointment with PC specialist if specially requested.
McCorkle et al 2015 USA	PC provided by different members of PC unit focusing on: monitoring patients' status, providing symptom, management, executing complex care procedures, teaching patients and family caregivers, clarifying the illness experience, coordinating care, responding to the family, enhancing QOL, and collaborating with other providers and discussing goals of care. Also received a Symptom Management Toolkit.	Led by advanced practice nurses, with access to PC unit (physician assistants, medical social workers), which met regularly to discuss patients' status and management strategies.	Did not receive the advanced practice nurse intervention. Received routine oncology care by a multidisciplinary team. Also received a Symptom Management Toolkit.
Tattersall et al 2014 Australia	Patients met with the PC nurse consultant member of the hospital PC team first. The nurse outlined available services and arranged referrals. The nurse also offered monthly telephone consultations.	PC nurse consultant with access to PC team	Referred to the PC service only if requested by the oncologist

Table 1. (Continued)

Study	Description of EPC	Team: Who is delivering the EPC	Control group procedures
Temel et al 2010 USA	Face to face palliative care consultations with PC team. General guidelines adapted from the National Consensus Project for Quality Palliative Care including physical and psychosocial. Specific attention to assessing physical and psychosocial symptoms, establishing care goals, assisting with treatment decision-making and coordinating care based on patients' needs	Five palliative care physicians and one advanced practice nurse delivering care (plus other members of PC team available)	No meeting with PC services unless requested. Received standard oncologic care.
Temel et al. 2017 USA	Patients met with member of a PC team and at least once a month until death. PC physicians phoned the patient when in-person visit was not possible.	PC team consisted of physicians, advanced practice nurses and the hospital team per the National Consensus for Quality Palliative Care guidelines. The hospital team observed inpatients during hospitalization.	Patients able to meet with PC physician upon request.
Vanbutsele et al 2018 Belgium	Introductory consultation with specialist nurse, a dietician and a psychologist. Follow-ups consultations were at the discretion of the patient. Access to PC physicians/team if required.	Standard Oncological Care by a multidisciplinary team (oncologists, other medical specialists, psychologists, social workers, dieticians, specialist nurses).	Standard Oncological Care included one introductory consultation with a specialist nurse, a dietitian and a psychologist at the start of their treatment. PC consultations assigned if requested by the patients or their physicians.
Zimmermann et al 2014 Canada	Face to face outpatient palliative care consultations Approach to care declared as multidisciplinary addressing physical, psychological, social and spiritual needs.	Palliative care physician and palliative care nurse (also available psychological support, physical therapy and occupational therapy).	No routine PC received but a referral initiated if requested.

FINDINGS FROM THE EPC TRIALS

The primary endpoint in all trials of EPC has been Health Related Quality of Life (HRQoL). Three studies used a composite primary endpoint with both HRQoL and symptoms intensity and resource use (Bakitas 2009), HRQoL and depression (Bakitas 2015), and HRQoL, symptoms, depression and distress (McCorkle).

Eight different instruments for measuring HRQoL were used:

- the Functional Assessment of Chronic Illness Therapy for Palliative Care, FACIT-Pal, in Bakitas 2009 and Bakitas 2015,
- the Trial Outcome Index, TOI, of the Functional Assessment of Cancer Therapy-Hepatobiliary, FACT-Hep, in Maltoni 2016,
- the Functional Assessment of Cancer Therapy-General, FACT-G, in Temel 2017, McCorkle2015,
- the McGill Quality of Life, McGill QOL, in Tattersall 2014 and Vanbutsele 2018 studies,
- the TOI of the Functional Assessment of Cancer Therapy-Lung, FACT-L, in Temel 2010,
- the Functional Assessment of Chronic Illness Therapy for Spiritual Well-Being, FACIT-Sp, in Zimmermann 2014.
- the Quality of Life at the End of Life, QUAL-E was also used in the Zimmermann study.
- and finally, the European Organization for Research and Treatment of Cancer Quality of Life Questionnaire (EORTC QLQ-C30) in the Groenvold 2017 and Vanbutsele 2018. In the Groenvold study the primary outcome was the change in each patient's primary need (the most severe of the seven QLQ-C30 scales).

Six studies undertook assessment of the primary endpoint at 12 weeks (Bakitas 2015, Maltoni 2016, Temel 2010, Temel 2015, Vanbutsele 2018, Zimmermann 2014) whilst two studies did a longitudinal assessment (Bakitas 2009, and Tattersall 2014), and finally in the Groenvold 2017 study the assessment of the primary endpoint was at 3 and 8 weeks, and in the McCorkle 2015 study at 1 and 3 months.

Results Regarding HRQoL

In four studies (Bakitas 2009, Temel 2010, Maltoni 2016, Vanbutsele 2018) there was a statistically significant improvement in HRQoL at 12 weeks after integration of EPC. In the Bakitas 2009 study the EPC group compared with the control group had a mean overall treatment difference of 4.6 (SE = 2) on the FACITPal overall QoL scale. In the Temel 2010 study, the EPC arm displayed significantly better HRQoL on the TOI of the FACT-L at three months with a mean of 59.0 (SD = 11.6 compared to 53.0 (SD = 11.5 for the control group. In the Maltoni 2016 study, using the TOI of the FACTHep, the EPC group has an estimated mean 84.4 (SD = 16.3) compared to 78.1 (SD = 21.3) for the control group. Finally, in the Vanbutsele 2018 study, using the EORTC QLQ C30, the EPC group had a score of 61.98

(95% CI: 57.02–66.95) and the control group a score of 54.39 (95% CI 49.23–59.56) with a difference of 7.60 (95% CI: 0.59–14.60; p=0.03).

In two studies, improvement in HRQoL was documented after 12 weeks (Zimmermann 2014, and Temel 2017). Zimmermann 2014 found a non-significant difference between groups in the score for the FACIT-Sp at 3 months, which was the primary endpoint, of 3.56 points (95% CI: 0.27-7.40, p=0.07) but a significant difference in QUAL-E of 2.25 (95% CI: 0.01-4.49, p=0.05). At 4 months, there were significant differences in change scores for both FACIT-Sp of 6.44 (95% CI: 2.13-10.76, p=0.006) and also QUAL-E 3.51 (95% CI: 1.33-5.68, p=0.003). In the Temel 2017 study, the mean FACT-G score for the control group at 12 weeks was 77.70 (95% CI: 75.77-79.63) and 80.10 (95% CI: 78.11-82.08) in the EPC group, with a mean difference of 2.40 (95% CI: -0.38-5.18), which was not statistically significant (p=0.091). At 24 weeks, the mean FACT-G score for the control group was 75.90 (95% CI: 73.59-78.21) and 81.26 (95% CI: 78.89-83.63) in the EPC group, with a mean difference of 5.36 (95% CI: 2.04-8.69), which was highly statistically significant (p=0.002).

Four studies showed no statistically significant benefit in HRQoL: Bakitas 2015, McCorkle 2015, Tattersall 2014 and Groenvold 2017. At three months, Bakitas 2015 reported a small but not significant difference on the FACIT-Pal with an estimated mean 129.9 (95% CI: 126.6-133.3) for the EPC arm and 127.2 (95% CI: 124.1-130.3) for the control (delayed EPC) arm. Equally at three months, McCorkle 2015 found no significant difference in FACT-G between the EPC group with an estimated mean 82.1 (SD=18.1) for the EPC group compared to 82.7 (SD=14.5) for the control group. Also, Tattersall 2014 could not identify any significant difference in HRQoL using the McGill QOL instrument with an estimated mean 5.2 (SD=0.8) for the EPC group compared to 5.2 (SD=0.7) for the control group. Finally, Groenvold using the EORTC QLQ-C30, and with the primary endpoint being the change in each patient's primary need (the most severe of the seven QLQ-C30 scales) at 8 weeks, showed no statistically significant difference in favour of the EPC group for the primary outcome of change in primary need: −4.9 points (95% CI −11.3-1.5; p = 0.14).

Results Regarding Depression

Three studies showed an improvement in depression / better mood (Bakitas 2009, Temel 2010, Temel 2017). Bakitas 2009 reported decreased depression measured with the CES-D for the EPC group (mean overall treatment difference of -1.8, SE=0.81). Temel 2010 reported that fewer patients in the EPC arm had depressive symptoms based on the HADS Questionnaire (16% vs 38%, p=0.01), whilst using the Patient Health Questionnaire-9 (PHQ-9) patients assigned to EPC had greater improvements in depression at 12 weeks (p=0.001)[17]. Temel 2017 showed that patients in the EPC arm had lower rates of depression at week 24, controlling for baseline scores, but there was no statistically significant difference at 12 weeks for the whole cohort. Furthermore, in this study, differences per cancer type were noted with lung cancer patients experiencing improvements in both HRQoL and depression at 12 and 24 weeks, whereas patients in the control group with lung cancer reported deterioration. Patients with GI cancers in both study groups reported improvements in HRQoL and mood by week 12.

Other studies, including Bakitas 2015 using the Center for Epidemiological Studies-Depression Scale (CES-D), Maltoni 2016 using the HADS-D questionnaire, McCorkle 2015 using the PHQ-9 and Vanbutsele 2018 using both the HADS-D and PHQ-9 questionnaires, showed no significant differences in depressive symptoms between groups at 3 months, whilst three studies (Tattersall 2014, Groenvold 2017 and Zimmermann 2014) did not examine depression.

Results Regarding Symptom Intensity/Severity

Results for symptom intensity/severity were again mixed. Two studies showed a benefit in symptom severity at three months; Temel 2010 showed a benefit for the EPC group in having a lower symptom intensity on the Lung-Cancer Subscale, LCS of the FACT-L at three months, as did Maltoni 2016, applying the HCS of the FACT Hep. Zimmermann 2014 found no significant differences with the Edmonton Symptom Assessment System (ESAS) between groups at 3 months but found improvement at 4 months ($p=0.05$).

Two studies showed a trend for improvement in symptom intensity; Bakitas 2009 showed a trend for lower symptom intensity as measured with the ESAS for the EPC arm ($p=0.06$), as did Bakitas 2015 but no statistically significant difference in symptoms severity using the symptom impact subscale of the QUAL-E ($p=0.09$).

Two studies showed improvement in some symptoms; in the Vanbutsele 2018 study, there was improvement in fatigue and diarrhoea at 18 weeks, whilst in the Groenvold 2017 study there was an improvement in nausea and vomiting in favour of the EPC group.

Finally, two studies showed no benefit at three months, McCorkle 2015 using the Symptom Distress Scale SDS, and Tattersall 2014, using the Rotterdam Symptom Checklist: Physical Symptoms, RSC.

Other Endpoints: Healthcare Utilization and Aggressive End of Life Care

Reduction in aggressiveness of care towards the EOL was seen in the Temel 2010 study [10], with a reduction in intravenous chemotherapy in the last 14 days before death [16] and a longer hospice stay [10]. In the same study, improved prognosis awareness was seen [26].

Maltoni 2016 reported a lower rate of chemotherapy in the last 30 days of life in the EPC arm, however with no difference during the last two weeks of life, as well as no difference for hospital admissions in the last 30 days before death and emergency department visits.

Equally Bakitas 2009 and Bakitas 2015 did not detect statistically significant differences between groups in number of days in the hospital, number of days in the intensive care unit (ICU) and number of emergency department visits [27]. No difference in chemotherapy use was seen in the Tattersall 2014 study and Zimmermann 2014 study. The McCorkle 2015, Temel 2017, Groenvold 2017 and Vanbutsele 2018 studies did not report measures of healthcare use or EOL care.

Better EOL communication was found in the Temel 2017 study, with a doubling of patients likely to discuss their wishes with their oncologist, if they were dying. Greater satisfaction with care was seen in the Zimmermann 2014 study.

Table 2. Study characteristics and results of randomized controlled trials (RCTs) included in the review

Study information	Study period	Participants	Cancer type, stage, prognosis and Performance Status (PS)	Data collection and tools used	Outcome
Bakitas et al., 2015 USA Randomization level: Patients Blinding: Yes Stratification: Yes Two sites	2010-2013	Eligible:1464 Total sample: 207 Total IG: Early intervention group: 104 Delayed intervention group: 103 Age: EG: 64.03 (10.28) DG: 64.6 (9.59) Gender: EG: 53.85% M DG: 51.46% M	Site: Lung 44.23%; GI tract 25%; Breast 9.62%; other solid tumour 9.62%; genitourinary tract 6.73%; hematologic malignancy 4.81% Metastatic: Yes Prognosis(T1): 6-24 months Median KPS=80.6	Endpoints: HRQoL, symptom impact and mood; One-year and overall survival, resource use and location of death Tool for HRQoL: FACIT-Pal	No difference in FACIT-Pal score, symptom impact or mood. Improvement in 1 year survival (p=0.038) No difference in resource use or aggressiveness of EOL care.
Groenvold et al., 2017 Denmark Randomization level: Patients Blinding: Yes Stratification: Yes Multiple sites	2011-2013	Eligible: 464 Total sample: 297 Total IG: 145 Age: IG: <50 7%, 50-59 19%, 60-69 45%, 70-79 24%, ≥80 5% CG: <50 10%, 50-59 16%, 60-69 38%, 70-79 29%, ≥80 6% Gender: IG: 43% M CG: 41% M	Site: Lung, digestive system, breast and other Stage: IV or cancer in the central nervous system grade III/IV Prognosis(T1): 12 MONTHS PS= WHO 0-2	Endpoints: primary need (the most severe of the seven QLQ-C30 scales), HRQoL, survival Tool for HRQoL: EORTC QLQ C-30	No difference on the primary outcome of change in primary need. No difference in EORTC QLQ C-30 scores at 8weeks except for nausea-vomiting. No difference in survival.
Maltoni et al., 2016 Italy Randomization level: Patients Blinding: No Stratification: NR Multiple sites	2012-1015	Eligible: NR Total sample: 207 Total IG: 100 Age: IG: Median = 67 (43-85) CG: Median = 66 (31-84) Gender: IG: 61.5% M CG: 52.8% M	Site: Newly diagnosed pancreatic cancer Metastatic: Yes Prognosis(T1): > 2months PS= WHO 0-2	Endpoints: HRQoL, mood, aggressiveness of EOL care, survival and relatives satisfaction with care Tool for HRQoL: FACT-Hep (Hepatobiliary) Trial Outcome Index (TOI): the combination of the physical, functional and Hepatic Cancer Subscale (HCS).	Improvement in HCS (p=0.013) and TOI score (p=0.041) No difference EOL care, depression / anxiety or survival.

Study information	Study period	Participants	Cancer type, stage, prognosis and Performance Status (PS)	Data collection and tools used	Outcome
McCorkle et al, 2015 USA Randomization level: Clinic Blinding: No Stratification: No One site	2010-2012	Eligible: 290 Total sample: 146 Total IG: 66 Age: 62.3% < 65 years, 37.7% 65 years and older Gender: 43.8% M	Site: Newly diagnosed lung, gynaecologic, head and neck and gastrointestinal Stage: Reported as "late-stage" Prognosis (T1): NR PS =0-2	Endpoints: HRQoL, symptom distress, health distress, depression, functional status, self-rated health, anxiety, uncertainty, self-efficacy. Tool for HRQoL: FACT-G	No difference in HRQol, symptom distress, depression, health distress, depression, functional status, self-reported health. At 1-3 months physical and emotional symptoms stable for both groups.
Tattersall et al, 2014 Australia Randomization level: Patients Blinding: No Stratification: No One site	2003-2005	Eligible: 141 Total sample: 120 Total IG: 60 Age: EPC: M = 63 (11.2) CG: M = 64 (11.1) Gender: IG: 53% M CG: 43% M	Site: Newly diagnosed Lung, gastrointestinal, gynaecological. breast Metastatic: Yes Prognosis (T1): 12 months	Endpoints: Symptom severity, HRQoL, feeling supported, place of death, survival. Tool for HRQoL: McGill QoL Questionnaire	No difference in HRQol, symptom severity. Trend for place of death for EPC group other than acute hospital. Trend for worse overall survival in EPC group (p=0.06) when adjusted for baseline characteristics.
Temel et al.[1] 2010 USA Randomization level: Patients Blinding: No Stratification: No One site	2006-2009	Eligible: 283 Total sample: 151 Total IG: 77 Age: IG: M = 64.98 (9.73) CG: M = 64.87 (9.41) Gender: 58.3% M IG:51% M CG: 45% M	Site: Newly diagnosed Non-small-cell lung cancer Metastatic: Yes Prognosis(T1): less than 1year PS = WHO 0-2	Endpoints: HRQoL, mood, use of health services and end-of-life care, Chemotherapy use, survival depression Tool for HRQoL: FACT-L	Improvement in FACT-L score, p=0.03 and depression p=0.01 Decrease in aggressive EOL care (p=0.05) [In Temel et al, 2010] Decrease in EOL chemotherapy (p=0.05) [In Greer et al.2012] Survival improvement [In Temel et al. 2010 p=0.02] PHQ-9 score (p<0.001) [In Pirl et al, 2012]

Table 2. (Continued)

Study information	Study period	Participants	Cancer type, stage, prognosis and Performance Status (PS)	Data collection and tools used	Outcome
Temel et al. 2017 USA Randomization level: Patients Blinding: No Stratification: Yes One site	2011-2015	Eligible: 480 Total sample: 350 Total IG:175 Age: M = 64.8 (10.88) IG: M = 65.64 (11.26) CG: M = 64.03 (10.46) Gender: 54% M IG: 52% M CG: 56% M	Site: Lung (NSCLC, small-cell, or mesothelioma) or non colorectal GI (pancreatic, oesophageal, gastric, or hepatobiliary) cancer Metastatic: Yes Prognosis(T1): NR PS= WHO 0-2	Endpoints: HRQoL, mood Tool for HRQoL: FACT-G	Improvement of FACT-G at 24 weeks p=0.01 (but not at 12 weeks which was primary endpoint) Improvement depression at 24weeks (p=0.048) Better patient doctor communication (p=0.004)
Vanbutsele et al, 2018 Belgium Randomization level: Patients Blinding: No Stratification: Yes One site	2013-2016	Eligible: 468 Total sample: 186 Total IG: 92 Age: IG: M = 64.5 (57.3-71.0) CG: M = 65.0 (57.0 – 71.0) Gender: IG: 64% M CG: 73% M	Site: Newly diagnosed advanced cancer (multiple types) Stage: Reported as advanced Prognosis(T1): 12months PS= WHO 0-2	Endpoints: HRQoL, wellbeing, mood, illness understanding overall survival Tool for HRQoL: EORTC QLQ C-30 and the McGill Quality of Life Questionnaire	Improvement in EORTC QLQ C-30 (p = 0.03) and in McGill (p = 0.0006) No difference in symptoms, mood, depression, anxiety, patients understanding, survival.
Zimmermann et al. 2014 Canada Randomization level: Patients Blinding: No Stratification: Yes Multiple sites	2006-2011	Eligible: 992 Total sample: 461 Total IG: 228 Age: IG: 61.2 (12.0) CG: 60.2 (11.3) Gender: IG: 59.6% M CG: 53.6% M	Site: Lung (24.1%) Gastrointestinal (32.5%) Genitourinary (11.8%) Breast (18%) Gynaecological (13.6%) (intervention) Metastatic: Yes Prognosis(T1): 6-24 months PS = WHO 0-2	Endpoints: HRQoL, symptom control, satisfaction with care, problems with medical interaction (Cancer Rehabilitation Evaluation System Medical Interaction Subscale CARES-MIS]) Tool for HRQoL: FACIT-SP, QUAL-E	Improvement at 3 months of QUAL-E (p=0.05) and satisfaction with care FAMCARE –P16 (p=0.0003) At 4 months improvement in HRQoL with FACIT-Sp, QUAL-E, symptom severity with ESAS and satisfaction with care with the FAMCARE-p16.

Overall Survival

Improvement in Overall Survival (OS) was seen in two studies (Temel 2010 and Bakitas 2015), with another study showing a trend in OS improvement (Bakitas 2009). One study showed worse survival (Tattersall 2014), which was not statistically significant when correction for imbalances between the two groups was made (adjusted for the oncologist's baseline estimate of likely survival, diagnosis, gender and time since diagnosis). Three studies (Maltoni 2016, Groenvold 2017, and Vanbutsele 2018) showed no difference in survival, whilst in other three studies (McCorkle 2015, Zimmermann 2014 and Temel 2017), no survival results were reported.

In Table 2, study characteristics and results are summarized.

DISCUSSION

In reviewing the results of these ten EPC trials, it is important to acknowledge that whilst overall there is a trend for better outcomes, especially in relation to HRQoL with EPC, the results are by no means uniform between different trials, whilst the magnitude of the benefit is small. There were similar conclusions from a Cochrane meta-analysis undertaken in 2017 of RCTs of EPC in patients with advanced cancer [27], which reviewed data in 7 trials (Bakitas 2009, Bakitas 2015, Maltoni 2016, McCorkle 2015, Tattersall 2014, Temel 2010 and Zimmermann 2014) with a total of 1054 patients. In the Cochrane meta-analysis, EPC improved HRQoL by 0.27 standardized mean deviations over Standard Oncology Care (SOC) and decreased symptom intensity by 0.23 standardized mean deviations; which by conventional criteria is a small difference. Furthermore there was no meta-analytical significant difference for survival or decreased depression. Whilst the investigators reported improved satisfaction with care and illness and prognosis understanding with the EPC intervention, they also noted that only two studies and a single study, respectively, provided evidence regarding the above.

The disparity in outcomes between different trials may be due to the different models of EPC used, the intensity of the intervention, other methodological issues, patients' issues (i.e., selection of appropriate patients for EPC trials), different timing in the disease trajectory of introducing the intervention and finally issues relating to the control arm: the so called Standard Oncology Care arm (SOC). We are going to refer to these issues in more detail below.

Different Models of SPC Used

There are important differences in the "intervention" arm in these trials; in fact, different models of SPC were used in the different studies. There were two predominant patterns of EPC delivery. The traditional model of PC delivery, with the intervention delivered by a PC team led by a specialist PC physician, with face to face consultations predominantly with the PC physician was used in the two Boston Temel studies, the Italian Maltoni study, the Canadian Zimmermann study and the Danish Groenvold study.

In contrast, in the other five studies a predominantly advanced / SPC nurse-led intervention was used (Bakitas 2009, McCorkle 2015, Tattersall 2014, Bakitas 2015 and Vanbutsele 2018). Furthermore, in the two studies by Bakitas et al. also called ENABLE II and III studies, there is an alternative model of delivery of SPC in that the nurse conducted predominantly an educational programme and this instead of being delivered face to face, was delivered via structured telephone consultations. In moving from ENABLE II to ENABLE III study, an initial visit with a PC specialist doctor was also initiated at the beginning, hence making the ENABLE III model move closer to the more traditional model of PC. In the McCorkle 2015 study, the intervention was carried by specialist nurses, physician assistants and social workers by face to face and telephone consultations. In the Australian Tattersall 2014 study and the Belgian Vanbutsele 2018 study, the intervention was initiated by the PC nurse, often via telephone in the Australian study but face to face in the Belgian study, and in both studies, following referral by the PC nurse, patients were also seen by a PC physician.

It is worth noting that with nurse-led EPC intervention trials, in terms of drug prescribing, those would be dependent, on primary physicians or oncologists, carrying out the prescription, and hence posing another barrier to effective symptom management, in contrast to PC physicians-led studies, where this would take place automatically.

Finally, another issue of the intervention arm in these trials, is the training of the staff delivering the intervention. By definition for a SPC intervention, these should be health care professionals, physicians or nurses with specialist PC training. In some studies, the manuscripts describe the staff delivering the care as PC physicians or PC nurses, hence can easily be classified as SPC. However, in some studies, where the intervention is delivered by advanced practice nurses, who may have training in PC, but their training and experience in PC cannot be verified, especially as this is not disclosed in the relevant publications. Of major concern regarding the adequacy of PC training and whether the advanced practice nurses have the required PC skills, is the study by McCorkle 2015 where the publication refers to advanced practice nurse (APN) training the clinic staff, who are other APNs, physician assistants and medical social workers as to the intervention process.

DIFFERENCES IN THE INTENDED INTENSITY OF THE EPC INTERVENTION

There were significant differences in the intensity of the EPC intervention, in relation to the number and frequency of visits and the duration of the intervention. A number of trials had fixed, at least monthly clinic face to face appointments (Temel 2010, Zimmermann 2014, Temel 2017, Maltoni 2016, Vanbutsele 2018) or telephone consultations (Bakitas 2009, Bakitas 2015, Tattersall 2014) until the patients died. In addition to this, some studies had an induction / more intensive initial period (Bakitas 2009 and 2015 with 4-6 weekly visits) prior to the monthly visits.

There were also studies with a fixed, initial period of EPC intervention, with no specified follow up arrangements, but patients would continue PC follow up according to their needs. The McCorkle 2015 study had a ten-week period intervention during which there were five (5) clinic visits and five (5) telephone consultations, whilst the Groenvold 2017 study had a fixed eight week intervention period, with the intensity of visits determined by the PC team as per local practice.

Table 3. Theoretical / intended EPC schedule and actual intensity of EPC delivery

Study	Intervention / Provided by	Theoretical / Intended EPC Schedule	Actual Intensity / Compliance
Bakitas et al. 2009	Advanced Practice Nurse (APN) (initial sessions and telephone consultations) PC physician and nurse appointments	Initial 4 sessions, then at least monthly until death. Telephone consultations at least monthly Monthly group shared medical appointments	113/161 completed >/ 1follow up assessment
Bakitas et al. 2015	PC physician and APN nurse.	After initial 6 weeks period, 1 PC physician visit then weekly APN telephone consults x6 monthly telephone calls	*88% completed > 3 sessions
Groenvold et al. 2017	PC team	8wk period, number of sessions determined by patients' need.	Only 74/145 (51%) had 2 or more face-to-face visits. 27/145 (18.6%) had > 5 telephone calls
Maltoni et al. 2016	PC Team with specialist physicians / nurses. PC physicians led.	Every 2-4 week until death.	Mean 5.1 (SD = 1.6) sessions up to 12 weeks Mean 8.9 (SD = 4.2) consultations up to the end of trial
McCorkle et al. 2015	Advanced Practice Nurse (APN)	10 week intervention APN coordinated care 5 clinic visits 5 telephone calls	Lost to follow up 30/66 in EPC arm and 24/80 in SOC arm. No information on actual visits per patient
Tattersall et al. 2014	PC nurse	First visit: face to face PC nurse then monthly telephone consultations	Several patients not ready for PC *5/60 >3 telephone contacts *3/60: 2-3 contacts *28/60: 1 contact *51/60 saw PC physician
Temel et al. 2010	PC team (board certified PC physicians and APN nurses)	Initial session and then at least monthly until death	Average 4visits
Temel et al. 2017	PC Team with specialist physicians / nurses	At least monthly clinic visits.	Average visits 6.54 by 24 weeks 56% had >/ 7 visits 24% had 5-6 visits 11% had 3-4 visits
Vanbutsele et al. 2018	PC nurses led. Access to PC physicians if required.	Initial session with PC nurse, dietician and psychologist. Then, follow-up as required.	71% (61 patients) compliance by 12 weeks. 89% (82 patients) > 1 consultation until 18 weeks 60% (50 patients) >/ 3 consultations by 24 weeks. 11% (10 patients) had no consultation. 27% (25 patients) > 1 consultation with PC physician by 12 weeks and 35% by 24 weeks.
Zimmermann et al. 2014	PC Team with specialist physicians and nurses / Led by PC physicians	At least monthly	35% had > 5 consultations 30% had 4 consultations

ACTUAL INTENSITY/COMPLIANCE WITH EPC INTERVENTION

There are some very interesting observations regarding the actual use / compliance with EPC intervention (Table 3). In three studies there are significant concerns regarding low use / compliance with the EPC intervention. In the Tattersall 2014 study, several patients commented that they were not ready for PC, with only 5/60 having more than 3 telephone contacts, 3/60 having 2-3 and 28/60 having only 1 telephone contact. In the McCorkle 2015 study there was a large number of patients lost to follow up, 30/66 in EPC arm and 24/80 in SOC arm, with no information on actual visits per patient provided in the manuscript. Finally in the Groenvold 2017 study, only 74/145 of the patients in the EPC arm, were seen more than once by the SPC teams. It is very interesting to note that these are the only three studies, where there was no improvement in HRQoL at any timepoint, except for the Bakitas 2015 study, which by design tested early versus late SPC.

DIFFERENT POPULATIONS OF CANCER PATIENTS

There were different cancer types allowed to participate in these ten studies. Only two studies concentrated on a single specific cancer type: lung cancer (Temel 2010), pancreatic cancer (Maltoni 2016). One study looked at lung and non-colorectal gastro-intestinal (GI) cancer (Temel 2017) and another study looked at lung, gynaecological, head and neck and gastrointestinal cancer (McCorkle 2015). The other six studies allowed all different cancer types.

As already mentioned in the findings section, the Temel 2017 study highlights a disparity in outcomes between the lung cancer and the non-colorectal GI cancer patients. It is therefore important to consider that patients with different cancer diagnoses, may have different symptom burden, and there may be differences in the benefit derived from EPC. Future EPC trials would need to be powered enough to allow to measure and account for the differences in symptoms and HRQoL between different cancer types, plus investigate how these individual symptoms are effectively palliated either by EPC or by other means.

METHODOLOGICAL ISSUES ABOUT TRIALS OF EPC

Studies of EPC come with several methodological challenges. A review of trials of EPC for patients with serious illnesses [28] has highlighted the fact that patients are usually referred or recruited by oncologists, rather than screened for eligibility. Therefore, selection bias may take place [27], given that patients are informed about PC, so it is likely that patients more open to PC participate in some of these trials. We have identified four studies (Bakitas et al., 2009; Temel et al., 2010; Vanbutsele et al., 2018; Zimmermann et al., 2014) with potential selection bias due to lack of allocation concealment. In Temel et al. (2017) allocation was concealed until after randomisation while Zimmermann et al. (2014) discuss the bias from randomizing clusters before consenting patients.

Most of the trials present high risk of performance bias because of lack of blinding procedures in terms of outcome assessment and participants (Bakitas et al., 2009; Groenvold et al., 2017; Maltoni et al., 2016; McCorkle et al., 2015; Tattersall et al., 2014; Temel et al., 2010; Temel et al., 2017; Vanbutsele et al., 2018). Only Zimmermann et al. (2014) cluster trial reported adequate blinding procedures. It is also of note that only Bakitas et al. (2015) reported blinding investigators. However, we agree with Haun et al. (2017) approach that blinding of investigators in the context of PC is most of the times not feasible. This is more important when considering that the ecological validity in EPC, like with any other complex intervention, is challenging [29].

There were also differences in randomisation and stratification factors used. Cluster randomisation was used in the Zimmermann 2014 and McCorkle 2015 studies. In the Zimmermann 2014 study there were 24 medical oncology clinics to be cluster randomized. In the McCorkle 2015 study the small number of clinics, only four disease-specific multidisciplinary clinics, did not allow for stratification per tumour type, potentially introducing bias, as there may be differences in PC needs and response to EPC for different cancer types. To avoid inter-correlations Bell and McKenzie [30] suggest using more than 4 sites.

Attrition is another serious methodological consideration. We have discussed this previously in a meta-analysis of cancer SPC trials [31] where we found attrition to be between 29.1%-46.6%. In most recent studies attrition ranged from 25.6% in the control group to 22.1% in the intervention group (Groenvold et al., 2017). In Vanbutsele et al. (2018) 29.3%, 28.9% and 28.1% were lost to follow-up at 12, 18 and 24 weeks respectively (excluding at each time-point those who were lost to death). Attrition is an important indicator of the acceptability of the intervention and compromises the robustness of results, so investigators need to consider minimizing the impact of attrition and reporting this adequately. Attrition can be serious when the intervention group shows higher rates than the control (Zimmermann et al., 2014) or when high rates are reported in both groups (Tattersall et al., 2014).

Instruments used for measuring primary and secondary end points need to be carefully considered. A large number of endpoints increases the risk of Type I error. It is expected that EPC trials will increasingly become published and therefore investigators will be informed by previous studies on which endpoints to prioritize. For example, in Vanbutsele et al. (2018) the large number of endpoints was recognized as a risk for Type I error, but these exploratory findings can inform future trials. The authors have also used two different tools to measure HRQoL because one provided the opportunity to capture additional domains of HRQoL like spiritual aspects.

Reporting in EPC trials' evaluations is important. An important consideration when reporting is to properly describe the intervention and control procedures and avoid referring to the latter as 'usual care' [31]. Moreover, other sources of bias were identified like significant baseline differences between intervention and control group (McCorkle et al., 2015), lack of power to detect cancer sub-type differences in HRQoL (Temel et al., 2017), dilution of intervention effect (Temel et al., 2017) and the fact that several trials were conducted in a single Centre (please see Table 2) limiting the generalizability of study findings. Overall, the certainty in the EPC trial evidence is compromised from high risk of bias in various studies and findings need to be interpreted with these biases in mind.

TIMING AND DEFINITION OF EPC

The concept of EPC originated with the Phase II, single arm, Temel [32] study from Boston for patients with advanced lung cancer where PC input was offered to patients at (or very close to) the time of diagnosis of metastatic disease.

The definition/timing of intervention of EPC at the time of diagnosis of advanced cancer has been adopted in most studies included in this review (Bakitas 2009, Temel 2010, Bakitas 2015, Tattersall 2014, McCorkle 2015, Temel 2017, Maltoni 2016, Vanbutsele 2018), with the exception of the Canadian and Danish trials. The time-intervals from diagnosis of advanced cancer to patient entry to the EPC trials has been defined as within 30-60 days (Bakitas 2015), within 8 weeks (Temel 2010; Temel 2017), within 12 weeks (Vanbutsele 2018) and finally within 100 days (McCorkle 2015).

Of great interest in terms of the timing of the EPC intervention are the findings of the ENABLE III study, where this was investigated within the two randomisation arms in order to determine the best timing to offer SPC after cancer diagnosis. In this study, the randomisation was into an immediate SPC group versus a delayed by 3 months SPC group, from the time of diagnosis. Of note that the earlier referral group had a statistically significant survival advantage from 11.8 months to 18.3 months (HR=0.72, p=0.003), however no statistically significant difference in patient reported outcomes was documented, which was in fact the aim of this study.

In terms of the point in the disease trajectory of the EPC intervention, information on prognosis as specified by the individual studies is useful: with five studies specifying a prognosis of about 1 year, two studies specified 6-24 months, one study > 2months, and two studies did not consider prognosis as an eligibility criterion.

The definition of EPC however is not absolute. Other definitions beyond the provision of SPC close to the diagnosis of metastatic, incurable cancer exist. For instance, EPC has been defined as being seen by a PC specialist greater than 3 months before death [33], or at the time of chemotherapy resistance (platinum resistance in ovarian cancer) [34].

Regarding the timing of SPC referral, it may be appropriate to consider other issues including the underlying cancer diagnosis, associated prognosis and availability/impact of effective systemic therapy, which may be interlinked with each other, which we are going to discuss in the following paragraphs.

IMPACT OF UNDERLYING DIAGNOSIS AND AVAILABILITY OF EFFECTIVE SYSTEMIC THERAPIES IN OUTCOMES OF EPC TRIALS

There comes an interesting observation from the Temel 2017 trial, where there is an imbalance in the lung cancer cohort between the rate of the Epidermal Growth Factor Receptor (EGFR) mutation positive patients in the SOC group (10 out of 96 patients) versus in the intervention, EPC group (19 out of 95 patients). The benefit of EGFR Tyrosine Kinase Inhibitors (TKI's) is well documented in patients with EGFR mutations, with response rates in most trials more than 70%, whilst a positive impact on HRQoL has also been established[35]. This may have contributed to the improvement seen in the HRQoL in the lung cancer patients in the EPC group. However, the wider issue, is that in the presence of effective systemic therapy, palliation of patients' symptoms and improvement in HRQoL is likely to come first from systemic therapy rather than EPC. Hence, we believe that patients with untreated activating EGFR mutations are not good candidates for EPC trials. Equally patients with other known oncogenic drivers and effective targeted therapy, or patients with endocrine responsive tumours, should not be included in EPC trials or for the practice of EPC.

How Standard/Appropriate Is the Standard Oncology Arm in EPC Trials?

In considering outcomes of EPC trials, we have focused quite a lot on the EPC intervention and how EPC can produce improvements in HRQoL, but we have not given enough attention to the comparator arm, which is Standard Oncology Care (SOC), and which is by no means standard. SOC should include both disease directed therapy and also best supportive care. A systematic review of Best Supportive Care (BSC) trials in 2015 showed that only one third of the studies offered a detailed description of BSC, whilst none documented evidence-based symptom management [36]. Finally, in another recent review regarding implementation of BSC in clinical trials with cancer patients, only 55 out of 73 studies provided some definition of SOC, whilst only two studies provided SOC that incorporated routine physical, psychological and social assessments including referral to SOC specialists [37].

This however goes beyond the definition of supportive care in the control arm, but it relates to both the philosophy and the actual content of SOC. The American Society of Clinical Oncology in a publication "Toward Individualized Care for Patients With Advanced Cancer" suggests that "consideration of disease-directed therapy, symptom management, and attention to quality of life are important aspects of quality cancer care" [9]. There are concerns regarding the imbalance of the care provided to patients, focusing predominantly on disease directed therapy, and neglecting to address patients' symptoms, consequences of disease and its treatment and HRQoL issues [38]. Furthermore, there are several studies, which show that oncologists often lack the necessary skills and fail to manage adequately even the simplest of the physical symptoms, that of pain even in the US [39, 40]. It is likely that we do even less well with psychological symptoms, spiritual and existential concerns of patients, with indirect evidence for this from a survey of Australian oncologists [41], where 92% of oncologists felt confident in the management of physical symptoms, compared to only 61.7% for psychological symptoms and 53.9% for existential distress. Equally in the European Society of Medical Oncology (ESMO) survey, respondents were involved more commonly in treating physical symptoms (pain 93%, fatigue 84%, nausea/emesis 84%), than in managing psychological symptoms such as depression/anxiety (65%) and existential distress (29%) [42].

Hence, it may be argued that the reason for the benefit seen with EPC, is that it provides for deficiencies in SOC, i.e., management of physical, psychological, social and spiritual problems of patients with advanced cancer. Furthermore, it is likely that deficiencies in management of these symptoms relate to inadequate PC training by oncologists [38]. Surveys of oncologists suggest the need for PC skills training; in the ESMO survey [42], 42% of respondents felt that they had not received adequate training in PC during their training and a similar proportion of 42% of Canadian oncologists recognize their limitations in terms of providing PC [43].

Ultimately with more effective PC training and oncologists becoming proficient to provide basic PC, there should be less difference in outcomes between the SOC arm and the EPC arm. This should inform the future study design of EPC trials.

GENERIZABILITY OF EPC TRIALS

There are significant limitations as to the generalizability of the findings from these studies. Firstly, these studies were done in Western, developed countries, most in the US (5) and one each in Canada, Australia, Italy, Belgium and Denmark, lacking diversity with respect to race and ethnic group. Furthermore, with the exception of the Italian and Danish studies, which were truly multi-centre trials, the rest were single centre trials (Boston, Toronto, Sydney, Yale New Haven, Ghent) and the ENABLE trials were undertaken in two centres in New Hampshire and Vermont. Finally, all these studies were undertaken in centres with tradition in the provision of PC, and in resource rich environments.

Hence, we lack data from non- western or developing countries, from multi-centre trials, and non -Caucasian patients, as well as in settings where PC services are not well developed.

CONCLUSIONS/SUGGESTIONS FOR FUTURE TRIALS

The findings of this review should not stop the oncology and PC community from doing EPC studies, but instead should encourage trials especially in different health care settings, and in different countries outside the USA / Canada, Western Europe and Australia.

An adequate follow-up period is required in EPC evaluations so that intervention effects can be detected. For example, Groenvold et al. (2017) argue that an 8-week period might not have been sufficient to detect the EPC effect. Whilst in Bakitas 2009, Temel et al. 2010, Maltoni et al. 2016 and Vanbutsele et al. 2018, a benefit was seen at 12 weeks, studies by Temel and colleagues in 2017 failed to detect an effect at 12 weeks but found one in 24 weeks, and Zimmermann et al. 2014 showed an improvement in HRQoL not at 3 but at 4 months. Therefore, the timing necessary for follow-up needs to be considered carefully.

Careful attention needs to be given to the patient eligibility criteria to select patients that are more likely to benefit from an EPC intervention. Untreated patients with endocrine responsive tumours or with known oncogenic drivers and where there is available systemic endocrine or targeted therapy, or even patients where first line therapy may be associated with high response rates (e.g., first line therapy of breast and bowel cancer) and whose symptoms are likely to be palliated with systemic therapy, should be excluded from entering EPC trials, at least in their current form, recruiting at the time of diagnosis of advanced disease.

Moreover, the "dose" and intensity of the EPC intervention needs to be carefully considered, with evidence from this review suggesting that intensity (at least monthly consultations with SPC team) matters. The intensity of intervention needs also to be clearly reported in future studies and as to what the planned and what the actual adherence to this was. Temel (2017) suggest identifying a balance between strictly manualizing and allowing physicians to provide personalized care by addressing patients' concerns. We recommend to researchers, policy makers and Journal Editors to:

a) Publish a detailed protocol with information on how the EPC was developed, what it entailed, the frequency of visits and theoretical assumptions, including any guidelines that may have been used or adapted.
b) The protocol also needs to explain with detail what the 'usual care' entails and comment on skills of Oncologist that provide basic PC to the control group.
c) Publish the adherence to the protocol parameters in the trial (e.g., actual delivery / intensity of SPC compared to the protocol)

There should be further distinction as to the aims and expected outcomes for future EPC trials according to the health care settings and quality of SOC as well as availability of SPC services. In countries where available SPC services are scarce, and where there may be concerns about the SOC, EPC trials should be undertaken to show the benefit of EPC to help shape local policy and influence allocation of health care resources towards PC services. These studies should help to make the case for more PC training for oncologists, with the aim to provide more effective symptom control and supportive and basic PC to our patients.

In countries where PC services are reaching integration and advancements have been made in the SOC, with oncologists receiving more PC training and developing an expertise in PC (e.g., Boston USA, Canada, UK / Europe, Australia), the natural progression of EPC trials in the future, would be to enrich these trials with the patients that DO need to be seen by SPC teams; those are likely to be patients with difficult to control / refractory symptoms, with poor systemic therapy options and those where there is more of a burden in psychological/ existential issues, where there would be a need for input from more health care professionals.

Areas for further research should include investigating further differences in symptom burden for different cancer types, considering which are the patients more likely to benefit from EPC, what the optimal EPC intervention and intensity of this intervention should be, as well as investigating the optimal timing of the integration of EPC into oncology care. Furthermore, future trials should provide guidance as to what standard oncology care should entail, and should strive to capture symptom management especially in the non-EPC arm, with the aim to identify deficiencies in the care we currently provide to our patients.

REFERENCES

[1] WHO 1990 *Cancer pain relief and Palliative Care*. Geneva, WHO: 11 technical report series: 801.
[2] Quill TE, Abernethy AP. Generalist plus Specialist Palliative Care — Creating a More Sustainable Model. *N Engl J Med* 2013; 368:1173-1175.
[3] Lamont EB, Christakis NA. Physician factors in the timing of cancer patient referral to hospice palliative care. *Cancer* 2002; 94: 2733–37.
[4] Osta BE, Palmer JL, Paraskevopoulos T, et al. Interval between first palliative care consult and death in patients diagnosed with advanced cancer at a comprehensive cancer center. *J Palliat Med* 2008; 11: 51–57.

[5] Reville B, Miller MN, Toner RW, et al. End-of-life care for hospitalized patients with lung cancer: utilization of a palliative care service. *J Palliat Med* 2010; 13:1261-6.

[6] Earle CC, Landrum MB, Souza JM, Neville BA, Weeks JC, Ayanian JZ. Aggressiveness of cancer care near the end of life: is it a quality-of-care issue? *J Clin Oncol* 2008; 26:3860-6.

[7] Neuss MN, Jacobson JO, Earle C, et al: Evaluating end of life care: The Quality Oncology Practice Initiative (QOPI) experience. *J Clin Oncol* 20:486s, 2006. (suppl; abstr 8573).

[8] Emanuel EJ, Young-Xu Y, Levinsky NG, et al: Chemotherapy use among Medicare beneficiaries at the end of life. *Ann Intern Med* 138:639-643, 2003.

[9] Peppercorn JM, Smith TJ, Helft PR et al. American society of clinical oncology statement: toward individualized care for patients with advanced cancer. *J Clin Oncol.* 2011; 29(6):755-60.

[10] Temel JS, Greer JA, Muzikansky A, et al: Early palliative care for patients with metastatic non-small-cell lung cancer. *N Engl J Med* 2010; 363:733-742.

[11] Bakitas M, Lyons KD, Hegel MT, et al: Effects of a palliative care intervention on clinical outcomes in patients with advanced cancer: The Project ENABLE II randomized controlled trial. *JAMA* 2009; 302:741-749.

[12] Smith TJ, Temin S, Alesi ER et al. American Society of Clinical Oncology Provisional Clinical Opinion: The integration of Palliative Care into Standard Oncology Care. *J Clin Oncol.* 2012; 10; 30(8):880-7.

[13] Ferrell BR, Temel JS, Temin S et al. Integration of Palliative Care Into Standard Oncology Care: American Society of Clinical Oncology Clinical Practice Guideline Update. *J Clin Oncol* 2017; 35 (1):96-112.

[14] Richardson WS, Wilson MC, Nishikawa J, Hayward RS. The well-built clinical question: a key to evidence-based decisions. *ACP J Club*. 1995 Nov–Dec; 123(3): A12–3.

[15] McGowan, J., Sampson, M., Salzwedel, D.M., et al. PRESS peer review of electronic search strategies: 2015 guideline statement. *Journal of clinical epidemiology* 2016; 75, 40-46.

[16] Greer JA, Pirl WF, Jackson VA et al. Effect of Early Palliative Care on Chemotherapy Use and End-of-Life Care in Patients with Metastatic Non–Small-Cell Lung Cancer. *J Clin Oncol* 2011; 30: 394-400.

[17] Pirl WF, Greer JA, Traeger L et al.Depression and Survival in Metastatic Non–Small-Cell Lung Cancer: Effects of Early Palliative Care *J Clin Oncol* 2012; 30:1310-1315.

[18] Bakitas MA, Tosteson TD, Li Z et al. Early Versus Delayed Initiation of Concurrent Palliative Oncology Care: Patient Outcomes in the ENABLE III Randomized Controlled Trial. *J Clin Oncol* 2015; 33:1438-1445.

[19] Tattersall MHN, Martin A, Devine R. et al. Early Contact with Palliative Care Services: A randomized trial in patients with newly detected incurable metastatic cancer. *J Palliat Care Med* 4: 170. doi:10.4172/2165-7386.1000170.

[20] McCorkle R, Jeon S, Ercolano E. et al. An Advanced Practice Nurse Coordinated Multidisciplinary Intervention for Patients with Late-Stage Cancer: A Cluster Randomized Trial. *J Pall Med* 2015; 18 (11): 962-969.

[21] Vanbutsele G, Pardon K, Van Bell S. et al. Effect of early and systematic integration of palliative care in patients with advanced cancer: a randomised controlled trial. *Lancet Oncol* 2018; 19: 394-404.

[22] Zimmermann C, Swami N, Krzyzanowska M, et al: Early palliative care for patients with advanced cancer: A cluster-randomised controlled trial. *Lancet* 383:1721-1730, 2014 1.

[23] Maltoni M, Scarpi E, Dall'Agata M et al. Systematic versus on-demand early palliative care: results from a multicentre, randomised clinical trial. *E J Cancer* 2016; 65: 61-68.

[24] Temel JS, Greer JA, El-Jawahri A, et al: Effects of early integrated palliative care in patients with lung and gastrointestinal cancer: A randomized clinical trial. *J Clin Oncol* 2017; 35 (8): 834-841.

[25] Groenvold M, Petersen MA, Damkier A et al. Randomised clinical trial of early specialist palliative care plus standard care versus standard care alone in patients with advanced cancer: The Danish Palliative Care Trial. *Palliative Medicine* 2017; 31(9): 814–824.

[26] Temel JS, Greer JA, Admane S, et al. Longitudinal perceptions of prognosis and goals of therapy in patients with metastatic non-small cell lung cancer: results of a randomized study of early palliative care. *J Clin Oncol* 2011; 29: 2319-26.

[27] Haun MW, Estel S, Rücker G, Friederich HC, Villalobos M, Thomas M, Hartmann M. Early palliative care for adults with advanced cancer. *Cochrane Database of Systematic Reviews* 2017, Issue 6. Art. No.: CD011129. DOI: 10.1002/14651858.CD011129.pub2.

[28] Davis MP, Temel JS, Balboni T, Glare P. A review of the trials which examine early integration of outpatient and home palliative care for patients with serious illnesses. *Ann Palliat Med* 2015;4(3):99-121.

[29] Movsisyan A, Melendez-Torres GJ, Montgomery P. Outcomes in systematic reviews of complex interventions never reached "high" GRADE ratings when compared with those of simple interventions. *Journal of Clinical Epidemiology* 2016;78:22–33.

[30] Bell, ML and McKenzie, JE, 2013. Designing psycho-oncology randomized trials and cluster randomized trials: variance components and intra-cluster correlation of commonly used psychosocial measures. *Psycho-Oncology*, 22(8), pp.1738-1747.

[31] Kassianos, AP, Ioannou, M, Koutsantoni, M, and Charalambous, H. 2018. The impact of specialized palliative care on cancer patients' health-related quality of life: a systematic review and meta-analysis. *Supportive Care in Cancer*, 26(1), pp.61-79.

[32] Temel JS, Jackson VA, Billings JA, et al. Phase II Study: Integrated Palliative Care in Newly Diagnosed Advanced Non–Small-Cell Lung Cancer Patients. *J Clin Oncol* 2007; 25:2377-2382.

[33] Amano K, Morita T, Tatara R, et al. Association between early palliative care referrals, inpatient hospice utilization, and aggressiveness of care at the end of life. *J Palliat Med* 2015;18:270-3.

[34] Lowery WJ, Lowery AW, Barnett JC, et al. Cost effectiveness of early palliative care intervention in recurrent platinum-resistant ovarian cancer. *Gynecol Oncol* 2013;130:426-30.

[35] Thongprasert S, Duffield E, Saijo N, et al. Health-Related Quality-of-Life in a Randomized Phase III First-Line Study of Gefitinib Versus Carboplatin/Paclitaxel in Clinically Selected Patients from Asia with Advanced NSCLC (IPASS). *Journal of thoracic oncology* 2011; 6(11):1872-80.

[36] Nipp RD, Currow DC, Cherny NI, et al. Best supportive care in clinical trials: review of the inconsistency in control arm design. *British Journal of Cancer* 2015; 113: 6-11.
[37] Lee RT, Ramchandran K, Sanft T, et al. Implementation of supportive care and best supportive care interventions in clinical trials enrolling patients with cancer. *Annals of Oncology* 2015; 26: 1838-1845.
[38] Charalambous H, Silbermann M. Clinically based palliative care training is needed urgently for all oncologists. *J. Clin. Oncol.* 2012; 30 (32):4042-3.
[39] Fisch MJ, Lee JW, Weiss M, et al: Prospective, observational study of pain and analgesic prescribing in medical oncology outpatients with breast, colorectal, lung, or prostate cancer. *J Clin Oncol* 2012; 30:1980-1988.
[40] Breuer B, Fleishman SB, Cruciani RA, et al. Medical oncologists' attitudes and practice in cancer pain management: A national survey. *J Clin Oncol* 2011; 29:4769–4775.
[41] Ward AM, Agar M, Koczwara B. Collaborating or co-existing: a survey of attitudes of medical oncologists toward specialist palliative care. *Palliat Med.* 2009; 23(8):698-707.
[42] Cherny NI, Catane R; European Society of Medical Oncology Taskforce on Palliative and Supportive Care. Attitudes of medical oncologists toward palliative care for patients with advanced and incurable cancer: report on a survey by the European Society of Medical Oncology Taskforce on Palliative and Supportive Care. *Cancer* 2003; 98(11):2502-10.
[43] Wentlandt K, Krzyzanowska MK, Swami N, et al. Referral Practices of Oncologists to Specialized Palliative *Care. J Clin Oncol* 2012; 10.1200/JCO.2012.44.0248.

BIOGRAPHICAL SKETCHES

Dr. Haris Charalambous

Dr. Haris Charalambous qualified from the Medical School of the University of Southampton in the UK, and subsequently trained in Internal Medicine and Clinical Oncology obtaining the Membership of the Royal College of Physicians and the Fellowship of the Royal College of Radiologists in the UK. He worked as a consultant clinical oncologist both in the UK (Poole and Newcastle upon Tyne hospitals) and currently working in Cyprus. He has a special interest in the treatment of Thoracic and Urological Cancers, and in the integration of Palliative Care concurrent with standard Oncology care for patients with advanced cancer. He is a member of the EORTC Lung Cancer group. He has received research grants from the Royal College of Radiologists in the UK, Schering Plough, Sanofi and MSD. Currently he is the principal investigator in a phase II maintenance trial of Pembrolizumab in patients who have not progressed after first line chemotherapy for metastatic Non-Small Cell Lung Cancer. He authored over 25 peer reviewed articles and 4 book chapters.

Dr. Angelos P. Kassianos

Dr. Angelos P. Kassianos received his PhD in Health Psychology from the University of Surrey in the UK. He then worked as a researcher in Imperial College London, the University of Cambridge, the University of Cyprus and the University College London. His research is related to cancer prevention, early diagnosis and palliative care. In 2015, he received a Fulbright Visiting Research Scholarship to work for four months at Harvard Medical School, Dana Farber Cancer Institute on patients' priotiries in palliative care. He also teaches in research methods, health psychology and psychometrics. Currently, he is funded by the UK Department of Health's Policy Research Unit in Cancer Prevention, Screening and Early Diagnosis. He authored over 20 peer reviewed articles and 7 book chapters.

In: Palliative Care
Editor: Michael Silbermann

ISBN: 978-1-53616-199-1
© 2019 Nova Science Publishers, Inc.

Chapter 16

THE ROLE AND IMPORTANCE OF RESEARCH IN PROMOTING PHARMACOLOGICAL MANAGEMENT OF CANCER RELATED PAIN

Elon Eisenberg[*], MD

Pain Research Unit, Institute of Pain Medicine, Rambam Health Care Campus, Haifa, Israel, and B. Rappaport Faculty of Medicine, Technion - Israel Institute of Technology, Haifa, Israel

ABSTRACT

Approximately two-thirds of patients with advanced cancer suffer moderate to severe pain caused by either the cancer itself or cancer treatment. Additionally, a considerable number of cancer survivors continue to suffer constant pain despite being cancer-free. Since pharmacotherapy is a cornerstone in the treatment of cancer related pain, further research on efficacy and safety of pharmacological analgesic-interventions is clearly indicated. This chapter provides the reader with essential information on research on cancer pain management. The first part of the chapter is more theoretical, reviewing the different types of published clinical studies, emphasizing the quality of evidence they produced. The second part present examples of studies and evidence for efficacy of existing treatments for cancer-related pain such as opioids, NSAIDs and cannabinoids, and of potentially newly introduced analgesic interventions.

Keywords: opioids, cannabinoids, World Health Organization, bone pain, chemotherapy, neuropathy

---

[*] Corresponding Author's E-mail: e_eisenberg@rambam.health.gov.il.; Fax: +972 4 7773505.

INTRODUCTION

Studies spanning the past three decades indicate that approximately two-thirds of patients with advanced cancer suffer moderate to severe pain. In the vast majority of these patients, pain is caused by the cancer either through direct invasion of surrounding tissues and nerves, or through the metastatic spread of the tumor to remote sites, commonly the bones.

Another major cause of pain in many patients is the cancer treatment itself. There is a host of "syndromes" of treatment-induced pain. Perhaps most common is the syndrome of chemotherapy-induced painful neuropathy, which is characterized by burning, shooting, or numb pain in a stocking and glove distribution. Another type of treatment-induced pain is postoperative pain, mostly caused by nerve injuries during surgery. A typical example is chronic pain after breast surgery known as post-mastectomy pain syndrome, but other types of surgery can also cause similar painful conditions. Hormonal therapies may cause joint pain; and radiation therapy, especially if co-administered with chemotherapy, may cause severe painful inflammation in the mouth, urinary bladder, and rectum, depending on the irradiated body region.

Importantly, due to advances in cancer therapy, many patients recover from their cancer. Unfortunately, a considerable number of these cancer free individuals have a constant reminder of their cured cancer in the form of chronic pain, which may last for months and even years.

This chapter is aimed to provide the reader with essential information on research in promoting cancer pain management. The first part of the chapter is more theoretical, reviewing the different types of published clinical studies with an emphasis on the quality of evidence presented. In the second part, examples of studies and evidence for efficacy of existing and potentially new analgesic treatments for cancer-related pain are presented.

QUALITY OF EVIDENCE

The practice of evidence based medicine (EBM) was defined by Sackett DL et al. (1996), in their well-cited BMJ paper as: "integrating individual clinical expertise with the best available external clinical evidence from systematic research, while taking into account patients' predicaments, rights, and preferences". Over the subsequent two decades, the perception of EBM has changed considerably. Nowadays it is defined as "an approach to medical practice intended to optimize decision-making by emphasizing the use of evidence from well-designed and well-conducted research. Although all medicine based on science has some degree of empirical support, EBM goes further, classifying evidence by its strength and requiring that only the strongest types can yield strong recommendations" (Accad, 2018). From a more practical standpoint, before recommending analgesic treatments to patients, caregivers should always ask - how effective is this treatment? Effectiveness refers to efficacy and to safely of any given therapeutic intervention. In other words, before prescribing an opioid to a patient with severe cancer related pain, the questions are do we have evidence for the efficacy and safety of this intervention, and what is the quality of the evidence?

A key issue for understanding quality of evidence is familiarity with the different types of studies and how they are conducted, because some studies produce highly reliable results, while others are far less trustworthy.

In some areas of medicine, no validated clinical trials have been conducted. In such cases clinical decisions are often made based on what is termed "expert opinion". This means that a group of experts in the discussed-field have made a recommendation about a specific intervention by consensus, based on their experience but without any supporting evidence drawn from clinical studies. Although "expert opinion" sounds convincing, it clearly represents the lowest level of scientific evidence.

The next level of evidence originates form case reports or case series. This is typically a description of one or a small number of patients to whom a treatment was administered, and the outcome reported.

Higher levels of evidence emerge from retrospective studies. Since prospective studies are time consuming and expensive, whenever there is a need to fill a gap in knowledge relatively quickly, this type of research is used. In such studies, medical records of patients - who received a certain treatment for a given medical condition - are studied retrospectively, and attempts are made to draw conclusions about the treatment effectiveness. The problem with these type of studies is that often physician notes vary considerably, thus enabling only a rough estimation of effectiveness. The scientific value of such studies remains limited at best.

Preferred studies are prospective. The simplest category of prospective studies are "open labeled" trials in which, typically, a small number of patients receive a well-defined treatment and are followed prospectively in a structured manner. These studies aim primarily to "prove a concept", rather than to provide strong evidence for effectiveness.

The following categories of prospective studies provide the best scientific evidence for effectiveness of treatments and should be regarded as complementary to each other. One group is termed "randomized controlled trials", and the other "large scale prospective studies" or "registries". Each approach has advantages and disadvantages. Typically the advantages of one are the disadvantages of the other.

Randomized controlled trials (or RCTs) aim to compare one treatment to another or to a placebo in a select group of patients. A strong evidence that treatment "A" is better than treatment "B" for a specific condition is typically based on one or more RCTs. While well conducted RCTs lead to high quality evidence, they also encounter some problems: (1) Cost – these studies are expensive; (2) The enrolled patients are selected to be as homogenous as possible. Hence, only patients with select characteristics enter such studies, generally only 10% of the patients with a given condition. The applicability of RCT results for the entire population of patients with the studied condition is therefore questionable; and (3) RCTs focus only on very specific questions and are not designed to address multiple aspects of a complexed medical condition.

In some areas of medicine, multiple RCTs have been conducted yielding consistent results. In other fields, results from different RCTs have not been congruent, and led to confusion in terms of treatments efficacy. Meta-analyses are supposed to solve the confusion by extracting the raw data from *all* relevant studies and re-calculating the effect of any given treatment.

Another category of prospective studies includes large-scale, open-labeled, prospective studies, sometimes termed registries. Registries are meant to overcome some of the RCTs' related problems. In contrast to RCTs, these generally lack exclusion criteria and all patients with a given medical condition (e.g., breast cancer) or all patients who receive a treatment (e.g., radiation therapy) enter the registry and are followed in the most structured way possible for extended time periods (typically months or even years). Registries aim to provide "real life" conclusions about predictors, effectiveness and outcomes of a condition or a treatment. Such studies are required in areas where large gaps in knowledge exist.

STRENGTH OF EVIDENCE

A second important issue in the context of guideline consistency is how quality of evidence and grade strength of recommendations are rated. The Grading of Recommendations Assessment, Development and Evaluation (GRADE) approach was developed to provide a system for rating quality of evidence and strength of recommendations that is explicit, comprehensive, transparent, and pragmatic (Guyatt et al., 2008). The GRADE system defines the following four levels of evidence quality:

High quality - Further research is very unlikely to change our confidence in the estimate of effect, as for example, when multiple high quality RCTs provide consistent and convincing results.

Moderate quality - Further research is likely to have an important impact on our confidence in the estimate of effect and may change the estimate. For example, when two high quality RCTs provided inconsistent or even conflicting results.

Low quality - Further research is very likely to have an important impact on our confidence in the estimate of effect and is likely to change the estimate. For example, when only one small scale RCT is available that has reported biases.

Very low quality - Any estimate of effect is very uncertain. For example, when only one case suggests an effect may exist.

STUDIES AND QUALITY OF EVIDENCE OF EFFECTIVENESS OF SPECIFIC THERAPEUTIC INTERVENTIONS FOR CANCER PAIN MANAGEMENT

Oral Opioids for Moderate to Severe Pain

Opioids are a cornerstone in the treatment of moderate to severe cancer pain, and have been used for this indication for more than three decades, since the publication of the WHO cancer pain guidelines (WHO, 1986). Nonetheless, a legitimate question is do we truly have scientific evidence to support continuously using opioids for moderate to severe cancer pain, and are they of high quality?

Oral morphine is commonly regarded as the opioid analgesic of choice for managing moderate to severe cancer related pain. This is for a good reason, since dozens of RCTs showed evidence for its efficacy in this patient population. A recent Cochrane review (Wiffen, 2017) consisting of 62 studies and 4241 participants who received oral morphine, showed that a standard of 'mild pain intensity at most' was achieved in the vast majority of patients. Seventeen of the studies found that 'no worse than mild pain' was achieved by 96% of 377 participants. Although the quality of the evidence was reported to be generally poor (studies were old, often small, and mainly reported equivalence between different formulations), the authors concluded that 'morphine is an effective analgesic for cancer pain'.

A more recent systematic review conducted by UK researchers tested the efficacy, tolerability and acceptability of oxycodone for cancer-related pain in adults (Schmidt-Hansen, 2018). The authors included 23 RCTs with over 2200 participants. Their meta-analyses found that oxycodone was equally effective to morphine. The authors' conclusion was "oxycodone can be used as an alternative to morphine".

Hence, in the case of oral morphine and oxycodone, we have large numbers of RCTs reaching the same conclusion. Although some of the studies present methodological challenges, together they produce a 'mass effect'; sufficient to say the effectiveness of these opioids has 'stood the test of time'.

Rapid Onset Opioids (ROOs) for Breakthrough Pain

Breakthrough pain is a transient exacerbation of pain that occurs either spontaneously or in relation to a specific predictable or unpredictable trigger despite relative stable and adequately controlled background pain. Breakthrough pain usually relates to background pain and is typically of rapid onset, severe in intensity and generally self-limiting within 30 minutes (intermittent spikes). Notably, other, transient cancer pain exacerbations (or pain flares) also exist. Breakthrough pain has traditionally been managed by the administration of supplemental immediate-release oral opioids (rescue medication) at a dose proportional to the total around-the-clock opioid dose (Davies, 2009). In recent years, new opioid formulations were developed to provide a rapid onset, short-lasting analgesia for breakthrough pain. New oral, buccal tablet and film, sublingual tablet, nasal spray, and a sublingual spray of fentanyl formulations—all termed rapid onset opioids (ROOs)—are now available. All have the common advantage of rapid entry into the systemic circulation via transmucosal absorption, thus avoiding hepatic and intestinal first-pass metabolism and allowing a rapid onset of action, similar to intravenous opioid injections. Vigorous research in recent years yielded at least 10 RCTs, all tested for their effect on breakthrough pain. The main outcome was change from baseline pain intensity relative to placebo at up to 60 minutes after the medication intake. At 30 minutes, all medications were superior to placebo with regard to immediate release, except morphine sulfate which showed efficacy over placebo only after 45 minutes. The intra-nasal fentanyl spray seemed to have a shorter onset of analgesia relative to the other ROOs (Zeppetella, 2014). Consequently, ROOs have changed the approach to managing breakthrough pain (Mercadente, 2017) and nowadays, once diagnosed, breakthrough pain should be treated by a ROO whenever available, rather than by a rescue dose of immediate-release oral opioid. This change is supported by high quality evidence.

Non-Steroidal Anti-Inflammatory Drugs (NSAIDs)

Non-opioid drugs are commonly used to treat cancer related pain, and are recommended for this purpose in the WHO cancer pain treatment ladder, either alone or in combination with opioids or other drugs (WHO, 1986). A 2017 Cochrane review (Derry, 2017) attempted to provide an updated estimate of the type and strength of evidence in support of using oral nonsteroidal anti-inflammatory drugs (NSAIDs) in adults with cancer related pain; their review included randomized, double-blind, single-blind, or open-label studies lasting one week or longer. Despite the long use of these drugs in cancer patients, only 11 trials met the inclusion criteria and provided data on more than 900 patients with mostly moderate or severe pain. Eight studies used a double-blind design, two a single-blind design, and one open-label. Most studies had methodological faults with high risk of bias for blinding, incomplete outcome data, or small size. The authors were not able to compare NSAIDs as a group with another treatment, or one NSAID with another NSAID, and judged all outcomes as very low-quality evidence. Their conclusion was there is no high-quality evidence to support or refute the use of NSAIDs alone or in combination with opioids for the three steps of the WHO ladder, and there is very low-quality evidence that some people with moderate or severe cancer pain can obtain substantial levels of benefit within 1-2 weeks.

TESTING DRUGS FOR SPECIFIC PAIN CONDITIONS: CHEMOTHERAPY INDUCED PERIPHERAL NEUROPATHY AND METASTATIC BONE-PAIN

Testing the effects of pharmacological treatments in any given field of medicine is usually conducted by one of the two following approaches. The 'top-down' approach principally tests existing treatments or interventions for new indications. It is therefore easier to adopt, although it often lacks solid scientific grounds in terms of underlying analgesic mechanisms. The 'bottom up' approach tries to introduce new molecules which were developed based on mechanism-derived understandings. There are numerous examples of using the 'top-down' approach in the context of cancer-related pain. One example is the challenging field of chemotherapy induced peripheral neuropathy (CIPN) which is often painful and where no therapies are currently available to prevent its occurrence (Gewandter, 2018). A review of the most recent RCTs on this topic reveals pharmacological trials on duloxetine - as a study protocol (Matsuoka, 2017), 8% capsaicin patch - with positive results (Filipczak-Bryniarska, 2017), pregabalin – with negative results (de Andrade, 2017) and minocycline – also with negative results (Pachman, 2017). Thus, although easier to adopt, this approach does not guarantee successful results.

The bottom-up approach, although based on solid scientific grounds and therefore expected to yield positive clinical results, sometimes also fails. One example relates to bone pain in patients with cancer, one of the most common pain syndromes directly related to a tumor (Portenoy, 2018). Existing analgesic therapies are non-specific. Major discoveries have recently been made during related-to-tumor-nerve interactions, and their contribution to cancer-related pain includes specific ion channels, signaling cascades operational at the tumor–nerve interface, gene regulation by tumor–nerve interactions and nerve-derived factors modulating tumor cells (Selvaraj, 2015). Thus, new potential targets for treatment have become available. Two such targets that have been tested in RCTs in patients with cancer with bone pain are worth mentioning: nerve growth factor and endotheline-1. Tanezumab is a nerve growth factor monoclonal antibody, which has shown signals of efficacy in patients with painful bone metastases. In one RCT testing the analgesic effect of intravenous injections of 10 mg tanezumab or placebo, the primary endpoint of study was not achieved. Post hoc analyses suggested that tanezumab had greater efficacy in patients with lower baseline opioid use and/or higher baseline pain, but the study population size (n = 59) was not large enough to yield significant positive results (Sopata, 2015).

A second trial (Fizazi, 2013) was a much larger phase III, multi-center RCT on more than 1000 patients with metastatic castration-resistant prostate cancer that investigated the efficacy and safety of zibotentan, an oral specific endothelin A receptor antagonist. Noteworthy, pain was only one of the secondary end points (the primary end point was overall survival). Unfortunately, no significant differences were observed in any of the primary or secondary endpoints between the active drug and the placebo groups.

CANNABINOIDS AND CANNABIS

Cannabinoids, the major active compounds of the cannabis plant, have a potential therapeutic effect on cancer symptoms such as pain and chemotherapy induced nausea. It is not surprising that cancer patients frequently use cannabis to reduce pain and other symptoms during the course of their illness (Reinarman, 2011; Waissengrin, 2015). In Israel, patients with cancer who request medical cannabis, quickly obtain authorization and receive treatment within a matter of days; whereas authorization for using medical cannabis for other indications can take many months. There are two reasons for this difference. Firstly, some patients with cancer pain, especially those with advanced cancer, may not survive many weeks and therefore need the medication quickly. Secondly, many people believe that medical cannabis is the solution for otherwise unrelieved cancer related pain at all stages of the disease and regard it almost as a "panacea" drug. What evidence do we have to support this notion?

Cannabis can be supplied in two different ways: cannabinoid based medications, which are either extracts of the cannabis plan, or synthetic compounds, primarily THC.

Reviewing the evidence regarding cannabinoid based medications reveals two RCTs, which tested the efficacy of the oral-mucosal spray nabiximols (2.7 mg THC, 2.5 mg CBD (Sativex). One trial demonstrated superiority of Sativex over placebo in reducing pain intensity by 30% at the end of a 2-week treatment period (Johnson, 2010), but the second multicenter trial, using the same criteria, failed to show a difference between two doses of Sativex and a placebo (Portenoy, 2012).

With regard to herbal cannabis, a literature search of smoking marijuana for the relief of cancer related pain failed to yield any RTCs. Only two small studies on orally consumed THC extracts from natural herbal cannabis by Noyes et al. (1975a,b) were published. One identified a correlation between THC doses and pain relief. The second study found a significant difference in pain reduction between THC and placebo. A recent survey from Israel, which included approximately 17,000 patients with cancer, found that nearly 2% received authorization for cannabis use from an institutional oncologist. Most of the patients had metastatic disease (i.e., advanced cancer). By the end of the first month of medical cannabis use, 50-70 percent of surviving users reported improved appetite, nausea, general well-being and pain with mild side effects (Waissengrin, 2015). This, however, was a 'snapshot' observational study, conducted at a single point of time, and therefore provided only very-low quality evidence. A second trial worth mentioning, also from Israel, analyzed data routinely collected as part of a program treating 2970 cancer patients with medical cannabis during 2015 - 2017. At the end of the six months follow-up period, one quarter of the patients died and nearly 20% stopped the treatment. Importantly, well over 90% of the remaining patients reported an improvement in their symptoms. The authors' conclusion was that cannabis as a palliative treatment for cancer patients seems to be well tolerated, effective and a safe option to help patients cope with their malignancy related symptoms (Bar-lev, 2018).

Several systematic reviews on this topic were published in recent years. A 2015 review in the Journal of the American Medical Association identified three studies on patients with cancer related pain. Although pain intensity was attenuated, the magnitude of average pain reduction was approximately half a point on a 10-point scale, which is not a considerable change (Whiting, 2015). A more recent systematic review and meta-analysis of cannabinoids in palliative medicine by a German group found no differences between medical cannabis and placebo in reducing pain intensity by 30%(Mücke, 2018). Importantly, a 30 percent decrease in pain is regarded as significant by most patients.

To conclude, results of published studies show that the average effect of medical cannabis on cancer pain does not appear to be robust. Secondly, a relatively small number of studies exist; therefore it is still difficult to draw firm conclusions concerning the efficacy of medical cannabis for cancer related pain. Yet, when analyzing the results of RCTs we need to take into consideration the fact that RCTs always refer to 'an average response'. There is always a spectrum of responses. So while some patients do not benefit from treatment, others experience dramatic pain reduction. Indeed, in a recent article entitled "integrating cannabis into clinical cancer care", Dr. Donald Adams (2016), a senior oncologist at the University of California in San Francisco, wrote: "Clinically, I have observed that many cancer patients benefit from adding cannabis to their pain regimen. Some sorts of cancer-related pain appear to respond to medical cannabis." When referring to patients at the most advanced stages of illness he adds, "Patients who have been put on high doses of opiates at the end of life by their well-meaning care team, frequently feel totally unable to communicate with their loved ones in their precious remaining time because of altered cognition. Many have successfully weaned themselves down or off of their opiate dose by adding cannabis to their regimen."

SUMMARY AND RECOMMENDATIONS

While some therapies for the management of cancer related pain, such as opioids for moderate to severe pain or ROOS for breakthrough pain, are supported by high quality evidence; only very poor quality evidence supports the use of other medications, cannabinoids for example. Many other treatments fall in between. The production of high quality evidence is a difficult task that requires considerable resources and efforts, and the results are not always guaranteed. What this means is that gaps in knowledge in various areas of cancer related pain continue, and that ongoing efforts to narrow these gaps should be made. Until this happens, the clinical practice should be based on best available evidence.

REFERENCES

Abrams DI. Integrating cannabis into clinical cancer care. *Curr Oncol.* 2016 Mar;23(2):S8-S14.

Accad M, Francis D. Does evidence based medicine adversely affect clinical judgment? *BMJ.* 2018 Jul 16;362:k2799.

Bar-Lev Schleider L, Mechoulam R, Lederman V, Hilou M, Lencovsky O, Betzalel O, Shbiro L, Novack V. Prospective analysis of safety and efficacy of medical cannabis in large unselected population of patients with cancer. *Eur J Intern Med.* 2018;49:37-43.

Davies AN, Dickman A, Reid C, Stevens AM, Zeppetella G; Science Committee of the Association for Palliative Medicine of Great Britain and Ireland. The management of cancer-related breakthrough pain: recommendations of a task group of the Science Committee of the Association for Palliative Medicine of Great Britain and Ireland. *Eur J Pain.* 2009;13(4):331-8.

de Andrade DC, Jacobsen Teixeira M, Galhardoni R, Ferreira KSL, Braz Mileno P, Scisci N, Zandonai A, Teixeira WGJ, Saragiotto DF, Silva V, Raicher I, Cury RG, Macarenco R, Otto Heise C, Wilson Iervolino Brotto M, Andrade de Mello A, Zini Megale M, Henrique Curti Dourado L, Mendes Bahia L, Lilian Rodrigues A, Parravano D, Tizue Fukushima J, Lefaucheur JP, Bouhassira D, Sobroza E, Riechelmann RP, Hoff PM; PreOx Workgroup, Valério da Silva F, Chile T, Dale CS, Nebuloni D, Senna L, Brentani H, Pagano RL, de Souza ÂM. Pregabalin for the Prevention of Oxaliplatin-Induced Painful Neuropathy: A Randomized, Double-Blind Trial. *Oncologist.* 2017 Oct;22(10):1154-e105.

Derry S, Wiffen PJ, Moore RA, McNicol ED, Bell RF, Carr DB, McIntyre M, Wee B. Oral nonsteroidal anti-inflammatory drugs (NSAIDs) for cancer pain in adults. *Cochrane Database Syst Rev.* 2017 Jul 12;7:CD012638.

Filipczak-Bryniarska I, Krzyzewski RM, Kucharz J, Michalowska-Kaczmarczyk A, Kleja J, Woron J, Strzepek K, Kazior L, Wordliczek J, Grodzicki T, Krzemieniecki K. High-dose 8% capsaicin patch in treatment of chemotherapy-induced peripheral neuropathy: single-center experience. *Med Oncol.* 2017 Aug 17;34(9):162.

Fizazi K, Higano CS, Nelson JB, Gleave M, Miller K, Morris T, Nathan FE, McIntosh S, Pemberton K, Moul JW. Phase III, randomized, placebo-controlled study of docetaxel in combination with zibotentan in patients with metastatic castration-resistant prostate cancer. *J Clin Oncol.* 2013;31(14):1740-7.

Gewandter JS, Brell J, Cavaletti G, Dougherty PM, Evans S, Howie L, McDermott MP, O'Mara A, Smith AG, Dastros-Pitei D, Gauthier LR, Haroutounian S, Jarpe M, Katz NP, Loprinzi C, Richardson P, Lavoie-Smith EM, Wen PY, Turk DC, Dworkin RH, Freeman R. Trial designs for chemotherapy-induced peripheral neuropathy prevention: ACTTION recommendations. *Neurology.* 2018 Jul 27.

Guyatt GH, Oxman AD, Vist GE, Kunz R, Falck-Ytter Y (2008). GRADE: an emerging consensus on rating quality of evidence and strength of recommendations. *BMJ* 2008;336:924–6.

Johnson JR, Burnell-Nugent M, Lossignol D, Ganae-Motan ED, Potts R, Fallon MT. Multicenter, double-blind, randomized, placebo-controlled, parallel-group study of the efficacy, safety and tolerability of THC:CBD extract and THC extract in patients with intractable cancer-related pain. *J Pain Symptom Manage.* 2010;39:167–179.

Matsuoka H, Ishiki H, Iwase S, Koyama A, Kawaguchi T, Kizawa Y, Morita T, Matsuda Y, Miyaji T, Ariyoshi K, Yamaguchi T. Study protocol for a multi-institutional, randomised, double-blinded, placebo-controlled phase III trial investigating additive efficacy of duloxetine for neuropathic cancer pain refractory to opioids and gabapentinoids: the DIRECT study. *BMJ Open.* 2017 Aug 28;7(8):e017280.

Mercadante S. New drugs for pain management in advanced cancer patients. *Expert Opin Pharmacother.* 2017;18(5):497-502.

Mücke M, Weier M, Carter C, Copeland J, Degenhardt L, Cuhls H, Radbruch L, Häuser W, Conrad R. Systematic review and meta-analysis of cannabinoids in palliative medicine. *J Cachexia Sarcopenia Muscle.* 2018;9(2):220-234.

Noyes R Jr, Brunk SF, Avery DA, et al. The analgesic properties of delta-9-tetrahydrocannabinol and codeine. *Clin Pharmacol Ther* 1975B;18:84-9.

Noyes R Jr, Brunk SF, Baram DA, et al. Analgesic effect of delta-9-tetrahydrocannabinol. *J Clin Pharmacol.* 1975A;15:139-43.

Pachman DR, Dockter T, Zekan PJ, Fruth B, Ruddy KJ, Ta LE, Lafky JM, Dentchev T, Le-Lindqwister NA, Sikov WM, Staff N, Beutler AS, Loprinzi CL. A pilot study of minocycline for the prevention of paclitaxel-associated neuropathy: ACCRU study RU221408I. *Support Care Cancer.* 2017 Nov;25(11):3407-3416.

Portenoy RK, Ahmed E. Cancer Pain Syndromes. *Hematol Oncol Clin North Am.* 2018;32(3):371-386.

Portenoy RK, Banae-Motan ED, Allende S, et al. Nabiximols for opioid-treated cancer patients with poorly-controlled chronic pain: a randomized placebo-controlled dose-graded trial. *J Pain.* 2012;13:438–449.

Reinarman C, Nunberg H, Lanthier F, Heddleston T. Who are medical marijuana patients? Population characteristics from nine California assessment clinics. *J Psychoactive Drugs.* 2011;43:128–35.

Sackett DL, Rosenberg WM, Gray JA, Haynes RB, Richardson WS. Evidence based medicine: what it is and what it isn't. *BMJ.* 1996;312(7023):71-2. Wikipedia 2018: https://en.wikipedia.org/wiki/Evidence-based_medicin.

Schmidt-Hansen M, Bennett MI, Arnold S, Bromham N, Hilgart JS. Efficacy, tolerability and acceptability of oxycodone for cancer-related pain in adults: an updated Cochrane systematic review. *BMJ Support Palliat Care.* 2018 Jun;8(2):117-128.

Selvaraj D, Kuner R. Molecular players of tumor–nerve interactions. *Pain.* 2015;156(1):6-7.

Sopata M, Katz N, Carey W, Smith MD, Keller D, Verburg KM, West CR, Wolfram G, Brown MT Efficacy and safety of tanezumab in the treatment of pain from bone metastases. *Pain.* 2015;156(9):1703-13.

Waissengrin B, Urban D, Leshem Y, Garty M, Wolf I. Patterns of use of medical cannabis among Israeli cancer patients: a single institution experience. *J Pain Symptom Manage.* 2015;49(2):223-30.

Whiting PF, Wolff RF, Deshpande S, Di Nisio M, Duffy S, Hernandez AV, Keurentjes JC, Lang S, Misso K, Ryder S, Schmidlkofer S, Westwood M, Kleijnen J. Cannabinoids for Medical Use: A Systematic Review and Meta-analysis. *JAMA.* 2015 Jun 23-30;313(24):2456-73.

Wiffen PJ, Wee B, Moore RA. Oral morphine for cancer pain. *Cochrane Database Syst Rev.* 2016 Apr 22;4:CD003868.

World Health Organisation (1986) *Cancer Pain Relief.* WHO, Geneva.

Zeppetella G, Davies A, Eijgelshoven I, Jansen JP. A network meta-analysis of the efficacy of opioid analgesics for the management of breakthrough cancer pain episodes. *J Pain Symptom Manage.* 2014;47(4):772.e5–785.e5.

BIOGRAPHICAL SKETCH

Prof. Elon Eisenberg

Prof. Elon Eisenberg graduated from Sackler School of Medicine, Tel-Aviv University in Israel. He completed a residency in Neurology, at Rambam Medical Center, Haifa, Israel, and Neurology - Pain Fellowship at Massachusetts General Hospital, Harvard Medical School in Boston, USA.

Prof. Eisenberg has been the director of the Institute of Pain Medicine at Rambam Health Care Campus, Haifa, Israel, and the President of the Israeli Pain Association. He is currently the director of the Pain Research Unit at the Institute of Pain Medicine, Rambam Health Care Campus. He is a Professor of Neurology and Pain Medicine and the Dean of the Faculty of Medicine, and holds the Otto Barth Family Academic Chair in Biomedical Science at the Technion - Israel Institute of Technology. His main areas of research include mechanisms and treatment of pain with special emphasis on neuropathic pain, CRPS, cancer pain, opioids and cannabinoids. Prof. Eisenberg has published about two-hundred articles, book chapters and abstracts in various areas of pain.

In: Palliative Care
Editor: Michael Silbermann

ISBN: 978-1-53616-199-1
© 2019 Nova Science Publishers, Inc.

Chapter 17

RESEARCH ON WHAT 'MEANING' REALLY MEANS FOR CANCER PATIENTS NEAR THE END OF LIFE: FINDINGS FROM A MIXED METHODS STUDY

Adi Ivzori Erel[1,2], *Lee Greenblatt-Kimron*[3] *and Miri Cohen*[4,*]

[1]The Ruth & Bruce Rappaport Faculty of Medicine, Technion - Israel Institute, Department of Family Medicine, Haifa, Israel
[2]Clalit Health Services, Haifa and Western Galilee District, Haifa, Israel
[3]Ariel University, Department of Social Work, Ariel, Israel
[4]University of Haifa, Faculty of Social Welfare and Health Sciences, Mount Carmel, Haifa, Israel

ABSTRACT

Background: The meaning of life plays a central role in every person's life, and becomes particularly pronounced when confronting highly stressful life circumstances. There is a dearth of research specifically addressing the meaning-making process, and its result - meaning-made - and their impact on quality of life among cancer patient near the end of life.

Objective: The study combined quantitative and qualitative methodologies; the primary aim was to expand the understanding of the role of meaning in life among cancer patients near the end of life and its effect on quality of life.

Method: A total of 150 questionnaires and 20 in-depth interviews were completed with cancer patients near the end of life, who received treatment in either a home hospice setting or the Oncology Department at Rambam Hospital.

Results: Regardless of place of treatment, nationality or religiousness, the participants reported moderate levels of overall quality of life and emotional distress, together with a very low physical quality of life, high meaning in life (meaning-made), and a low level of involvement in a current search for meaning (meaning-making process). In addition, only the meaning-made variable was associated with a higher quality of life. The content analysis of the in-depth interviews suggests that the search for meaning occurs at earlier stages along the disease pathway. Towards the end of life, the

---

* Corresponding Author's E-mail: mcohen2@univ.haifa.ac.il.

participants' experience of life and its meaning is focused on the most intimate relationships and important elements - family, faith and, ultimately, the physical comfort and the possibility of enjoying the small and simple things in life, which each participant described according to his/her own personal preferences and inclinations.

Conclusions: This study is one of the first to examine meaning in life, thus expanding the current understanding of the experience of meaning at the end of life, and the various roles that meaning-making and meaning-made play near the end of life. Both the quantitative and qualitative studies propose that, in contrast to meaning-made, the meaning-making process is a coping strategy seldom used by cancer patients near the end of life, and is unrelated to quality of life.

Keywords: meaning-focused coping, end of life, advanced cancer patient, palliative care, depression, anxiety, quality of life

INTRODUCTION

Cancer is among the leading causes of death worldwide. In 2012, there were 14 million new cases and 8.2 million cancer-related deaths worldwide [1]. Advanced cancer is a formidable source of stress, due to the imminent threat to life and bodily integrity. It also has many implications regarding all aspects of life, and requires coping with severe symptoms that cause physical and mental suffering. The treatment usually given at this stage is palliative care. *Palliative care* is defined as an overall therapeutic approach aimed at ensuring the highest possible quality of life for patients with advanced diseases. It is aimed at preventing or reducing the patients' suffering by identifying and treating physical, mental, spiritual and social problems, while giving meaning to life and treating death as a natural process without precipitating or prolonging the dying process [2]. In this sense, *meaning in life* is defined as a subject that is an integral part of the quality of life of cancer patients approaching death. Notwithstanding this definition, few studies have examined the role of the meaning of life among this population.

MEANING IN LIFE

A sense of meaning in life is the most important and profound concern of human existence. Throughout the ages, philosophers, psychologists, writers, and religious leaders have tried to answer the question: "What is the meaning of life?" Nonetheless, despite the numerous attempts to define meaning in life, a single, all-encompassing definition of the concept still does not exist [3, 4]. In philosophical literature, the concept of *meaning in life* is defined as an internal commitment that a person develops toward life in the context of his beliefs. For this reason, various interpretations have been proposed. Religious models claimed, for example, that the meaning of life derives from God; others argued that meaning in life derives from the very existence of man (Alexis, 2011).

Despite the various approaches to understanding the meaning of human life, there is a consensus that this is a central issue and that meaning in an individual's life is a source of strength, particularly when coping with difficult life experiences. Towards the end of the twentieth century, research on meaning began to expand in additional directions, including the investigation of the effects of perceptions of meaning in life on adaptation when experiencing difficult life events [5, 6, 7, 8]. *Meaning-made*, in the wake of stressful events, is a central axis in the theories of adaptation to stressful events [9]. This has been highlighted and developed in recent years through the new coping approaches presented by Park and Folkman, who emphasize the meaning-making and meaning-made processes [6, 10, 11].

THE MEANING-MAKING MODEL OF COPING WITH LIFE STRESS

Individuals create perceptions of meaning for themselves that represent beliefs, goals, and subjective feelings regarding their existence in the world [12]. These perceptions accompany a person throughout his life; however, when an unexpected traumatic event occurs, which contradicts the individual's perceptions of general meaning, these meanings are undermined [12, 13]. For example, a perception of trust in human beings may be undermined due to a harmful event experienced by the individual or a significant other.

Folkman [24] defined *meaning-focused coping* as searching for new goals and planning goal-oriented actions, using measures such as reassessment of reality (e.g., redirecting life goals from career to family) or emphasizing beliefs and spiritual experiences (e.g., strengthening religious beliefs). Meaning-focused coping is not intended to change the stress factor, and it does not directly reduce the negative emotions or distress resulting from one's reaction to the stress situation. Instead, it is aimed at adjusting the way the individual assesses the situation.

Park [11] broadened the concept of meaning-focused coping, which distinguishes between *meaning-making* as a *process* and *meaning-made* as a *result*, which specifically refers to searching for and finding meaning in relation to coping with health and illness-related threats.

The meaning-making process is defined as the overall effort to create and/or increase the individual's understanding of the significance of the stressful event. Meaning-making is considered a common way of adapting to stressful events [15] and can lead to re-evaluation, which may enable the individual to create new meaning and adapt to the stressful situation.

Coping with cancer generates patients' needs to reassess the meaning of their situation. Along the pathway of coping with cancer, patients deal with different interpretations in the process of searching for logic to somehow explain the traumatic occurrences and their consequences [16]. Studies on the relationship between meaning-focused coping and the adjustment of cancer patients have found inconsistent results, sometimes indicating a good adjustment and, at other times, an increase in distress as observed in a survey conducted by Park and her colleagues [17].

Meaning-made refers to the outcome of reinterpreting the event (in this case, the illness), while altering or not altering the individual's previous perceptions. The reinterpretation aims to achieve cognitive consistency between the meaning the individual held until he experienced the crisis, and the meaning he attributed as a result of the crisis [11], in an attempt to reduce the gap between them. Reducing this gap helps create new perceptions after the trauma and, in the end, nurtures a realistic perception of the situation. It therefore operates as an auxiliary factor in the adjustment process.

MEANING-MAKING AND COPING WITH CANCER AT THE END OF LIFE

The number of studies that examined meaning-focused coping at the end of life is very small [18, 19, 20]. Moreover, in most studies in the field of palliative therapy that deal with meaning in life, the meaning-making process in life was not measured as a variable in itself; instead, it was included as a measure of psychological well-being [21, 22, 23]. However, meaning in life is one of the most affected psychological structures at the end of life [18, 24, 25, 26]. Researchers have shown that dealing with meaning is common among cancer patients in the advanced stages of the disease. It was found that towards the end of life, patients reported that issues related to meaning in life preoccupied them more than physical symptoms, physical well-being, and social support [21], and they perceived meaning as an important factor in their emotional well-being [18, 27, 28, 29]. In addition, patients at the end of life reported the existence of meaning and the motivation to create meaning more than healthy individuals. Also, end of life patients also mentioned great suffering combined with the use of coping strategies that were focused mainly on meaning [23].

Wrubel [30] and her colleagues argued that a life with meaning among patients with terminal diseases at the end of their lives was likely to contribute to their psychological well-being, even more than the given death. Moreover, meaning in life at this stage is not evaluated/measured by major existential issues, but rather, as Frankel argued, by the specific meaning an individual attributes to life at a given time [31]. Indeed, different sources of meaning can have a different effect on emotional well-being among cancer patients at the end of life. Thus, it was found that among end of life patients, the existence of personal relationships, the ability to preserve culture and tradition, and taking an interest in society are associated with low levels of depression [32].

It is especially complex to conceptualize and examine meaning-making and meaning-made processes [11, 17], and there are very few studies in this field. Therefore, the purpose of this study was to examine meaning-focused coping processes among end of life cancer patients, and the associations of patients' emotional well-being and quality of life. Since the field of research on meaning – that focused on the end of life cancer patients - is limited, this study examined issues which, to date, have barely been previously examined. The study specifically examined the roles of the meaning-making process and meaning-made near the end of life, and their impact on quality of life.

In light of the above, and in order to gain a better understanding of the structure of meaning in life among cancer patients near the end of life, we perceived the need to use a mixed-methods research model, in order to increase the breadth and depth of the data.

The primary aim of our research was to expand the understanding of the role of the meaning-making process and meaning-made in relation to the well-being and quality of life of cancer patients near the end of life, from different cultural and religious backgrounds. Due to the complexity of meaning processes, we approached this issue using both quantitative and qualitative research methods. *The quantitative part of the study used structured questionnaires and attempted* to examine the direct and indirect relations between meaning-focused coping (the meaning-making process and meaning-made, and quality of life measures). *The qualitative study used in-depth interviews to* examine the ways in which cancer patients near the end of life experience and perceive their special situation in regard to meaning-making process and meaning-made. This was done in order to examine these processes from the phenomenological perspective, in an attempt to attain an in-depth understanding of the essence of the phenomenon, especially in a multicultural context.

The study was approved by the Helsinki Communities of Clalit Health Services and the Rambam Medical Center, as well as by the University of Haifa's Ethics Committee. All the participants signed an informed consent form.

QUANTITATIVE STUDY

Methods

Method: One hundred and fifty cancer patients, 18 years old or above, defined by the treating professionals as 'patients at the end of life' (prognosis of up to six months left to live and not receiving any curative treatment) participated in the study. The patients were recruited consecutively from two main care facilities: the Oncology Institute at the Rambam Medical Center or home hospice operated by the main health services clinic in Israel (Clalit Health Services, Haifa and the West Galilee districts). During the period of the study, 214 patients were interviewed, of whom 150 participated; the rest were unable to participate due to their condition, refusal or because they died in the days between the telephone call and the date set for the visit.

Participants completed several questionnaires:

The Meaning-Making and Meaning-Made Questionnaire [33]

A five-item questionnaire to evaluate the meaning-making process, and five items to evaluate meaning-made in life.

McGill Quality of Life Questionnaire [34]

Originally a 17-item questionnaire consisting of four sub-scales: physical quality of life; psychological quality of life; existential welfare; and a sense of meaning in life, and a single item for measuring general quality of life. The questionnaire is designed to study the quality of life of patients defined as dying in various dimensions. Three items were used in this study: a. a General Quality of Life item; b. an item that examines the quality of physical life in the past week; and c. the participants were asked to indicate three physical symptoms they had experienced as 'most difficult' in the past week, and to rate the intensity of each of the indicated symptoms.

The BSI-18, Brief Symptom Inventory [35]

A shortened version of the BSI questionnaire that includes 53 items evaluating nine groups of psychiatric symptoms [58]. The shortened questionnaire includes three dimensions: depression, anxiety, and somatization. The present study did not use the section that examined symptoms of somatization, in light of the many physical symptoms associated with cancer at the end of life. The questionnaire therefore included 12 items that examined emotional distress (anxiety and depression).

All of the questionnaires were validated and had acceptable internal reliability (Cronbach's alpha <0.75).

RESULTS

Participants were between the ages of 30-93 (mean (M) = 65.08; standard deviation (SD) =1.15). The number of women was slightly higher than the number of men, with no significant difference between the groups (53.3% women versus 46.7% men). Most of the participants were married (67.3%). Participants had a wide range of levels of education, between 0 and 20 years of education (mean 12.7; standard deviation 3.6). The participants were Jews (78%) and Arabs (22%); most of the participants, both Jews and Arabs, described themselves as secular (50%) and traditional (30%).

All participants in the study were diagnosed with metastatic cancer (except for one participant who had been diagnosed with an unplanned anaplastic astrocytoma and his prognosis by doctors was less than 6 months left to live). Most of the participants in the two groups rated themselves as 'needing help in all activities' or were confined to bed; about 30% reported needing partial help only. The initial diagnosis among the participants ranged from months to years, with the average being just over five years. In terms of the types of treatment patients received during the course of the disease, the four most common treatments for the disease were surgery, chemotherapy, radiotherapy and biological treatments. Seventy-eight percent of the participants received more than one type of treatment and 60% of the patients underwent three or more treatments.

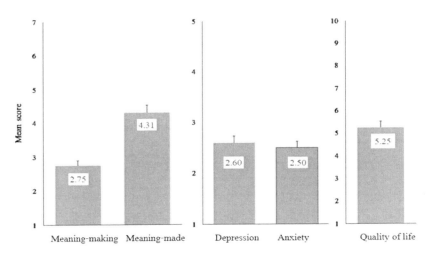

Figure 1. Means of the study variables.

Figure 1 describes the averages of the study variables. It is possible to see that the mean of meaning-making was significantly lower (SD=2.05 M=2.75) than the mean of meaning-made (SD= 1.7 M=4.31). Accordingly, the participants reported a strong existence of meaning, and the degree of dealing with significance and meaning-making was much lower. Although they were at the final stage of the disease, they reported, on average, a high quality of life (SD=2.36 M=5.25), while in a specific reference to physical quality of life, it was lower (SD=2.05 M=3.34). By means of the BSI, levels of anxiety and depression were examined, and were found to be at the center of the scale, indicating moderate levels of symptoms of depression (SD=1.09 M=2.60) and anxiety (SD=1.13 M=2.42). These levels were similar and without significant differences.

CORRELATIONS AMONG THE RESEARCH VARIABLES

Table 1 describes the correlations among meaning-making, meaning-made, quality of life, and symptoms of depression and anxiety with background variables. Pearson correlation tests showed that meaning-making processes and meaning-made were related differently to the background variables. Participants who experienced poorer economic conditions and poorer functional status were less likely to undergo meaning-making processes, while meaning-made was associated with a lower age and more children. Depression was associated with a better functional state, while anxiety was associated with younger age and higher economic status. Specifically, participants with a lower functional level experienced higher levels of depression, while younger participants and those with a higher economic status experienced more anxiety, when quality of life was not associated with any of the research variables.

With regard to the correlations among and between the research variables, as can be seen in Table 1, the meaning-making process and meaning-made were found to have a positive correlation: the more people deal with meaning-making, the more they report having meaning in their lives. Meaning-made was associated with higher levels of quality of life and lower levels of anxiety and depression. Therefore, the variables contributing to better quality of life were examined using multiple regression tests.

Table 1. Correlations among the research variables

	1	2	3	4	5	6	7	8	9
1. Age	1								
2. Economic situation	-0.07	1							
3. Number of children	0.07	**0.22****	1						
4. Functional situation	**0.28****	-0.05	-0.08	1					
5. Meaning-making	-0.12	**-0.16***	-0.06	**-0.15***	1				
6. Meaning-made	**-0,18***	-0.06	**0.15***	-0.13	0.03	1			
7. Overall quality of life	0.04	-0.04	0.07	-0.13	0.13	**0.38****	1		
8. Depression	-0.07	0.12	-0.03	**0.21***	-0.03	**-0.48****	**-0.53****	1	
9. Anxiety	**-0.18***	**0.16***	-0.04	0.11	0.14	**-0.19****	**-0.21****	**0.54****	1

$p < 0.01$* $p < 0.001$.**

The following background variables - age, economic status, and functional status - were included in the regression analysis, but because the association with quality of life was found to be non-significant, these background variables are not presented. In the first step, meaning-making and meaning-made variables were entered. A positive significant correlation was found only with quality of life; therefore, the higher the perception of meaning (meaning-made) in one's life, the higher the individual's perceived quality of life. In the second step, levels of depression and anxiety were added. In this step, only the depression variable was found to be negatively associated with quality of life; thus, the correlation with meaning-making became insignificant. This is in light of the strong association with depression, which indicates that depression actually mediates the relationship between meaning-making and quality of life, such that the more the individual experiences meaning-made, the lower his level of depression, and consequently the higher his perceived quality of life.

Table 2. Multiple regression for predicting quality of life
(adjusted for background variables)

Variable	Model 1 B	SE	β	Model 2 B	SE	β
Meaning-making	.15	.20	.13	.14	.08	.12
Meaning-made	.52	.11	.39*	.21	.11	16.
Depression				-.20	.04	.51*-
Anxiety				.21	.18	.10
R^2	.19			.34		
F (df)	4.78*(5,144)			8.0* (7,144)		

*p<.001.

In conclusion, the findings of the quantitative study indicate that meaning-made among cancer patients near the end of life has a strong positive association with quality of life, such that the higher the perception of meaning, the higher the individual's perceived quality of life. In contrast, the meaning-making process was not found to be associated with quality of life among cancer patients near the end of life.

THE QUALITATIVE STUDY

Method

The objective of the qualitative study is to understand the ways in which cancer patients near the end of life experience cope with their situation. The qualitative study specifically focused on the meaning-making and meaning-made contexts, in an attempt to examine the concepts from a phenomenological perspective, which strives to understand the essence of the phenomenon, especially in a multi-cultural context.

The sample included both Jews and Arabs - 10 patients in a home hospice care setting and 10 patients in a hospital. All of the participants had a very low level of daily functioning and needed assistance in most or all daily living activities. In terms of gender, 11 women and 9 men between the ages of 31-77 were interviewed; the number of years of education ranged between 12 to 20. Marital status was varied: 11 participants were married, 3 were divorced, 3 were widowed and 3 were single. A total of 12 participants were native Israelis. The level of religiosity reported by participants ranged from secular to ultra-Orthodox. Nine participants defined themselves as secular, 1 of which reported she had previously been religious, 5 who said they were observant, 5 who reported being religiously observant, and 1 who had previously been secular and was now religious. Except for one, all participants died within 10 days to 6 months after the interview. All the interviewees' names are fictitious.

The study was approved by the Helsinki Communities of Clalit Health Services, and Rambam Medical Center, as well as by the University of Haifa's Ethics Committee.

Participants in the qualitative part of the study did not participate in the quantitative part; their interviews were partially conducted in parallel with the quantitative data collection and partially after the completion of the quantitative research. In addition, an attempt was made to interview cancer patients at the end of life from various backgrounds - different ages, religion, economic status and marital status - in order to provide a diverse and comprehensive picture representing the theoretical and scientific knowledge of coping with cancer according to the theoretical sampling method [82]. The study's qualitative data collection was conducted through semi-structured, in-depth interviews. The interview provides a source of learning about and understanding the participants' experiences and was conducted based on the interview guide. The interview guide includes significant key areas; however, it is flexible and enables a dialogue with the interviewees. It also ensures a "safe" space which allows patients to express their experiences in their own words. The interviews were conducted in the natural environment where patients receive treatment. Questions included in the interview: interviewees' perception of life and meaning of life before the illness; the patient's perception of the disease, and coping with it at various stages, with an emphasis on the current stage; family and social relationships and other support factors; as well as questions related to meaning-making and meaning-made.

All interviews were conducted by the researcher (A.I.E) and were recorded. The interviews were transcribed by the researcher (A.I.E), word-for-word, indicating breaks and non-verbal communication in the interviews. The interviews were conducted in a flexible manner, and not all interviews dealt with every subject. The order of the subjects differed from interview to interview. The interviews were analyzed using content analysis. In order to identify and encode key themes and patterns, in the first stage all of the interviews were read, the main topics raised in the interview were identified, and sub-categories were created. Next, a search was conducted in order to identify associated topics and to further group sub-categories into secondary categories. In the last stage, the main themes were identified, which represent the main points of the study [36].

FINDINGS FROM THE QUALITATIVE RESEARCH

>"Meaning is a matter of philosophy; I just want to be healthy without any philosophy"

The theme focuses on ruminations about meaning and the disputation of meaning; elements that give meaning to life and meaning-making; the roles of religion, faith and culture in relation to sense of meaning in life versus the sense of a lack of meaning; and finally, the question of fulfilment as the acceptance of death and the summary of accomplishment in life.

At the stage during which the interviewees participated in the study, all of them, without exception, were dealing with issues related to the present meaning and/or lack of meaning in their lives; yet, they hardly mentioned the meaning-making process. Instead, the participants dealt with topics that had previously defined meaning for them, such as family roles, work, status, social roles, etc., as well as the meaning and lack of meaning these topics have for them today. Most participants mentioned the way in which the understanding that their time is limited, which results in a separation from their former roles, and the connection to what seemed significant to them during other periods of their life. It seemed that most participants did not mourn the loss of their professional roles. In contrast, they expressed loss mainly about the things they could no longer do on the personal and family level.

The participants' definition of *meaning* in relation to the past was based on what they defined as their main role in life: parent, manager, grandfather/grandmother, etc. The reference to the past as a point of comparison usually did not negate the importance of these roles when they were healthy, but the participants were preoccupied with questions about the current significance of these roles. According to the participants, when death approaches and people face the reality of the end of their lives, they do not deal with questions such as: 'What significant roles have I performed in my life? How much money did I earn? or What have I studied?' Instead, individuals relate to the people and activities that can still make them happy.

At the point in time when I met the participants, they were not occupied with reassessing the meaning of their situation, and they fully understood the consequences of the disease. From their words, it is evident that in the earlier stages of the disease pathway, they were busy evaluating their lives and trying to find new meaning in relation to their current situation. Some participants expressed a sense of "missed opportunities" in their lives and regretted the meaning they could have had: If they had known they would get sick, they would have taken advantage of opportunities or allowed themselves to develop more or differently. The feeling of missed opportunities was described as a very painful feeling associated with a lack of meaning or as the recognition that their earlier lives had not been sufficiently meaningful. In all of the interviews, reflecting on the life that was and that which was not was fraught with great difficulty. Some participants lapsed into a fantasy in which it was still possible to try and realize some of their unfulfilled dreams. These fantasies, however, were always accompanied by a painful awakening.

When the participants referred to the present and the very near future, it appeared that their perspective was clearer and, in some respects, more focused on the things that were important to them today. In comparison, their attitude toward the past was characterized by ambivalence and tended to shift back and forth - between their insights as healthy people and their current insights as people with a terminal illness. Most of the participants intuitively answered the question of what is meaningful to them today, and the interviews show that as one's physical condition deteriorates, meaning is reduced to self-related issues, and ultimately to the most basic experience of physical comfort. The diminution of the world is often described in comparative terms: past versus present.

It seemed that the new meaning in the lives of most of the interviewees was reflected in what the interviewees described as "the small things." Many interviewees used this expression to describe the meaning of their current lives. In the first reading of the interviews, this theme was labelled as signifying a lack of meaning, but further examination of these materials led to the deeper understanding that this was not the intention at all; the patients were trying to convey a particular insight. The definition of "the small things" that most of the participants spoke about had different meanings related to the participants' condition or deepest desires and inclinations. However, it may be suggested that recreation with family and a positive physical feeling were the most common things mentioned. There appear to be no differences in relation to meaning between the patients receiving treatment in a home hospice setting and the patients receiving treatment in a hospital setting.

In contrast to most of the participants, a *sense of a total absence of meaning* was found among very few participants.

Religion and faith play a very prominent role in the discourse of meaning, and were mentioned in interviews as both providing meaning and undermining it. Perhaps because the theological conceptions about the meaning of life in the three major monotheistic religions - Christianity, Islam, and Judaism - were guided by the belief in the existence of one God, no differences were found in the way participants related to religion and faith. In their testimonials, most of the religious interviewees referred to God, to their prayers and praying, and to the security they feel in the fact that *"everything is written ..."* or *"from the writings"* ("Machtov"). No differences were found among the different religions. It seemed that the participants who defined themselves as believers did not abandon their faith, and were unwilling to dispute their fate (the fate of a terminal disease). They held onto their beliefs, which strengthened them and, in some cases, liberated them from taking responsibility for their situation – *"whatever He decides ..."* Some of the interviewees mentioned their reconciliation with religion, as a result of their situation. Several participants described how, because of the disease, they felt closer to God and their faith.

Fulfillment and Acceptance of Death

The subject of the meaning of life also arises with regard to the question of fulfillment and acceptance of death, and the ability to sum up one's activities in life. Although all of the study participants referred to the fact that they were dying in one of three forms - open and direct speech, indirect speech, or nonverbal communication - only a small number of interviewees mentioned active preparations they had made for separation from the world. From the reports of those who discussed these issues, it appeared that the separation itself became the main meaning driving their lives. These preparations included activities such as the preparation of albums, writing farewell letters or the detailed planning of their funeral and what would be written on their gravestone. Six of the participants who spoke openly about separation were secular with a moderate-to-high level of education; all but one of them died shortly after the interview. The interviews that related to active separation clearly showed the great significance attributed to it: *"I already know what will be written on my tombstone ..."* Another interviewee said: *"... I decided to write a book about the history of my life, so I wrote a 120-page book ..."* It seems that the preoccupation with death lends patients a certain sense of control over the future. Although most of the interviewees dealt with the topic of death, it does not appear that they necessarily accepted it or prepared for it. In some cases, they accepted their fate; some were successful in asking questions that directly concerned them, while others asked questions that revolved around these issues. Many of the interviewees expressed the wish that it would all just end - whether because of their emotional and physical difficulties, their difficulty in seeing the pain of those close to them, or simply out of acceptance and a genuine desire to end their difficult journey.

In summary, at the end of life, the assessment of life and its meaning become focused on the most basic elements: one's environment, family and faith, and finally, physical comfort. Along with these things is the possibility of enjoying the small and simple things, as described by each of the participants, according to their individual preferences – the things that are close to their hearts. Last, but not least, meaning in life also includes the presence of meaning that each participant had before they became ill, together with the knowledge of their impending death. The meaning of *faith* in these stages is reflected in the hope that the God they believe in will prolong their lives or give them a good death and/or eternal life. The acceptance of death and making active preparations for it was reported by a minority of the participants. However, it appears that many of the patients were more interested in *talking* about their imminent death, their fears, and about preparations they would like to make, rather than actually making these preparations. The interviewees comprehended my willingness to listen to their experiences related to life and death, and some spoke of these topics for the first time. Due to the nature of the research and the one-time encounter with the patients, I did not encourage discussion of this topic, for fear they would have no one with whom to continue the conversation or that engaging this subject for too long would cause distress. This was in spite of my feeling that all of the people in the study felt relieved to be able to talk about life in the shadow of death, and a large portion of them expressed this openly at the end of the interview.

DISCUSSION

In this chapter, we showed that both Jewish and Arab patients near the end of live report a moderate level of overall quality of life and emotional distress, together with a very low level of physical quality of life. Jewish and Arab participants reported high levels of meaning in their life (meaning-made), but a low level of involvement in a present search for meaning (meaning-making). In addition, only the meaning-made variable was strongly correlated with higher quality of life. In the qualitative section of the study, participants were able to discuss perceptions and feelings related to coping with the end of life and its meaning, which they could not express in a structured questionnaire. The participants described the changes in the meaning they gave to roles in different areas of their lives - from the time of the disease's diagnosis. The subject of meaning in life in the present and the very near future did not include philosophical questions about the essence of life. The participants' point of view becomes very clearly focused on the small things that are important to them today.

From the analysis of the interviews in the study, it emerged that the meaning of life at the end of life exists midway between clear realizations about the "lived life" and knowledge of imminent death. Therefore, a certain acceptance of the situation exists, alongside a certain amount of denial, and those dealing with advanced disease swing back and forth between the two pillars of these complex structures.

In contrast to previous studies conducted mostly among healthy populations or among women who survived breast cancer (e.g., [37, 6, 38]), our study showed that people at the end of life who found some meaning in their lives are not intensively engaged in meaning-making processes. Therefore, meaning-making does not constitute a widespread coping strategy for patients at the end of life. Our findings confirm and expand Park's [11] model, which separates the meaning-making process from its result - meaning-made, and relates to the different roles of each stage of the process.

Shmotkin and Shrira [39, 40, 41, 42] argued that the search for meaning (meaning-making) has an adaptive role in mitigating the negative effects of difficult life events, and the associations or lack of associations between meaning-making and subjective well-being variables are dependent on their initial closeness to events of suffering and distress. In line with our findings that the existence of meaning (meaning-made) is related to quality of life, they suggest that subjective well-being and meaning in life may empower and strengthen each other when coping with situations of threat and distress. In these difficult situations, a higher level of subjective well-being is accompanied by a higher level of meaning-made. It is therefore possible that individuals with advanced cancer - for whom a long period has passed since the initial stressor (the diagnosis), and who have often and closely scrutinized the meaning of their condition - the existence of meaning in their lives is perceived more strongly and clearly; thus, they do not need to reassess it. The clear meaning of their lives contributes to positive coping with the condition [34]. The results of the qualitative part of the present study support the quantitative findings, which show that the vast majority of participants are not engaged in meaning-making processes at this stage in life. It seems that their understanding of the meaning of life – regarding both the positive and negative parts - are clear to them and directly influence the way they experience life at this stage.

In line with the findings of the study, both theorists and researchers found that towards the end of life, meaning and purpose in one's life were found necessary for the creation of personal well-being, even more so than physical symptoms, well-being or support [18, 21, 43, 44, 45]. Possible explanations for the associations between the meaning of life and quality of life, in general, and at the end of life in particular, can be found in Victor Frankel's [5] writings. Frankel refers to a sense of meaning in extreme situations. According to him, even when an individual cannot change his/her situation, the individual can change his/her outlook, even if there is no perspective of time in his life. Frankel argues that the individual can rise above external conditions. The natural tendency of people in any situation is to find meaning that will yield insights into their situation, and give them the feeling that their life was valuable, even if it is about to end. Frankel adds that this sense of existential meaning is directly related to low mental distress, and a general sense of life's value, regardless of the source of suffering [31]. Another explanation of the association between meaning and quality of life at the end of life can be found in the writings of Maslow [62], the father of the humanistic approach, although according to his theory of needs, Maslow argues that a sense of meaning and self-realization in life will be difficult to achieve unless one's basic physiological needs are met. According to Maslow, under certain conditions of disease or extreme physical conditions, it would be enough to satisfy certain basic needs in order to advance to the next level in the needs hierarchy [62]. This is because a sense of security in treatment, along with feelings of belonging and love, all serve to create a sense of respect and appreciation. These feelings can act as a moderator in the absence of basic needs, and help individuals achieve self-fulfillment and a sense of meaning in their life, which is necessary in order to feel satisfaction in life. At the same time, Maslow [62] argued that in physiologically extreme situations, meaning and realizations about life will, in most cases, be associated with the physiological and biological needs that enable survival (the need to breathe, drink, eat, sleep, and reproduce). Therefore, it can be assumed that the sick individual will redefine his concept of quality of life in a very different way from a person whose basic needs are fulfilled, and thus are not perceived as a significant concern. In his writings, Maslow [62] reiterates that he does not perceive the meaning of life as fundamentally different from other concepts related to quality of life. According to him, self-realization, satisfaction with life, and perceiving life as meaningful do not differ from one another; therefore, there is clearly a strong association among these variables. To sum up, scholars of science and research, who examined the concept of finding meaning in life - regardless of whether it was analyzed, perceived as a separate concept from other quality of life concepts, related to death or dependent on other circumstances - always perceived it as a top priority, in relation to life and quality of life. The present study reinforces this notion about the importance of a sense of meaning in life, even in close proximity to death.

The findings of the qualitative study broaden and deepen the understanding of meaning-making processes and meaning-made at the end of life. The participants described the feeling of "hanging between life and death" and the experiences they undergo, as well as their relationships, the meaning they give to their bodies, and the role of treatments in their lives. They feel they are constantly moving back and forth between the experience of life and the experience of death. The complexity of the participants' experience which, on the one hand, requires them to "adhere to life," whilst simultaneously "preparing for death," is referred to as the "intermediate area" experience in the psycho-oncology literature [47, 48, 49]. Being in this area makes it possible to simultaneously contain the duality of life and death, without trying to resolve it or having to choose between hope and perhaps denial or between acceptance and separation [47]. According to psychoanalytic theories, this duality exists throughout life. However, it takes on a more central role when the experience of life is threatened and the person himself is aware of his imminent death, and receives further confirmation of such from the environment, whether in words or behavior. Salander and Lilliehorn49 specify the existence of an "intermediate zone" of partial awareness, ambiguity and hope, which allows cancer patients to continue to live, despite the knowledge of their imminent death. They describe in depth how patients with advanced lung cancer cope with a real threat to their lives. Apparently, the knowledge that medicine cannot cure metastatic lung disease does not eliminate the hope of prolonging life, of relieving suffering and enjoying the remaining time; thus, these contrasts simply coexist. Winnicott [50] also wrote about the existence of an intermediate area where "manipulations" and "cover stories" exist, meaning, people "pretend" or tell themselves "stories," due to the difficulty of coping with a particular reality. People suffering from life-threatening illnesses play with reality by engaging in a sort of self-deception: although patients are well aware of their actual medical condition, they choose to swing back and forth between reality and fantasy, because it makes their lives easier [51].

The painful emotional experiences that accompany cancer patients at the end of life touch upon the cornerstones of human existence, and raise issues related to the meaning and/or meaninglessness of life [52, 53]. Many participants described the changes in the meaning they give to roles in different areas of their lives from the perspective of the pre-/post-diagnosis of the disease, up to their current stage. When their immediate future seems final, the focus shifts to the here and now, to enjoying the simplest everyday pleasures and the people closest to them. It is possible that for those whose time in the world is limited for various reasons, the understanding of the fragility of life influences their choices and social goals, regardless of age or culture [54, 55]. In these situations, individuals' goals and motivations change completely; they minimize their social networks and relations, and focus on their closest and most meaningful relationships [54, 55]. Accordingly, the participants did not discuss the need for meaning-making in their lives at this stage, but several participants described the meaning-making process that characterized their coping with earlier stages of the disease; for example, coming closer to God and even becoming religious, acquiring new hobbies, and planning trips for when they are healthy.

The participants' reference to the subject of meaning in the context of the present and the very near future did not include philosophical questions about the essence of life, and their point of view became clearly focused on the small things that were currently important to them. Spending time with family and very close friends and a physical feeling of well-being were mentioned as the most common desires. This finding is consistent with the findings of studies indicating that relationships with family and significant others are a particularly important source of meaning in life among patients with advanced cancer [19, 32, 55]. The discussion on meaning was characterized by the constant transition between the meaning things have today, and/or which they had in the past, and the meaning they will have in a future, in which the participants will not share. The discussion related to attributing meaning to one's life and death; sometimes the participants talked about meaning that included plans for the future and the meaning of their imminent death in the same sentence. Acceptance of death and active preparation for death were discussed by a minority of the participants. It is clear that those who had dealt with the issue of separation turned both the separation and the preparation into something that gave meaning to their lives. I got the feeling that most patients would have liked to talk more about their upcoming deaths, about their fears and the preparations they would like to make. They touched upon these issues in conversation alongside fantasies about life events they would still be privileged to take part in. The general impression from the discussion with the participants was that even when it was clear that they had completely accepted their situation, the acceptance of death was coupled with a certain denial of the situation.

Religion and faith play a very prominent role in the discussion of meaning, and were mentioned in interviews mainly as sources that provide meaning, but also undermine it. It is possible that since the theological conception of finding meaning in life in the three major monotheistic religions - Christianity, Islam, and Judaism – were all guided by the belief in the existence of one God, there was no difference in the ways the patients in the study related to religion and belief. All of the religious participants, along with some of the secular participants, described *faith* as a significant resource that helps provide hope and meaning at this stage. The participants described their conversations with God, prayers of strength and the experience of coming closer to religion, alongside questions about the world to come. Qualitative research that deals with the spiritual needs of cancer patients at the end of life [56] found that, at this stage, spiritual needs, and in particular embracing religion, are closely related to purpose and meaning in life, and that many patients change their definition of spirituality and their original feelings about religion with reference to God and religious symbols. It was also found that embracing religion in times of crisis may provide an opportunity for people to discover purpose and meaning in their lives [57]. In addition to the strengthening and positive aspects described by the participants, one of the participants recounted an ongoing state of conflict with regard to faith. In another interview, the belief in the world to come resulted in anxieties related to reward and punishment, as well as to questions of what might be awaiting one after death. Accordingly, studies that examined spiritual and existential coping strategies among advanced cancer patients found that while some participants' level of religiosity related to meaning-made and a high level of quality of life, for others it was related to questions about their belief, which they felt was being tested - and lower meaning-made levels [55, 58].

The Meaning of the Body: All participants referred to the physical changes they underwent: extreme thinness, hair loss, great weakness, loss of internal and external organs, etc.; the centrality of the body in the context of meaning in life was very noticeable. Similar to the descriptions given in this study regarding the influence of body image and changes - which were sometimes described as a betrayal of an external object, and at other times as mourning over the loss of one's internal identity - studies show that body depletion and poor body image were found to be major causes of psychological distress, and are related to the perception that life is lacking in value and low in meaning [59, 60].

RECOMMENDATIONS FOR PRACTICE

The present study has a number of practical implications for professionals in multi-disciplinary fields who treat cancer patients at the end of life. The large number of deaths from cancer worldwide indicates growing populations of advanced-stage cancer patients. Therefore, knowledge about these patients' ability to cope is of crucial importance to healthcare workers seeking to adapt their professional assistance to the patient's needs, especially when there are no more treatments to offer and the role of medical care is limited.

Although the prevailing tendency in the literature is to relate to the near end of life as a period that emphasizes a sense of meaninglessness and lack of purpose in life [4, 20], most of the participants in the study reported a high level of meaning in their lives and a low level of meaning-making. The findings of the present study indicate a strong correlation between meaning-made and quality of life, thus supporting prior studies that examined meaning-focused treatment programs [18, 52, 61]. However, the understanding that the meaning-making process is apparently not a widespread coping strategy among cancer patients at the end of life emphasizes the importance of focusing these programs on strengthening the existing sense of meaning, rather than on activities that encourage meaning-making processes and the improvement of a sense of meaning. In other words, it is necessary to strengthen the values and beliefs that the patient feels encourage him to continue to treasure life. Nietzsche [63] wrote: "He who has a why to live can bear almost any how." Strengthening the "why," means that the goal of life - as declared by the patient at the end of his life, whatever it is - will strengthen the patient, so that he can withstand the terrible "how" of his existence. Therefore, individual and group treatments in this field should focus mainly on the experience itself - what the patient receives from life at the moment - the things he finds beautiful and true, the connections with the people he loves, existence alongside objects that are dear to his heart, and strengthening the values he believes in, rather than new or additional meaning-making, as some of the meaning-making-focused programs suggest [48]. Additionally, the existing meaning-focused programs require a relatively long group or individual intervention (8 weeks) - a very long period of time for cancer patients near the end of life. Therefore, it is recommended to build short-term programs of two or three sessions, focused on the existing meaning as mentioned above, and on individual programs that can take place both in home and hospital settings.

The current study emphasizes the importance of the physical component of the growing-ever-nearer-to- death experience (the tribulations of the body during the course of the disease), a central issue that influences the creation of a sense of meaning at this stage, and suggests that meaning-focused programs should also include aspects that deal with the meaning patients attribute to the experience of body changes and deterioration. Therapy with a sensory dimension that includes pleasant physical experiences, such as foot or scalp massage, can also allow patients to feel positive physical experiences. The combination of family members or other close individuals in therapy, together with positive sensory elements, may allow the integration of two sources of meaning that most patients indicated as having meaning, in addition to providing an intimate experience that has been noted as lacking.

The intimate relationships built in a very short time period with the patients at these stages of life often enables the occurrence of certain processes which, in a normative situation, would take a long time. Professional and responsible use of work with meaning at these stages can be a meaningful experience for family members and therapists, as described in the attached reflection.

A Personal Reflection (Written by Adi Ivzori -Erel)

For the past 18 years, I have been working as a social worker with end-of-life patients. Over the past decade, my focus has been specifically on oncology patients. My initial working assumption was that the best place to live and die, at the end of life, is at home; that the home would be the center of meaning during the final stage of life, and that people at this stage would find it difficult to find meaning and be engaged in adapting their previous beliefs to a new situation. Moreover, I was also sure I would discover that the most important task of accompanying patients at the end of life would be to help them separate from their loved ones.

I approached this study with the conviction that I wanted to deepen my knowledge of theories that deal with the care of these patients, as well as gain a deeper understanding of the experiences they undergo. I approached a subject which I thought I understood, as a lecturer and therapist with past knowledge and experience. I was, therefore, extremely surprised to discover that many of the study's conclusions differed from my initial beliefs and assumptions, and from the significant body of knowledge I had accumulated over the course of my work, which was in line with the accepted knowledge in the literature review.

In every interview I conducted and in every meeting during the study, I discovered new insights and gained further understanding and knowledge about meaning of life at the end of life. At first, when I asked questions in a weak and apprehensive voice, the answers I received were also weak and apprehensive. I felt that people were afraid to allow me to enter into the realm of their real experience with the end stage of cancer - in which the rules change, meanings change, the external environment changes, the personal environment (the physical body) changes, and thoughts change. The first few times I asked the participants to share the meaning of their home as a place of care for them, I was surprised to hear their answers: "... the meaning of home has changed for me, I no longer feel that I belong to it"; "... my body has become foreign to me"; "all of the things that were important to me in the past seem meaningless today."

The meaning of the reference to time is another insight that emerged from the study. Previously, my work with patients had mostly been based on past understandings - the patients' need to summarize the life that was, and part from their significant others. However, during and after this study, the new discussions that emerged were fascinating, and along with the new understandings, my therapeutic sessions quickly changed their frame of reference - from a major preoccupation with what had *been*, to a common attempt to understand what was happening *now*. I became preoccupied with new questions: *What has changed? How does life continue with such a short "expiration date"?* I have studied and am still learning this new language - a language that swings back and forth from knowledge to denial, which perceives a harsh continuum of contrary processes that cannot be separated from one another. During the period preceding death, the present and the future continue to exist relentlessly side by side, despite the patient's clear knowledge of the disease's inevitable progression and the cognitive, social and psychological difficulties the patients experience. Moreover, patients have difficulty understanding what is occurring - to them and around them - often experiencing a lack of familiarity with what is happening to their bodies and souls, in their family, and in their immediate surroundings. I found myself drawing maps with the patients to help them orient themselves, in an attempt to make sense of their chaos. I tried to let them lead me towards those things which were meaningful to them. There were long conversations about personal objects from the past: a doll they had loved in childhood, a dog that had accompanied them through life, imaginary friends from childhood who had now returned and shared their inner conversations – and with whom chaotic and confused dialogues, reflecting their inner turmoil, could be conducted.

In the therapeutic sessions, when I "speak their language," with the words they choose to describe their situation, the word "death" rarely comes up in conversation. Sometimes, veiled references are made, such as "when the silence comes" or "in the end"; but more often than not, death is not mentioned at all, as if there is no need to talk about it directly. As one patient told me: "We do not talk all the time about the fact that we are alive; there is no need to talk about the fact that we are dying all the time ... When you say *future*, you mean the future in which you live, but when I say *future,* I mean the future in which I am dead."

The number of therapeutic meetings with my dying patients are few, too few ... three sessions, more or less. We do not determine ahead of time whether the next meeting will happen or not, so every therapeutic session includes a beginning, a middle and an end; the sessions often last about two hours. The same question opens every session: "Tell me what's important to you, so that I can get to know you, and will be able to accompany you in the process you are going through now." Another question I now include in light of insights I gained from the study is: "What do you want us to focus on in this meeting: about what happened (in the past), about what is happening now (in the present) or about what will happen (in the future)?" This question opens up the possibility of talking about the experiences of the present and the future, and these questions, almost without exception, enabled a discussion that was led by the patient. During the sessions with the patients, I regularly put in writing almost every word that was said. At some point, the patients begin to speak more slowly. No one ever asked me not to write. In most of the following meetings, if there was one, we would read some of what was written down in the previous meeting, discuss it, add to it, and sometimes we arranged it as a present to give to a loved one.

With parents of young children, I often write a story for the children, a story that focuses on the good and on strengthening shared experiences. These stories provide reinforcement, a sense of pride and great love. The aspect of missing out on the life that was not lived is not mentioned in these stories, but it does have a place in most of the counseling sessions in various ways. During these sessions, the discourse about the life that was, and the life that will not be, reveal a sense of missed opportunities – about events that were incomplete or missed experiences. This was especially noticeable among parents of young children.

Over the years, I have had the unique opportunity to work with patients from different cultures and religions, including Jews, Christians, Muslims, Druze and Bedouins. Each culture has its own special emphasis, but the general discussion during these life stages is universal; the same questions apply to everyone. While the answers differ from person to person, they are also amazingly similar. However, there are certain differences. The issue of meaning in life in the Arab society in Israel focuses more on family honor and personal dignity, concerns like: 'What will be said about me after my death?' Therefore, a question I often asked Arab patients is: "What would a close person tell me about you that would help me get to know you?" I might actually then ask a family member or close friend to tell me about the patient, so that I can get to know him/her. These words are transcribed for the purpose of talking with the patient, but relatives also give testimonials, as this may be a first-time opportunity to say, out loud, what they think of their father/mother and so on.

In conclusion, there is a tremendous advantage to learning coping methods and experiencing a disease at the end of life, firsthand from those who are dealing with it. These firsthand accounts provide therapists with the ability to observe and adapt the real needs of these patients in the context of demographic and environmental conditions, the weakened body, social and internal relations, and the complex dual meaning of a life that is ending, but still wants to burn bright. The research and therapeutic experience of working with these patients emphasizes the need to expand the theoretical and empirical knowledge and understanding of the complexity of palliative treatment at the end of life. I feel these encounters are a great privilege, and that we still have much to learn about the meaning of life and coping with terminal illness at the end of life.

REFERENCES

[1] National Cancer Institute. (2018). *NCI Cancer Statistics.* Retrieved from https://www.cancer.gov/about-cancer/understanding/statistics.

[2] World Health Organization. (2008). *The World health report: 2008: Reducing the risks, promoting healthy life.*

[3] Park, C. L. (2010). Making sense of the meaning literature: an integrative review of meaning making and its effects on adjustment to stressful life events. *Psychological Bulletin, 136*(2), 257.

[4] Park, C. L. (2017). Unresolved Tensions in the Study of Meaning in Life. *Journal of Constructivist Psychology, 30*(1), 69-73.

[5] Janoff-Bulman, R. (1992). *Shattered Assumptions: Towards a New Psychology of Trauma.* New York, NY: Free Press.

[6] Park, C. L., & Folkman, S. (1997). Meaning in the context of stress and coping. *Review of General Psychology*, *1*(2), 115-144.

[7] Steger, M. F. (2012). Experiencing meaning in life: Optimal functioning at the nexus of well-being, psychopathology, and spirituality. In P. T. Wong (Ed.), *The human quest for meaning: Theories, research, and applications* (2nd ed., pp. 165-184). N Y: Taylor & Francis Group, LLC.

[8] Wortman, C. B., & Silver, R. C. (1987). Coping with irrevocable loss. In American Psychological Association Convention, In VandenBos G.R., Bryant B.K., (Eds.), *Catactysms, Crises, and Catastrophes Psychology in Action* (pp. 185–235). Washington, DC: American Psychological Association.

[9] Affleck, G., & Tennen, H. (1991). Social comparison and coping with major medical problems. In J. Suls & T. A. Wills (Eds.), *Social comparison: Contemporary theory and research* (pp. 369–393). Hillsdale, NJ: Erlbaum.

[10] Folkman, S. (1997). Positive psychological states and coping with severe stress. *Social Science & Medicine*, *45*(8), 1207-1221.

[11] Park, C. L. (2011). *Meaning, coping, and health. Oxford handbook of stress, health, and coping*, (pp. 227-241). Oxford: Oxford University Press.

[12] Reker, G. T., & Wong, P. T. (2012). Personal meaning in life and psychosocial adaptation in the later years. In P. T. Wong (Ed.), *The human quest for Meaning: Theories, research, and applications* (2nd ed., pp. 433-456). New York, N.Y: Taylor & Francis Group, LLC.

[13] Reker, G. T., & Wong, P. T. (1988). Aging as an individual process: Toward a theory of personal meaning. In J. E. Birren., & V. L. Bengston (Eds.), *Emergent theories of aging* (pp. 214–246). New York, N.Y: Springer.

[14] Folkman, S. (2008). The case for positive emotions in the stress process. *Anxiety, Stress, and Coping*, *21*(1), 3-14.

[15] Gillies, J., & Neimeyer, R. A. (2006). Loss, grief, and the search for significance: Toward a model of meaning reconstruction in bereavement. *Journal of Constructivist Psychology*, *19*(1), 31-65.

[16] White, C. A. (2004). Meaning and its measurement in psychosocial oncology. *Psycho-Oncology*, 13(7), 468-481.

[17] Park, C. L., Edmondson, D., Fenster, J. R., & Blank, T. O. (2008). Meaning making and psychological adjustment following cancer: the mediating roles of growth, life meaning, and restored just-world beliefs. *Journal of Consulting and Clinical Psychology*, *76*(5), 863-875.

[18] Breitbart, W., Rosenfeld, B., Pessin, H., Applebaum, A., Kulikowski, J., &Lichtenthal, W. G. (2015). Meaning-Centered Group Psychotherapy: An Effective Intervention for Improving Psychological Well-Being in Patients with Advanced Cancer. *Journal of Clinical Oncology*, *33*(7), 749-754.

[19] Bentur, N., Stark, D. Y., Resnizky, S., & Symon, Z. (2014). Coping strategies for existential and spiritual suffering in Israeli patients with advanced cancer. *Israel Journal of Health Policy Research*, *3*(21).

[20] Rosenfeld, B., Saracino, R., Tobias, K., Masterson, M., Pessin, H., Applebaum, A., ... & Breitbart, W. (2017). Adapting Meaning-Centered Psychotherapy for the palliative care setting: Results of a pilot study. *Palliative Medicine, 31*(2), 140-146.

[21] Cohen, S. R., Boston, P., Mount, B. M., & Porterfield, P. (2001). Changes in quality of life following admission to palliative care units. *Palliative Medicine, 15*(5), 363-371.

[22] Morita, T., Murata, H., Kishi, E., Miyashita, M., Yamaguchi, T., &Uchitomi, Y. (2009). Meaninglessness in terminally ill cancer patients: a randomized controlled study. *Journal of Pain and Symptom Management, 37*(4), 649-658.

[23] Lethborg, C., Aranda, S., Cox, S., & Kissane, D. (2007). To what extent does meaning mediate adaptation to cancer? The relationship between physical suffering, meaning in life, and connection to others in adjustment to cancer. *Palliative & Supportive Care, 5*(4), 377-388.

[24] Rodin, G., Lo, C., Mikulincer, M., Donner, A., Gagliese, L., & Zimmermann, C. (2009). Pathways to distress: the multiple determinants of depression, hopelessness, and the desire for hastened death in metastatic cancer patients. *Social Science & Medicine, 68*(3), 562-569.

[25] Wilson, K. G., Chochinov, H. M., McPherson, C. J., LeMay, K., Allard, P., Chary, S. & Feininger, R. L. (2007). Suffering with advanced cancer. *Journal of Clinical Oncology, 25*(13), 1691-1697.

[26] Wright, S. T., Breier, J. M., Depner, R. M., Grant, P. C., & Lodi-Smith, J. (2017). Wisdom at the end of life: Hospice patients' reflections on the meaning of life and death. *Counselling Psychology Quarterly*, 1-24.

[27] Breitbart, W., Rosenfeld, B., Gibson, C., Pessin, H., Poppito, S., Nelson, C., ... & Olden, M. (2010). Meaning-centered group psychotherapy for patients with advanced cancer: a pilot randomized controlled trial. *Psycho-Oncology, 19*(1), 21-28.

[28] Hernandez, D. (2017). Life Meaning in Patients Diagnosed With End-Stage Liver Cancer: An Interpretive Phenomenological Approach. *Paper presented at Sigma Theta Tau International's 28th International Nursing Research Congress. STTI.*

[29] Kaufman, S.R. (2005). *And a time to die: How American hospitals shape the end of life.* New York, NY: Scribner.

[30] Wrubel, J., Acree, M., Goodman, S., & Folkman, S. (2009). End of living: Maintaining a life world during terminal illness. *Psychology and Health, 24*(10), 1229-1243.

[31] Frankl, V. E. (1985). *Man's search for meaning.* New York, N.Y: Simon and Schuster.

[32] Scheffold, K., Mehnert, A., Müller, V., Koch, U., Härter, M., &Vehling, S. (2013). Sources of meaning in cancer patients–influences on global meaning, anxiety and depression in a longitudinal study. *European Journal of Cancer Care*, 23, 472–480.

[33] Steger, M. F., Frazier, P., Oishi, S., & Kaler, M. (2006). The meaning in life questionnaire: Assessing the presence of and search for meaning in life. *Journal of Counseling Psychology, 53*(1), 80-93.

[34] Cohen, S. R., Mount, B. M., Strobel, M. G., & Bui, F. (1995). The McGill Quality of Life Questionnaire: a measure of quality of life appropriate for people with advanced disease. A preliminary study of validity and acceptability. *Palliative Medicine, 9*(3), 207-219.

[35] Derogatis, L. R. (2001). *BSI 18, Brief Symptom Inventory 18: Administration, scoring and procedures manual.* NCS Pearson, Incorporated.

[36] Shkedi, A. (2003). *Words that try to touch: qualitative research - theory and practice.* Tel Aviv: Ramot - Tel Aviv University. (from Hebrew).

[37] Park, C. L., & George, L. S. (2013). Assessing meaning and meaning making in the context of stressful life events: Measurement tools and approaches. *The Journal of Positive Psychology*, 8(6), 483-504.

[38] Levkovich, I., Cohen, M., Pollack, S., Drumea, K., & Fried, G. (2016). Cancer-related fatigue and depression in breast cancer patients postchemotherapy: Different associations with optimism and stress appraisals—CORRIGENDUM. *Palliative & supportive care*, 14(5), 596-596.

[39] Shmotkin, D., & Shrira, A. (2012). On the distinction between subjective well-being and meaning in life: Regulatory versus reconstructive functions in the face of a hostile world. In P. T. P. Wong (Ed.), *The human quest for meaning: Theories, research, and applications* (2nd ed., pp. 143-163). New York, NY: Routledge.

[40] Shmotkin, D., & Shrira, A. (2013). Subjective well-being and meaning in life in a hostile world: Proposing a configurative perspective. In J. Hicks and C. Routledge (Eds.), *The experience of meaning in life: Classical perspectives, emerging themes, and controversies* (pp. 77-86). New York, NY: Springer.

[41] Shrira, A., Palgi, Y., Ben-Ezra, M., & Shmotkin, D. (2011). How subjective well-being and meaning in life interact in the hostile world? *Journal of Positive Psychology*, 6, 273-285. doi:10.1080/17439760.2011.577090.

[42] Shrira, A., Shmotkin, D., Palgi, Y., Soffer, Y., HamamaRaz, Y., Tal-Katz, P., Ben-Ezra, M., & Benight, C. C. (2015). How do meaning in life and positive affect regulate adaptation to stress? The case of firefighters following the Mount Carmel forest fire. *Israel Journal of Psychiatry and Related Sciences*, 52(3), 68-70.

[43] Breitbart, W., Poppito, S., Rosenfeld, B., Vickers, A. J., Li, Y., Abbey, J., & Cassileth, B. R. (2012). Pilot randomized controlled trial of individual meaning-centered psychotherapy for patients with advanced cancer. *Journal of Clinical Oncology*, 30(12), 1304-1309.

[44] Mok, E., Lau, K. P., Lai, T., & Ching, S. (2012). The meaning of life intervention for patients with advanced-stage cancer: development and pilot study. *Oncology Nursing Forum*, 39 (6), 480-488.

[45] Guerrero-Torrelles, M., Monforte-Royo, C., Rodríguez-Prat, A., Porta-Sales, J., & Balaguer, A. (2017). Understanding meaning in life interventions in patients with advanced disease: A systematic review and realist synthesis. *Palliative Medicine*, 31(9), 798-813.

[46] Maslow, A. (1962). Toward a psychology of being. Princeton, NJ: D. Van Nostrana Company, Inc.

[47] Hales, S., Lo, C., & Rodin, G. (2010). *Managing Cancer and Living Meaningfully (CALM) treatment manual: an individual psychotherapy for patients with advanced cancer*. Toronto, Canada: Princess Margaret Hospital, University Health Network.

[48] Salander, P. (2012). Cancer and "playing" with reality: Clinical guidance with the help of the intermediate area and disavowal. *Acta Oncologica*, 51(4), 541-560.

[49] Salander, P., & Lilliehorn, S. (2016). To carry on as before: A meta-synthesis of qualitative studies in lung cancer. *Lung Cancer*, 99, 88-93.

[50] Winnicott, D. W. (1986). *The theory of the parent-infant relationship. Essential papers on object relations*, NYU Press, 233-253.

[51] Basch, M. F. (1983). The perception of reality and the disavowal of meaning. *The Annual of Psychoanalysis*, 11, 125-153.

[52] Breitbart, W., & Heller, K. S. (2003). Reframing hope: Meaning-centered care for patients near the end of life. *Journal of Palliative Medicine*, 6(6), 979-988.

[53] Diaz-Frutos, D., Baca-Garcia, E., García-Foncillas, J., & López-Castroman, J. (2016). Predictors of psychological distress in advanced cancer patients under palliative treatments. *European Journal of Cancer Care, 25(4),* 608-615.

[54] Carstensen, L. L. (1995). Evidence for a life-span theory of socioemotional selectivity. Current *Directions in Psychological Science*, 4(5), 151-156.

[55] Kissane, D. W., Lethborg, C. E., & Kelly, B. (2012). Spiritual and religious coping with cancer. In Grassi, L., &Riba, M. (Eds.), *Clinical Psycho-Oncology: An International Perspective* (pp. 281-295). West Sussex, UK: John Wiley & Sons Ltd.

[56] Hermann, C. P. (2001). Spiritual needs of dying patients: a qualitative study. *Oncology Nursing Forum*, 28(1), 67-72.

[57] Steger, M. F., & Frazier, P. (2005). Meaning in life: One link in the chain from religiousness to well-being. *Journal of Counseling Psychology, 52*(4), 574.

[58] Blinderman, C. D., & Cherny, N. I. (2005). Existential issues do not necessarily result in existential suffering: lessons from cancer patients in Israel. *Palliative Medicine, 19*(5), 371-380.

[59] Diaz-Frutos, D., Baca-Garcia, E., García-Foncillas, J., & López-Castroman, J. (2016). Predictors of psychological distress in advanced cancer patients under palliative treatments. *European Journal of Cancer Care, 25(4),* 608-615.

[60] Vehling, S., Lehmann, C., Oechsle, K., Bokemeyer, C., Krüll, A., Koch, U., & Mehnert, A. (2012). Is advanced cancer associated with demoralization and lower global meaning? The role of tumor stage and physical problems in explaining existential distress in cancer patients. *Psycho-Oncology, 21*(1), 54-63.

[61] Chochinov, H. M. (2003). Thinking outside the box: depression, hope, and meaning at the end of life. *Journal of Palliative Medicine*, 6(6), 973-977.

[62] Maslow, A. (1962). Toward a psychology of being. Princeton, NJ: D. Van Nostrana Company, Inc.

[63] Nietzsche, F. (1889). Maxims and arrows. Twilight of the Idols, Aziloth Books. 23-27.

BIOGRAPHICAL SKETCHES

Adi Ivzori-Erel

Dr. Adi Ivzori-Erel is the Director of the Psycho-Social field in the Division of Family Medicine, and Associate Lecturer of Medical Education in the Ruth & Bruce Rappaport Faculty of Medicine at the Technion, Israel Institute of Technology. Adi received her BSW in Social Work in 1995 and her MSW in 2003 from the University of Haifa, Israel. She received her PhD in 2018 from the University of Haifa, Israel, in the area of psycho-oncology: "The Role of Sense of Place and Personal Resources in Meaning Making and Meaning Made and their Relationships with Quality of Life in Cancer Patients near the End of Life: A mixed methods approach." This study is one of the first to examine sense of place in relation to the treatment setting. As a result, this study expands the understanding of the meaning of the treatment setting at the end of life, and adds to what is known about the meaning-making process and meaning-made at the end of life.

She has 24 years of clinical experience as a social worker. She has worked in a geriatric assessment clinic treating a wide range of geriatric patients and their families, including Holocaust survivors, and has many years of experience guiding therapeutic and educational groups.

Adi has been working for over 10 years as a social worker in the Hospice Care Unit for Continued Treatment, Clalit Health Services, Haifa and Western Galilee, treating patients near the end of life and their family members.

She is also an Associate Lecturer and teaches medical students and interns in family medicine, courses on doctor-patient communication, end of life communication and palliative care, and plays a central role in promoting communication skills among family physicians and medical students.

Dr. Ivzori Erel was awarded a grant for her PhD dissertation from the National Insurance Institute and the Minister/Ministry of Welfare in Israel.

Her main areas of research are Medical Education, Psycho-Oncology, Communication and Multicultural aspects of Medical Education. She has published an article in *Medical Education Journal* and is currently writing several additional articles. She has presented numerous papers in conferences in Israel, and presented a number of papers in international medical education conferences.

Lee Greenblatt-Kimron

Dr. Lee Greenblatt-Kimron teaches in the Department of Social Work at Ariel University. She received her BSW in 1999 and her MSW from the School of Social Work, Haifa University, in 2009. She received her PhD in 2017 from the Gerontology Department, Haifa University, dissertation title: Heart Rate Variability, Physical and Mental Health among Holocaust Survivors: The Mediating Role of Cognitive Processes and Coping.

Lee Greenblatt-Kimron has 18 years of clinical experience as a social worker. She has worked in the health services field, treating a wide range of patients including oncology patients, victims of terror, and war and burn patients. She has also treated Holocaust survivors for several years, many of them in their homes, due to their deteriorating physical condition. She has volunteered in a running group for war veterans suffering from post-traumatic stress disorder, and established a walking group for Holocaust survivors. She has also treated victims of sexual trauma in a municipal sexual trauma clinic. Lee's main areas of clinical experience and research are psychological trauma, posttraumatic stress disorder, posttraumatic growth, gerontology, Holocaust survivors, stress and coping, health conditions and psycho-oncology diseases. She has published articles in international journals in these areas and has presented numerous papers in conferences in Israel.

Miri Cohen

Professor Miri Cohen is the Head of the School of Social Work, Faculty of Social Welfare and Health Sciences, University of Haifa. She received her BSW in Social Work from The Hebrew University of Jerusalem, Israel, in 1973 and her MSW from Haifa University in 1986. She received her PhD in 2000 from the Faculty of Medicine, the Technion, Israel, in the area of psycho-neuro-immunology. Between the years 2006- March 2012, she served as the Head of the Gerontology Department.

She is the current president of the Israel Psycho-Oncology Society, a board member of the Israeli Oncology Council, a board member of the journals *Psycho-Oncology* and *The Journal of Research in Social Work Practice* and a former Associate Editor of *Quality of Life Research*.

Miri Cohen has been awarded various grants, including The Israel Science Foundation, Israel Cancer Association, Müllerska Foundation and the Royal Swedish Academy of Sciences.

Her main areas of research are gerontology, Psycho-Neuro-Immunology (PNI), psycho-oncology, stress and coping, multicultural aspects of psycho-social and health care using advanced research methodologies.

She has published more than one hundred papers in refereed journals and several books and chapters in edited books. Many of her papers have been published in leading journals such as *Cancer, Breast Cancer Research and Therapy, International Journal of cancer, Psycho-Oncology, Journal of the Geriatric American Association,* and *Gerontologist*.

In: Palliative Care
Editor: Michael Silbermann

ISBN: 978-1-53616-199-1
© 2019 Nova Science Publishers, Inc.

Chapter 18

IMPORTANCE AND EFFECT OF RESEARCH FINDINGS ON THE OUTCOME OF CLINICAL PRACTICE OF PALLIATIVE CARE

Azar Naveen Saleem[1,*] *and Azza Adel Hassan*[1,2,†]
[1]National Center for Cancer Care and Research, Hamad Medical Corporation, Doha, Qatar
[2]Cancer Management & Research, Medical Research Institute, Alexandria University, Alexandria, Egypt

ABSTRACT

Palliative care began with a focus on the care of the dying. Dr. Cicely Saunders first articulated her ideas about modern hospice care in the late 1950s based on careful observation of dying patients. She advocated that only an interdisciplinary team could relieve the "total pain" of a dying person, and the team concept is still at the core of palliative care [3]. This observation of Dr. Saunders was the first research which paved the way for modern palliative medicine.

Supportive and palliative care has been recognized as an important component of quality health care for all patients with advanced or incurable diseases. The last 25 years have witnessed tremendous research in the field of palliative and end of life care. This has greatly improved our understanding of the impact of life limiting diseases on patients, their families, physicians and other members of the health care team. It has also shown that palliative interventions can improve patient and family outcomes and significantly reduce health care costs.

In recent times, research in palliative care has become quite exciting. It has brought substantial recognition and benefits to the field of palliative care around the globe. It has also contributed significantly towards improving clinical practice and has been translated into effective patient care.

There has been increasing awareness over the years about the concept of research in palliative medicine. However, it is known that there is still a significant gap which can be

---

* Corresponding Author's E-mail: azarnavin@gmail.com.
† Corresponding Author's E-mail: newazza@gmail.com.

filled by quality research and its application. Unlike other specialties, palliative care faces a lot of unique challenges which has hindered the growth of research. Palliative care researchers constantly face distinctive ethical problems and hindrances that extend far beyond those of standard research projects. Practical difficulties in palliative medicine research include high rates of loss of follow up due to physical inability, mental disability or death. Data collected from primary care givers (patient surrogate) may be subject to bias and other limitations. Funding allocation for research in palliative care has traditionally been quite limited, even in developed countries. In spite of all these limitations, research in palliative care has a bright future.

Future research in palliative care should focus on collaborative multi center studies, advanced research methodologies, policies and procedures. The future researches in palliative medicine should also focus its vison towards the geriatric population.

Keywords: Palliative care, end of life, research, quality of life

1. INTRODUCTION

Palliative care is defined by the World Health Organization as

"an approach that improves the quality of life of patients and their families facing the problem associated with life-threatening illness, through the prevention and relief of suffering by means of early identification and impeccable assessment and treatment of pain and other problems, physical, psychosocial and spiritual" [1].

The last 25 years have witnessed tremendous research in the field of palliative and end of life care. This has greatly improved our understanding of the impact of life limiting diseases on patients, their families, physicians and other members of the health care team. It has also shown that palliative interventions can improve patient and family outcomes and significantly reduce health care costs.

There has been a pattern change in the field of research in medicine which has moved away from the conventional speculative perceptive pattern towards evidence-based medicine (EBM). The multifarious issues of palliative care and terminal care involves considerations of the patient's social, physical, psychological and religious needs. Hence statistically significant benefits may be minimal in the field of palliative medicine and may not be related to health significance. The characteristic treatment *versus* placebo comparison required by the benchmark methodology of randomized controlled trials (RCTs) is not always satisfying. Also, the field of palliative care covers a diverse group of chronic and non-curable diseases and is no longer limited to malignancy. One of the major challenges in palliative care research is the difficulty in achieving adequate sample sizes; this can then affect the validity of the study. It is difficult to use controls in a dying patient and high patient turnover rates due to death results in short follow up durations. Compared to standard EBM protocols, palliative care needs specific tools to address its unique challenges. Non-RCT approaches of comparable value, rationality and magnitude steered by shared research networks using a 'mixed methods approach' are likely to pose the correct clinical questions and derive evidence-based yet clinically relevant outcomes [2].

Superior palliative and end of life care shall be best established by excellent research work that can provide a powerful and substantial proof. Developing such a proof is necessary to understand and adapt new changes into usual clinical practice. It is also vital that research outcomes in palliative and end of life care should be consistent, legitimate, and applicable.

2. HISTORY OF RESEARCH AND ITS IMPACT IN PALLIATIVE CARE MEDICINE

Numerous studies have been conducted all over the world in the field of palliative care medicine. In this chapter, we shall look at the history and impact of research in the field of palliative care around the globe. Palliative care began with a focus on the care of the dying. Dr. Cicely Saunders first articulated her ideas about modern hospice care in the late 1950s based on the careful observation of dying patients. She advocated that only an interdisciplinary team could relieve the "total pain" of a dying person in the context of his or her family, and the team concept is still at the core of palliative care [3]. The observation of Dr. Saunders itself was the first research which paved the way for modern palliative medicine. There is still a great need for effective research in the field of palliative care, in order to identify existing gaps and improve care for the dying and those in pain.

In 1997 the Institute of Medicine report "Approaching Death: improving care at the end of life" (M. I. Field and C. K. Cassel, editors) documented glaring deficiencies in end-of-life care in the United States [3]. At the time, this held true globally and it paved the way for multiple ground breaking research studies.

In 2010 a landmark study by Temel et al. looked at the benefit of early referral to palliative care for best supportive care plus standard oncology care vs standard oncology care alone. It gained widespread attention as it demonstrated improved survival and quality of life among lung cancer patients who received palliative care in addition to standard oncology care. Although the study was not powered for survival as the primary outcome, the results were unambiguous. The findings are unlikely to represent a type I error given that this experimental design supports earlier observational population-based studies [4]. This study had a great impact in the field of palliative medicine and created significant awareness about the necessity for early referral to palliative care.

Usual types of research seen in palliative care are retrospective studies, file and chart reviews, cross sectional studies, case reports and case-control studies. A major limitation of palliative care research is the difficulty in implementing longitudinal designs. Most interventional studies, especially randomized clinical trials, require longitudinal data. Regrettably, these studies have their limitations in applicability with respect to the field of palliative care. Studies involving patients with terminal illnesses are intrinsically limited by a short period of observation. Often it is only possible to monitor a specific outcome of interest within this short timeframe (e.g., Do Not Attempt to Resuscitate (DNAR) decision, existence of advance directives). Compared with other areas of clinical and behavioral research, use of surrogate or proxy respondents is very prevalent in terminal care research. Often, data is gathered from patient's families or caregivers. This reflects the fact that many dying patients are unable to participate in crucial methods of data gathering.

Over the last decade various organizations have called for the development of palliative care teams with the necessary skill and expertise to organize and conduct biomedical, clinical, behavioural and health services research for patients with serious and chronic illness. This has been stated in the reports of the Institute of Medicine in 1997, 2001 and 2003; the Research Task Force of the American Academy of Hospice and Palliative Medicine in 2003; and the National Institute of Health's (NIH) State of the Science Conference on End-of-Life Care in 2004. This will help to establish research networks and conduct multi-site studies to develop the knowledge base of the field and contribute to the goal of bringing an evidence-based approach to palliative care practice [7].

3. THE CHALLENGES IN PALLIATIVE CARE RESEARCH

Palliative care researchers face distinctive ethical problems and obstacles that extend far beyond those of standard research studies. Other limitations include the fragile population from which study subjects are enrolled and the patient and family's emotional distress. There are ethical challenges involved in using a medication or treatment on a trial basis in patients who wish only for comfort care. Practical difficulties in palliative medicine research include high rate of loss of follow up due to physical inability, mental inability and death.

There is a general consensus that end-of-life care must focus on the dying patients as well as their families. Dying patients typically desire that their families play a dominant role in end-of-life care decisions (Hopp 2000; Puchalski et al. 2000). For these reasons, it is appropriate to include family members in end-of-life care research.[5] In most studies conducted in terminal or dying patients, often the data source is the primary care giver. Data collection in this situation has limitations due to a lack of defined rules for gathering data from the patient's care giver rather than the patient. Often proxies may be the source of data even in situations where patients are capable of participating in data gathering. Almost totally absent are clear descriptions of justification for selection of the data source when there are more than one eligible primary care giver or family member. Most research in palliative care, especially those involving terminal or dying patients, is based on the contentment of patient's care givers and family members and not on the evaluations of patients themselves.

In studies where data has been collected from both patients and their care givers, significant disparity has been noted in reporting intensity of symptoms and comfort levels. This was especially notable with respect to pain, sleep patterns, gastrointestinal symptoms, appetite and bowel movements. This finding was reinforced in the study of Higginson and McCarthy 1993; Hinton 1996b; Layde et al.1995 [5]. Some studies suggest that there is a difference in perception of symptoms between the patient and caregiver, with typically lower quality of life and higher discomfort reported by family members. Nurses' ratings of patient symptoms, pain, and distress are typically more compatible with those of patients than family members' ratings.

A review of research funding in palliative care indicates that funding for palliative care research has been quite limited even in the developed countries. Each year, an estimated 19 million people need palliative care worldwide.

The UK is considered a worldwide leader in palliative care, end of life care and research and a nation with positive influence towards end of life care around the globe. Palliative care is a significant component of the UK National Health Service (NHS) and health care services in many other developed nations. Palliative care professionals in UK have already expressed serious concerns about lack of research in this field and underuse of existing research.

Research in this area remains underfunded in the UK compared to other specialties. Less than 0.3% of the £500 million spent on cancer research is allocated to palliative care, with funding for non-cancer conditions likely to be even less [6]. Moreover, there are studies which suggest that medical care for patients with advanced illness is characterized by inadequately treated physical distress, fragmented care systems, poor communication between doctors, patients, and families and enormous strains on family and support systems.

4. A BRIEF OVERVIEW OF SOME LANDMARK RESEARCHES IN PALLIATIVE CARE

There has been an increasing focus on palliative care research over the last two decades. It has brought substantial recognition and benefits to the field of palliative care around the globe. It has also contributed significantly towards improving clinical practice and has been translated into effective patient care.

This section shall focus on some of the ground breaking researches in palliative medicine looking at the influence of an early referral process, symptom assessment, symptom management, the impact of psychological support, the impact of social support, the benefits of communication and quality of end of life care.

A study with the research question "Is the quality of palliative care provided by dedicated palliative care units better than that of palliative care consultation teams?" (The Optimal Delivery of Palliative Care, Jaclyn Yoong, and Peter Poon, 2008) [8] was conducted at 77 inpatient facilities in the United States and Puerto Rico, with both palliative care consultation services and palliative care units. The results of the study showed that end-of-life care provided by dedicated palliative care units was rated better than that of palliative care consultation teams by bereaved family members of deceased patients. The study also shows that regardless, either palliative care model can play a key role in end-of-life care.

A 2016 meta-analysis of some clinical trials on early palliative care in adults with advanced cancer looked at the evidence for the effects of early palliative care on quality of life, survival, depression, and symptom intensity in people with advanced cancer. The meta-analysis included seven published studies and 20 ongoing studies. Most of the studies included participants older than 65 years of age on average, diagnosed with different tumor types and receiving treatment in tertiary care centers in North America. These studies compared early palliative care with standard oncological (cancer) care. All studies were funded by government agencies. The results of the meta-analysis and systematic review of the trials indicates that early palliative care interventions may have more beneficial effects on quality of life and symptom intensity among patients with advanced cancer than among those given usual/standard cancer care alone. It was also found that there is better family satisfaction with early palliative care [9].

There are many quality research studies which have focused on symptom assessment and management.

A 2015 study published in The American Academy of Hospice and Palliative Medicine journal aimed to validate the numerical rating scale (NRS) versions of Edmonton Symptom Assessment System (ESAS) and its revised version (ESAS-r). The study also looked at additional symptoms of constipation and sleep (CS) and assessed patient preference for either version. Sleep disturbance is common in patients with cancer but is not currently included in the ESAS. Outpatients with advanced cancer (N = 202) completed three assessments during a single clinic visit: ESAS-CS with an added time window of "past 24 hours"; ESAS-r-CS with a time window of "now" and symptom definitions; and the Memorial Symptom Assessment Scale (MSAS). Internal consistency was calculated using Cronbach's alpha. Paired t-tests compared ESAS-CS and ESAS-r-CS scores; these were correlated with MSAS using Spearman correlation coefficients. The results of the study showed that the ESAS-CS and ESAS-r-CS NRS versions are valid and reliable for measuring symptoms in this population of outpatients with advanced cancer. Although the ESAS-r-CS was preferred, patients favored the 24-hour time window of the ESAS-CS, which may also best characterize fluctuating symptoms [10].

A study looking at spirituality, religiosity, and spiritual pain among caregivers of patients with advanced cancer was published in the year 2012 in the American Journal of Hospice and Palliative Medicine. Caregivers (n = 43) of patients with advanced cancer in a palliative care outpatient clinic were interviewed with pre-determined demographic characteristics, religious affiliation and relationship to the patient. Levels of spirituality, religiosity, and spiritual pain were self-reported using numeric rating scales (0 = lowest; 10 = highest). The participants completed various validated questionnaires to assess sleep disturbance, psychosocial distress, coping skills and quality of life (QOL). The results showed that the majority of caregivers of patients with advanced cancer considered themselves spiritual and religious. Despite this, there is a high prevalence of spiritual pain in this population. Caregivers with spiritual pain experienced worse psychological distress and worse QOL. These findings support the importance of spiritual assessment and spiritual support for caregivers in this setting. The findings are of great significance as palliative care relies heavily on family and caretaker involvement [11].

End of life care is a very important pillar in palliative medicine. There have been many quality studies conducted in this area. A significant study titled "Factors considered important at the end of life by patients, family, physicians, and other care providers" was published in JAMA in 2000. It was a cross-sectional random stratified national survey conducted in March-August 1999. The study included four groups of respondents: seriously ill patients; recently bereaved family; physicians; and other care providers like nurses, social workers, chaplains and hospice volunteers. The results of the study showed that twenty-six items were consistently rated as being important across all four groups, with the main ones being pain and symptom management, preparation for death, achieving a sense of completion, decisions about treatment preferences, and being treated as a "whole person."

Eight items received strong importance ratings from patients but less from physicians (P < .001), including being mentally aware, having funeral arrangements planned, not being a burden, helping others, and coming to peace with God. Ten items had broad variation within as well as among the four groups, including decisions about life-sustaining treatments, dying at home, and talking about the meaning of death. Participants ranked freedom from pain most important and dying at home least important among nine major attributes [12].

5. THE FUTURE DIRECTION OF PALLIATIVE CARE RESEARCH

Research in palliative care medicine is multifaceted and has many inherent limitations. Future research in palliative care should be directed at addressing present gaps and bringing valuable improvement to the specialty. Researchers should give due consideration to appropriate case selection, stringent eligibility criteria, accurate recording of the process of care and detailed measurement of outcomes.

Researchers looking at patient experiences should make every effort possible to gather concerned data directly from patients. Data collection from primary care givers or family members, in necessary situations, should be restricted to visible activities of the patient. Information pertaining to the assessment of patient's symptoms and distress cannot be accurately obtained from the primary care givers or family members. Research protocols involving family members or caregivers should be based on well-framed criteria addressing concerns including:

(a) Why data is to be collected from the primary care giver and not the patient.
(b) What kind of information can be obtained from the primary care giver or the family member, and
(c) What are the circumstances under which information about the patient is obtained from the primary care giver.

Researchers should also develop and examine meaningful research questions and research domains, incorporate rigorous study designs that address potential limitations, mitigate bias or error, ensure quality control and support the formation of teams of transdisciplinary researchers.

The field of palliative medicine has been growing rapidly and is now in its seasoned phase, however research in the field has not kept up the pace and lags far behind.

There have been many positive changes over the last 25 years in palliative care research which has helped many people with life limiting illness.

Worldwide, the geriatric population has been growing steadily and is projected to rise further in the future. This will create an ever-increasing demand for palliative care in the geriatric population. Geriatric patients tend to have a myriad of chronic ailments, functional limitations, frailty and cognitive impairment. Consequently, they represent a high need group who are not well served in the current health care system. Future research in palliative care should also look towards addressing the unique needs of the geriatric population.

CONCLUSION

The current dearth of high quality research in palliative medicine compared to other specialities demands appropriate action to develop the knowledge base of palliative medicine and improve the standard of care for patients suffering from all life limiting illnesses. In order to improve the quality of research, researchers can benefit from collaborative multicentre studies so as to overcome the limitation of small numbers of eligible patients in a particular centre. Developing new palliative care policies and pathways to improve patient care and satisfaction should be based on sound research. The researches should be a logical examination done with a clear determination, based on noticeable experience in a neutral manner, guiding to the potential or credible answer to the exploratory question. Future studies should be a source of expanding our existing knowledge in palliative medicine and provide a better understanding of palliative care itself.

> "You matter because you are you, and you matter to the end of your life. We will do all we can not only to help you die peacefully, but also to live until you die."
> - Cicely Saunders

REFERENCES

[1] World Health Organization. *WHO Definition of Palliative Care* 2015 [cited 2015 16.05.2015]. Available online: http://www.who.int/cancer/palliative/definition/en/.

[2] Claire Visser, Gina Hadley and Bee Wee. Reality of evidence-based practice in palliative care. *Cancer Biology & Medicine*. 2015 Sep; 12(3): 193–200. doi: 10.7497/j.issn.2095-3941.2015.0041 PMC4607825, https://www.ncbi.nlm.nih.gov/pmc/articles/PMC4607825/.

[3] American Society of Haematology (ASH), *Palliative Care: An Historical Perspective*, Matthew J. Loscalzo: doi: 10.1182/asheducation-2008.1.465 ASH Education Book January 1, 2008 vol. 2008 no. 1 465. http://asheducationbook.hematologylibrary.org/content/2008/1/465.full.

[4] D C Currow, K Foley, S Y Zafar, J L Wheeler, and A P Abernethy., The need for a re-evaluation of best supportive care studies reported to date. *Br J Cancer*. 2011 Feb 1; 104(3): 390–391.

[5] Linda K. George. The Gerontologist: Research Design in End-of-Life Research. *The Gerontologist*, Vol. 42, Special Issue III, 86–98, https://academic.oup.com/gerontologist/issue/42/suppl_3.

[6] Higginson IJ. Research challenges in palliative and end of life care. *BMJ Supportive & Palliative Care* 2016;6:2-4. https://spcare.bmj.com/content/6/1/2.

[7] *National Palliative Care Research center* http:// www.npcrc.org/ content/ 15/ About-Palliative-Care.aspx#tabs-2453.

[8] Yoong, J., & Poon, P. (2018-04). *The Optimal Delivery of Palliative Care*. In (Ed.), 50 Studies Every Palliative Care Doctor Should Know. Oxford, UK: Oxford University Press, Retrieved 20 Sep. 2018, from http://oxfordmedicine.com/view/10.1093/med/9780190658618.001.0001/med-9780190658618-chapter-5.

[9] Haun MW, Estel S, Rücker G, Friederich H, Villalobos M, Thomas M, Hartmann M. Early palliative care for adults with advanced cancer. *Cochrane Database of Systematic Reviews 2017*, Issue 6. Art. No.: CD011129. DOI: 10.1002/14651858.CD011129.pub2 https://www.ncbi.nlm.nih.gov/pubmed/28603881 (PUBMED).

[10] Modified Edmonton Symptom Assessment System including constipation and sleep: validation in outpatients with cancer. *J Pain Symptom Manage*. 2015 May;49(5):945-52. doi: 10.1016/j. jpainsymman. 2014.10.013. Epub 2014 Dec 15. https://www.ncbi.nlm.nih.gov/pubmed/25523890 (PUBMED).

[11] Marvin Omar Delgado-Guay. Spirituality, Religiosity, and Spiritual Pain among Caregivers of Patients with Advanced Cancer. *The American Journal of Hospice and Palliative Medicine*, https://doi.org/10.1177%2F1049909112458030.

[12] Steinhauser KE1, Christakis NA, Clipp EC, McNeilly M, McIntyre L, Tulsky JA. Factors considered important at the end of life by patients, family, physicians, and other care providers *JAMA*. 2000 Nov 15;284(19):2476-82. https://www.ncbi.nlm.nih.gov/pubmed/11074777.

BIOGRAPHICAL SKETCH

Azza Hassan

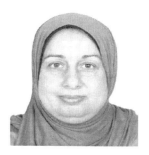

Program Director, Head of Supportive & Palliative Care Section
Medical Oncology, National Center for Cancer Care & Research
Assistant Professor of Clinical Medicine, Weill Cornell Medical College
Doha, Qatar

Medical Credentials
M.B.B.Ch.
Master's Degree in Clinical Oncology
Doctorate Degree in Clinical Oncology
American Board of Hospice and Palliative Medicine (ABHPM)

Dr. Azza Adel Hassan completed her Medical education in 1986 from Alexandria University, Egypt. She obtained her Master and Doctorate degree in Clinical Oncology. She got the certification of American Board of Hospice and Palliative Medicine (ABHPM) in 2003. Currently, she is Program Director of Supportive & Palliative Care Section at National Center for Cancer Care and Research, Hamad Medical Corporation, Doha, Qatar. She is also an Assistant Professor in Medical Research Institute, Alexandria University, Egypt.

She has several publications in the field of Clinical Oncology and Palliative Medicine in peer-reviewed Journals. She is an active member of Supportive And Palliative Care Working Group of European Society for Medical Oncology (ESMO), Middle East Cancer Consortium (MECC) and MASCC (Multinational Association of Supportive Care in Cancer).

In: Palliative Care
Editor: Michael Silbermann

ISBN: 978-1-53616-199-1
© 2019 Nova Science Publishers, Inc.

Chapter 19

THE IMPORTANCE OF PALLIATIVE CARE RESEARCH IN A CLINICAL SETTING: IDENTIFYING BARRIERS AND IMPLEMENTATION STRATEGIES

Tahani H. Al Dweikat[*]
Oncology/Hematology Unit, Sheikh Khalifa Medical City,
Abu Dhabi, United Arab Emirates

ABSTRACT

With the tremendous development of cancer care and palliative care environments, healthcare providers (HCPs) are constantly challenged to provide comprehensive and effective treatment to patients diagnosed with cancer and undergoing palliative care. The importance of research to translate findings into evidence-based clinical strategies has been identified as a crucial need and priority to promote excellence in patient care. Research has been the focus for the last decades, although resistant attitudes of nurses towards participating in clinical research in varied hospitals in different countries were identified as the biggest barrier to promoting excellence in palliative care and implementation strategies. Special consideration is needed while training clinicians who care for cancer patients and provide palliative care. Evaluation is required to ensure that the importance of implementing evidence-based practices is well established. Nurses' engagement in research must include conducting clinical trials as part of their work, so that results provided can be implemented. The challenges involve complementary therapies, together with integration of conventional and traditional medicine (CTM), besides the need to understand patients' cultural diversity and beliefs.

Keywords: palliative care, evidence based practice, cultural diversity, inpatient, ambulatory, outpatient, research, measurement, complementary, alternative, traditional therapies

---

[*] Corresponding Author's E-mail: tahanidweikat@live.com.

INTRODUCTION

Generally, nurses express positive attitudes towards providing palliative and end- of-life care. However, there is a lack of research-based practice toward various therapies which patients add to their conventional therapies, including complementary and traditional therapies (CTM) or complementary therapies. They have been defined by medical organizations, however their general definition includes regional therapy used to treat symptoms or manage side effects, which involve homemade remedies (herbal) or products made by private companies (Kaptchuk, 2001).

Despite nurses' positive attitude to involvement in research for populations such as cancer patients who undertake palliative therapy as part of their treatment, challenges are two-fold: firstly, the professional challenges (of stakeholders), secondly, the clinical challenges (of healthcare providers (HCP) regarding willingness to dedicate time to participate in studies. These are barriers to the development of palliative care research, and clinical implementation of research studies (Wohleber, 2003).

Complementary therapies and alternative medicines (CAM) have been widely and actively used among cancer patients undergoing chemotherapy and palliative care. Here the main use for complementary therapy has been in symptom and pain management and to improve quality of knowledge. The lack of existing research has had a negative effect on patients' quality of care and affect nurses' knowledge with regard to the use of such therapies on patients who receive conventional therapies (McKitrick & Davis, 2011). Furthermore, Karlawish discussed the importance of the ethical responsibilities for HCPs who work to promote proper quality of care grounded on evidence-based practice of research studies.

The World Health Organization (WHO) predicts a 50% increase of newly diagnosed cancer cases, from 10 million in 2000 to 15 million in 2020. Moreover, malignant tumors were the attributed cause of death of 12% worldwide (WHO, 2003). The increased prevalence of cancer throughout the world highlights the importance of research development in cancer and palliative care.

This chapter will identify two important factors that retroactively affect the development of palliative care research. These include the barriers to such research and its implementation strategies, a lack of knowledge related to the use of complementary therapy along with palliative care, finally, the importance of integrating palliative care research and measurement of outcomes into the clinical setting of the inpatient, ambulatory, home-based, and long-term care.

BARRIERS TO RESEARCH DEVELOPMENT

Barriers were identified in different articles, including that published by Ben-Arye and colleagues in a study involving sixteen Middle East countries in 2015. Here some primary barriers included physicians' skepticism and low participation in research, along with their failure to establish a clear of path of integrating complementary and traditional medicine into conventional therapy. In conclusion, the impact of insufficient participation and collaboration in palliative care research affected the improvement of patient outcome and quality of care.

Communication is another barrier identified in one of Ben-Arye's studies, wherein a questionnaire was distributed to HCPs regarding physicians' communications on complementary therapies. Its results revealed physicians' skepticism concerning integrating complementary therapies with conventional treatments due to lack of scientific evidence-based research to support the integration (2016).

For the past 17 years, research growth has been tracked through medical journal databases, which include a MEDLINE database search for the key term "palliative care." For example, the total number of palliative care articles published from 2000 to 2017 was 43,581. However the total of randomized controlled trials (RCTs), which are considered the gold standard of research, was limited to 1,295 articles (3% of the total RCTs published in such articles since 2000) (MEDLINE 2018). However, that does not reflect the growing number of research studies in palliative care (DC Currow,(2011 though it confirms the importance of conducting more palliative care research in all locations.

Some challenges were clearly identified in different studies. Ethical and clinical issues, which were the highest priorities discussed in Addington-Hall (2002) and Rhondali and colleagues (2014), highlighted that 75% of HCPs reported on difficulties in conducting palliative care research. Reasons included the vulnerabilities of the population due to weakness and changes in their condition, fluctuations in their willingness to participate and stay involved, and moreover, unprotected time for the HCPs also presented. Even though nurses were positive about involvement in research and participated, their willingness was affected by the recruitment time needed for patients, or the HCPs might not be supported by their institutions. Lack of support leads to staff losing interest in active or continuing participation. Despite the interest displayed, unethical barriers such as unprotected time may negatively impact or lead to delays in treatment and in providing patient care.

Challenges mainly consist of ethical considerations, time expenses, resources, study design and methodology and, moreover, stakeholders' support is crucial for research development. Because stakeholders thoroughly analyze financial expenses, this central challenge was clearly acknowledged in various studies, and is often addressed as an important consideration in the research development workload.

LACK OF RESEARCH TO SUPPORT CLINICAL PRACTICE

Despite the tremendous development and growth of cancer treatment in management of symptoms and side effects, patients tend to seek different approaches during or in conjunction with their treatment. Here they are exposed to less developed and supported scientific research without the evidence-based practices that guide the use of complementary therapies in palliative care, as the latter may be useful for symptom management, enhance quality of life or boost immunity, enabling patients to physically cope with fatigue and risk of infection. It is often a tempting option for patients with limited economic support to use complementary therapies as alternatives or as additions to conventional treatment Due to the lack of research to support the use of complementary therapies in conjunction with active treatments, the majority of patients rely on referrals from family, friends, on social media, and on single business practices which mix products together and sell them, or on random internet searches.

Furthermore, some safety-related risks of administering complementary therapies to patients were explained in a study of "Potential risks associated with traditional herbal medicine use in cancer care: A study of Middle Eastern oncology health care professionals." This study explained that the use of traditional herbal therapies depended on most patients' perceptions that herbs are natural and safer than chemical drugs, which may expose them to pharmacokinetic effects. When used with conventional therapies in sixteen Middle Eastern countries, some studies clearly addressed negative aspects of the adjunct use of herbal and traditional medicine with conventional therapies, such as efficacy and safety (Ben-Arye, 2015). Sparreboom and colleagues also advocated refraining from using herbal remedies during active chemotherapy, because of potential effects on the drug metabolism by the drug-metabolizing enzyme cytochrome P450 (CYP450) system, of which CYP3A4 is the responsible enzyme for drug metabolism in the liver and intestines.

Another definition was given by the National Center for Complementary and Integrative Health (NCCIH), which defined complementary medicine as a non-mainstream practice used together with conventional medicine (2017). The use of complementary therapy in cancer is viewed as a worldwide practice based on patients' religious and spiritual beliefs and socioeconomic status (Abuelgasim et al. 2018), as well as their level of education and the courage to share information with HCPs. However, the herbal usage in cancer patients in the United States during their active chemotherapy treatment was recently reported as above 35%. However it was reported that between 20% to 70% of patients worldwide were reluctant to disclose this to HCPs (Ben-Arye, 2015).

An example of patients' perception and beliefs in one of the Middle Eastern countries where most people shared the same beliefs was the prevalence of using complementary therapies in one of the Gulf States which was rated between 33 to 93.3%. Saudi Arabia had the highest prevalence in such practices compared to other countries (Jazieh, 2012). In this regard complementary therapies are divided into two sectors: religion based and dietary based. Patients practice certain religious beliefs mentioned in the Holy Quran (the central religious text of Islam), however, these are not supported by evidence-based research. Those commonly used in cancer diagnosed patients include; the act of supplication and recitation of drinking the Zamzam water (water from holy Mecca) as healing water, or regular water over which the Holy Quran was recited, as well as drinking honey, camel milk and camel urine. In addition, some types of herbs were also mentioned such as black seeds, garlic, olive oil and others, which are also widely used in Saudi Arabia and other Middle Eastern regions (Alrowais & Alyousefi, 2017).

In 2014, with the increased use of camel products in conjunction with active treatment, camel products (milk or urine) were linked to respiratory infection that was recently related to the endemic spread of brucellosis and Middle East respiratory syndrome coronavirus (MERS-CoV). As a result, cancer patients died during the viral outbreaks, but patients in the region continued to use camel products as complementary therapies notwithstanding the lack of evidence and research development (Alrowais & Alyousefi, 2017).

BARRIERS TO RESEARCH IMPLEMENTATION STRATEGIES

Despite the need for more evidence-based findings, the established ones for palliative care and the use of complementary therapy guidelines present some barriers for HCPs, which affect the implementation of research results into clinical areas. These factors can be focused into two main categories, namely "access" and "competency."

Access is mainly focused on the HCP's ability to access established research findings and use them as evidence-based practice in patient care, which includes HCP access to research findings such as journals and databases on complementary therapies, training, skill of research participation and access to protected research time. Poor access to funding was highlighted in 2001, when only 0.085% ($850,000) of approximately one billion dollars of National Health and Medical Research Council research funds was allocated to complementary therapy research (Bensoussan & Lewith, 2004). Results were that few trained HCPs were up-to-date with research, there was a lack of access to proper research findings related to complementary therapies. In addition, there were fewer opportunities for training and education of nurses and primary physicians as frontline care providers. These factors have an impact on the quality of care of patients undergoing chemotherapy treatments and using complementary therapies.

Competency refers to HCPs competency and skills in conducting and developing research in an evidence-based way and to publishing the findings through accessible databases.

CONCLUSION

While complementary therapies still require more research development, and there are many barriers to overcome before results are implemented, some recommendations emerge. Stakeholders must support and encourage HCPs in their research and practice. This includes training and fellowship opportunities, protected time for research, embedding the latter as part of comprehensive training for all clinicians in all cancer service providers' institutions worldwide, improving access to research, and an evidence-based practice database. Time must be allocated for physician-patient counselling which allows discussion or divulging information on using complementary therapies to identify potential risks to patient's health. Thus HCPs can identify the gaps and undertake a well-coordinated research effort that will assist in integrating evidence-based research in implementation of complementary therapies in patient care.

REFERENCES

Abuelgasim, K. A., Alsharhan, Y., Alenzi, T., Alhazzani, A., Ali, Y. Z., & Jazieh, A. R. (2018). The use of complementary and alternative medicine by patients with cancer: a cross-sectional survey in Saudi Arabia. *BMC Complementary And Alternative Medicine*, (1), doi:10.1186/s12906-018-2150-8.

Addington-Hall, J. (2002). Research sensitivities to palliative care patients. *European Journal of Cancer Care*, 11(3), 220–224.

Alrowais, N. A., & Alyousefi, N. A. (2017). Review: The prevalence extent of Complementary and Alternative Medicine (CAM) use among Saudis. *Saudi Pharmaceutical Journal*, 25306-318. doi:10.1016/j.jsps.2016.09.009.

Ben-Arye, E., Samuels, N., Goldstein, L. H., Mutafoglu, K., Omran, S., Schiff, E., & Silbermann, M. (2016). Potential risks associated with traditional herbal medicine use in cancer care: A study of Middle Eastern oncology health care professionals. *Cancer*, (4). 598.

Ben-Arye, E., Popper-Giveon, A., Samuels, N., Mutafoglu, K., Schiff, E., Omran, S., & Silbermann, M. (2016). Communication and integration: a qualitative analysis of perspectives among Middle Eastern oncology healthcare professionals on the integration of complementary medicine in supportive cancer care. *Journal of Cancer Research and Clinical Oncology*, 142(5), 1117-1126. doi:10.1007/s00432-016-2120-9.

Bensoussan, A., & Lewith, G. T. (2004). Complementary medicine research in Australia: a strategy for the future. *The Medical Journal of Australia*, (6). 331.

Blum, D., Inauen, R., Binswanger, J., & Strasser, F. (2015). Barriers to research in palliative care: A systematic literature review. Progress in *Palliative Care*, 23(2), 75. doi:10.1179/1743291X14Y.0000000100.

Currow, D. C. (2011). Special Section: The PRISMA Symposium: The PRISMA Symposium 3: Lessons From Beyond Europe. Why Invest in Research and Service Development in Palliative Care? An Australian Perspective. *Journal of Pain And Symptom Management*, 42505-510. doi:10.1016/j.jpainsymman.2011.06.007.

Chrystal, K., Allan, S., Forgeson, G., & Isaacs, R. (2003). The use of complementary/alternative medicine by cancer patients in a New Zealand regional cancer treatment centre. *The New Zealand Medical Journal*, 116(1168), U296.

Duke, S., & Bennett, H. (2010). A narrative review of the published ethical debates in palliative care research and an assessment of their adequacy to inform research governance. *Palliative Medicine*, 24(2), 111–126.

Jazieh, A. R., Al Sudairy, R., Abulkhair, O., Alaskar, A., Al Safi, F., Sheblaq, N., & ... Tamim, H. (2012). Use of complementary and alternative medicine by patients with cancer in Saudi Arabia. *Journal of Alternative And Complementary Medicine* (New York, N.Y.), 18(11), 1045-1049. doi:10.1089/acm.2011.0266.

Kaptchuk, T. J., & Eisenberg, D. M. (2001). A taxonomy of unconventional healing practices. *Annals of Internal Medicine*, (3). 196.

Karlawish, J. H. (2003). Conducting research that involves subjects at the end of life who are unable to give consent. *Journal of Pain & Symptom Management*, 25(4), S14–S24.

Keim-Malpass, J., Mitchell, E. M., Blackhall, L., & DeGuzman, P. B. (2015). Evaluating Stakeholder-Identified Barriers in Accessing Palliative Care at an NCI-Designated Cancer Center with a Rural Catchment Area. *Journal of Palliative Medicine*, 18(7), 634-637. doi:10.1089/jpm.2015.003.

Kirsh, K. L., Walker, R., Snider, S., Weisenfluh, S., Brown, G. M., & Passik, S. D. (2004). Hospice staff members' views on conducting end-of-life research. *Palliative and Supportive Care*, 2(3), 273–282.

National Center for Complementary and Integrative Health. *Alternative or Integrative: What's in name?* https://nccih.nih.gov/health/integrative-health#cvsa. Last accessed 29 Oct 2017.

Nyatanga, B., Cook, D., & Goddard, A. (2018). A prospective research study to investigate the impact of complementary therapies on patient well-being in palliative care.

Complementary Therapies in Clinical Practice, 31118-125. doi:10.1016/j.ctcp.2018.02.006.

Rhondali W, Berthiller J, Hui D, et al. Barriers to research in palliative care in France *BMJ Supportive & Palliative Care* 2014;4:182-189.

Sait, K. H., Anfinan, N. M., Eldeek, B., Al-Ahmadi, J., Al-Attas, M., Sait, H. K., & ... El-Sayed, M. E. (2014). Perception of patients with cancer towards support management services and use of complementary alternative medicine--a single institution hospital-based study in Saudi Arabia. *Asian Pacific Journal of Cancer Prevention: APJCP*, 15(6), 2547-2554.

Sparreboom, A., Cox, M. C., Acharya, M. R., & Figg, W. D. (2004). Herbal remedies in the United States: potential adverse interactions with anticancer agents. Journal of Clinical Oncology: *Official Journal of the American Society Of Clinical Oncology*, 22(12), 2489-2503.

The Use of Complementary and Alternative Medicine in the United States: About CAM. https://nccih.nih.gov/research/statistics/2007/camsurvey_fs1.htm. Last accessed 29 Oct 2017.

World Health Organization. (2003) *The World Health Report* 2003. WHO, Geneva.

BIOGRAPHICAL SKETCH

Tahani Dweikat

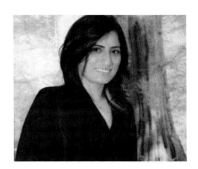

Tahani Dweikat, RN, BSN, EMHCA, OCN®, Charge Nurse in Oncology from the United Arab Emirates in Abu Dhabi, at Sheikh Khalifa Medical City (SKMC) Hematology Department.

Completed Bachelor of Nursing Science and holds a Master degree in "*Executive Masters in Healthcare administration (EMHCA)*" Zayed university, Ab Dhabi.

Holds national credentials as Oncology certified Nurse (OCN) through the Oncology Nursing Certification Corporation (ONCC).

Been active member in Oncology Nursing Society (ONS) and International Society of Nurses in Cancer care (ISNCC), has leadership roles within ONS where currently serves as the President of the Oncology Nursing Society (ONS) International Affiliate: UAE. For 2 years.

Currently actively involved in organizing and teaching educational study days for hematology and oncology courses, and in projects for the improvement of patient care.

In: Palliative Care
Editor: Michael Silbermann

ISBN: 978-1-53616-199-1
© 2019 Nova Science Publishers, Inc.

Chapter 20

PROMOTING RESEARCH AND PRACTICES IN PALLIATIVE CARE IN AN ISLAMIC MIDDLE-INCOME COUNTRY: OMAN AS AN EXAMPLE

Zakiya Al Lamki[*]
Pediatric Hematology and Oncology Unit, Department of Child Health,
College of Medicine and Health Sciences,
Sultan Qaboos University, Muscat, Sultanate of Oman

"Medicine does not have the armamentarium to address all the components of suffering induced by disease. Suffering in advanced cancer patients cannot be eliminated, but if adequate relief is achieved, then coping and personal growth can occur."
Sandy Macleod [1].

ABSTRACT

Oman, like other neighboring middle eastern countries of emerging economies, face an increasing risk of seriously Life Limiting Diseases (LLD) as a result of the ageing population, improvement in the standards of living and changes in lifestyle. It is internationally recognized for its highly efficient cure- oriented (biomedical) model of healthcare system where preventive and curative procedures are prioritized ahead of palliative care. However, since patients with chronic conditions and terminal illness have evolving complex physical, psychosocial and spiritual needs throughout their disease trajectory, such problems present a significant challenge necessitating change of the current system to one that will improve the quality of life of these patients. Therefore, palliative care ought to be integrated as the standard of care and developed to respond to the need of the rising numbers of people with LLD. Similar to some countries of the region, Oman is adopting pain management as a main aspect of palliative care. However, being a collective society holding to ancient traditions and taboos, it will need to pursue a biopsychosocial approach with greater emphasis on the psychosocial, cultural and spiritual relevance of palliative care. The aim of this chapter is to highlight factors which

---
[*] Corresponding Author's E-mail: zakiya.allamki@gmail.com.

will strengthen the practice including concerted efforts in training, education as well as development of research in the area, all of which are likely to consolidate palliative care in the country. This can subsequently reduce healthcare costs for LLD when initiated early. However, issues on response to the dying and grief works as well as non-allopathic healing practices under Graeco-Arabic (Islamic) medicine need to be contemplated if palliative care is to be more meaningful.

Keywords: practices and research, palliative care, islamic middle-income country

INTRODUCTION

With the improvement in the standards of living and changes in lifestyle among societies in transition such as the Middle East, there is a major surge in the number of the elderly population and seriously ill patients with life-limiting diseases (LLD). This is compounded with climbing incidence of chronic non- communicable diseases also known as 'diseases of affluence' including cancer [2]. For years, the World Health Organization (WHO) has been advocating for improved palliative care throughout the world which it describes as an approach that improves the quality of life of patients and their families facing the problems associated with life-threatening illness, through the prevention and relief of suffering by means of early identification and impeccable assessment and treatment of pain and other problems, physical, psychosocial and spiritual [3]. Accordingly, the treatment of these new trends of health problems still points out to the highly specialized driven cure-oriented (biomedical) model of health care rather than improvement of patients' quality of life (QoL) [4]. Cancer pain relief is ubiquitous but neglected public health problem in many of these countries where only a fraction of the population receives the relevant treatment. Like the rest of the developing countries, where more than half of the world's cancer patients live, majority present late at the time of diagnosis and thus late reporting of pain [5]. In fact, curative procedures are often prioritized ahead of palliative care and pain relief is hardly offered to the seriously ill patients.

It should be realized that palliative care is not an alternative to other models of healthcare but should be an integral part of a comprehensive healthcare services. This is currently lacking in many developing countries including countries of emerging economies. At its broadest, palliative care is an excellent symptom management and at the same time, facilitate excellent patient, family, and intra professional communication regarding illness, hopes, goals and expectations for treatment over time, toward the goal of creating a patient-centered plan of care [6].

Patients with cancer have complex physical, psychosocial, and spiritual needs that evolve throughout their disease trajectory. As they survive longer, the need grows for addressing the morbidity due to the underlying illness as well as treatment-related adverse events [7]. Whether for people with cancer or for others with chronic illness, palliative care is therefore an essential part of any health care system. Besides providing the best possible quality of life the aim is also for people approaching the end of life and for their families and carers. All too often, both health care professionals and the public, associate palliative care exclusively with end-of-life and hospice care. However, for several reasons it is not recognized in many government plans.

Palliative care is every day; it cannot be neglected in the efforts to provide greater accessibility to more curative drugs and technical therapies. Its integration throughout cancer treatment ought to be the standard of care and thus some developing countries are already advancing in such an agenda [8]. In spite of the concept of multiple domains, as per the practical implementation, palliative care is more accentuated towards the physical aspect; whilst the psychosocial aspects are mostly disregarded, due to which patients with terminal illness endure a significant psychological and social distress [9]. Although pain control is central to the concept of palliative care, it is well recognized that patient's major anguish is psychological distress; consideration therefore has to be taken into the emotional, psychological and spiritual needs as well as physical needs. It is a holistic approach to care and support.

The existing models of palliative care approaches in developing countries were initially developed to respond to the needs of people with cancer and have expanded to include people with HIV. Besides treatment to relieve pain and psychological distress, this includes home care. However, there seem to be an increasing awareness of the importance of spiritual care. Therefore spiritual, psychological, social, emotional and physical care should have equal footing in palliative care and should be a team-based care. Besides psychotherapeutic interventions and techniques used in clinical practice, spiritual and staff support are an integral part of all aspects of psychosocial care, using the expertise of physicians, nurses, and social workers as the core elements of a team, together with religious and community leaders, pharmacists, mental health practitioners, financial counsellors and front desk staff who observe family dynamics that are often unapparent to health practitioners [10, 11, 12].

Although palliative care is not new to health care or to practice of oncology, oncologists and oncology nurses still struggle to maximize the value of this type of care across the entire care continuum and across the patient's trajectory of illness [13]. Training for health workers and public education, understanding of what palliative is, and training to carry it out, are therefore necessary for policy makers, health professionals and families.

Intrinsic to palliative care is the recognition of the family as the unit of care and their support and education are therefore vital. The cancer diagnosis is a situation that affects not just the patient but also family members, producing great degrees of psychosocial distress. All parties involved have several unmet needs. The interplay of the relationships involved produces a lot of moral obligations and responsibilities. In addition, there are emotional and physical stresses affecting the patient and his family members as well as caregiver. This is more pronounced in many developing nations where palliative care is still at the stages of infancy, and the full complement of multidisciplinary team and support services are grossly inadequate or lacking. To achieve good palliative care, good psychosocial care is imperative [14]. Presently, care of the cancer patient is moving from the patient-centered approach to the 'whole-system approach' that encompasses the patient's interpersonal and family relationships as well as the best of medical and social care, in order to optimize the quality of life for such patients [11].

A patient is treated not only as an individual with problems and symptoms but also as a family member whose reactions interlock with the support system. As such, it is important to involve family members as colleagues in discussions and plan of care. In palliative care, the creation of a safe space for families to talk is important. Families need help as most of the time the patient either withdraws, or wants constant attention. The diagnosis of terminal illness is traumatic for everyone and knowledge and understanding of the crisis is important as everyone's realities change within seconds. All that was once certain becomes uncertain and the emotional and physical resources of the entire family are threatened. On the other hand, care offered to the patient and family is incomplete without considering the children, for whom parents usually require extra support and reassurance. An understanding of loss, grief and bereavement is necessary for all who work in palliative care. The journey through life-threatening disease is marked by loss; some come early and others later in the disease process. Grief is the reaction to loss and if patients and their families are helped to express this, they usually cope more effectively with the disease process. Fear often builds fear and a regular consultation with a trusted professional can often break this vicious circle. Honest reassuring discussion, to normalize fear, is usually sufficient. [15, 16].

SELF-LIMITING DISEASES IN OMAN

Oman is one of the middle-income countries situated at the south-eastern tip of the Arabian Peninsula. Like its neighbors, it has been observed that its ageing 4.6 million population and the sedentary lifestyle changes, face increasing risks of cancer and other seriously life-limiting diseases (LLD) [2]. Life expectancy at birth, which was less than 60 years four decades ago, has now risen to nearly 77 years [17]. The incidence of LLDs is common among the adult population but there are indications that these new assortment of health problems are occurring much earlier in life, affecting even young children and adolescents [18, 19, 20]. Besides the non-communicable diseases, Oman is also not immune to other conditions that are known to contribute to disability, such as HIV/AIDS. Although there are no formal studies capturing the magnitude of HIV/AIDS, it is known for having a low prevalence of HIV/AIDS [21]. A study suggests that Oman has a significant number of people with LLD due to genetic factors as a result of the cultural practice of consanguineous marriage [22]. The exponential growth in the incidence and prevalence of these conditions therefore present a significant challenge to its healthcare system and as such, necessitates to reequip itself with a new system to deal with the rising percentage of the LLD-afflicted population [23, 24]. According to Violan et al. multimorbidity increases the risk of premature death, hospitalizations, polypharmacy, loss of physical functioning, depression, and worsening quality of life, translating into a substantial economic burden for health systems [23]. Patients face loss at every level — long life expectancy, physical health, independence, career and status, normal family life, predictability and future, motivation and meaning, To the best of our knowledge, there are no data on the magnitude of such frailty and dependency in Oman; however anecdotal observations suggest that the country is gripped with a rising number of such individuals. LDD therefore has become a cross-demographic feature in Oman and is likely to surge further potentially causing long-term disability and dependency which will have repercussions on the allocation of resources in order to safeguard the well-being of its population [26].

Athough Oman has one of the most efficient healthcare systems in the world [27], it requires to shift its well-established public health programs from prevention and cure oriented for which it has been internationally lauded, to one that will improve quality of life for the patients [28, 29]. One such health care approach in societies in transition like Oman is culture-sensitive palliative care. So far, most of the discussions in Oman have been geared towards addressing the unmet or existing 'physical cure' for people with LLD and the country's health care system is officially adopting the new thrust towards pain-management. Most tertiary hospitals in the country are trying to make it an essential part of their standard patient care [30, 31]. However, like its neighboring countries, the least discussed are the psychosocial, cultural and spiritual approaches in the palliative care. The complex challenge of LLD would need to be confronted with approaches in psychosocial relevance and Oman will be better off if it pursues using a biopsychosocial approach, with greater emphasis on the cultural aspect of care. The goal in providing culture-sensitive care is to be sensitive and aware of the beliefs, values, traditions and practices of others and to respect them when providing care even if they are quite different from one's own [32]. Many people regard religion and spiritual as interchangeable terms but an appreciation of the difference is important when working in the palliative care setting. Spiritual care is recognized as much broader than religious concerns. The spiritual dimension is common to us all and is concerned with a search for meaning and enhances the sharing of beliefs and values. It assists the patient to be at peace.

As part of the required paradigm shift to address the unmet needs for people with LLD in Oman, the aim of this chapter is to highlight factors, including research, that are likely to consolidate the development of palliative care in the country where until recently has received scant attention [33]. There is the unsubstantiated view that palliative care is a 'luxury' of the rich industrialized countries of the west. The biopsychosocial philosophy of palliative care is finding resistance from the core of the modern medical fraternity. Their resistance is understandable because the current biomedical model of healthcare, hardly a half century old, is well equipped to cope with acute medical conditions and has been implemented successfully so far. This has been solidified by the increased standards of living. The trend in Oman substantiates the well-known McKeown hypothesis, that is, economic development invariably shapes the health of a population [34,].

The fact that the family is a central identity for people in Oman makes it important to understand how the family functions in a traditional society in transition. Like in the rest of the Arab world, the Omani society is characterized by large families. For Omanis, the extended family has been central to their individual identity and support. However, as in other societies in transition, there are indications that globalization, acculturation, and urbanization are fast replacing the old social order. As the extended family becomes eroded with the trend towards nuclear families, an inevitable consequence of urbanization, the traditional social network that had defined the individual identity is also weakening [35, 36]. The decline of such a powerful social order is likely to affect its most vulnerable members, such as those with LLD.

Omani families, like other societies in transition, owe their origins from ancient times. Each member's life is 'enmeshed' with that of the rest of the family. Oman's society appears to function as a collective rather than individualistic orientation where individuals are required to be obedient and loyal to the family or tribal values. The individual patient therefore has little autonomy and the involvement of the family in palliative care may implicitly contravene ethical practices that is intimately tied to biomedical care. When Omanis succumb to LLD, the extended family 'takes over' and shares the responsibility for their wellbeing as a society of interdependence, where sickness or disability is shared by the community. Thus, unlike the western society, the Omani philosophical orientation might be incompatible with views on informed consent, patient autonomy, confidentiality and open communication, as the family members take over the welfare and decision-making of the persons with LLD. In support of this view, there is an anecdotal observation in Oman that a patient tends to refuse to sign, for example, an informed consent. According to Silbermann [37], in reference to cancer, '…a diagnosis of cancer in many Middle Eastern countries is associated with a social stigma and misperceptions related to its incurability; and physicians, although many of them are trained in Western countries, still practice the truth disclosure policy that respects some of the historical and cultural misperceptions about cancer; and they frequently tell the truth about the condition to one of the family members and try to conceal it from the concerned patient.' Association with a particular cultural, ethnic or religious group may influence: expression and meaning of pain, suffering and attitude towards disclosure and awareness. If palliative care is going to grow in societies in transition like Oman, it would be essential to tailor-make it to be congruent with the expectation of the society [38]. Amidst these changes, the question is how much of the traditional family structures will remain and how far they can be relied upon as one of the bases for palliative care of the future. Studies on how the family in Oman is evolving in the light of modernization are urgently needed. The need for interdisciplinary palliative care is beyond the scope of the current ultra-specialized biomedical model of disease and healing that is adopted by the country's health care system.

MANIFESTATIONS OF LIFE LIMITING DISEASES

It has been well documented that LLD tends to impact the mental state or integrity of psychological functioning which, in turn, triggers adverse emotions, compromised cognition, and leads to overt maladaptive behaviour. People with LLD and emotional problems have been reported to be more vulnerable to early death [39]. There is an increasing awareness of the rising tide of psychological distresses. Although anxiety or depression has been shown to be widely prevalent in people with LLD [40], there is a gap in the treatment of mental health in individuals with LLD [41]. Depression is an emotional state and a form of psychological distress that commonly occurs in patients with life- threatening illness. Causes of depression include knowledge of a life-threatening diagnosis, presence of physical symptoms like pain and nausea, side effects from medical treatments, and loss of independence and functionality. Others are changes in family relationships, concern for dependents and changes in bodily function [42, 43, 44, 45]. During the years of my clinical practice, I came upon a number of patients with terminal illness whose major concern was not pain but fear of leaving behind their dependents namely wives and small children. The question here is how psychological distresses manifest in people with LLD in societies in transition?

Palliative care is not just vital in controlling symptoms of the patient's disease condition, but also aims to extend the patient's life, giving it a better quality. It includes treating physical symptoms as well as addressing psychosocial and spiritual needs. The negative effect of adverse emotional states in people with LLD raises the importance of the psychological component of care in the biopsychosocial model. Unlike biomedical intervention, palliative care aspires to include both social and psychological dimensions of care. However, several times in the course of management, the psychosocial impact of cancer, HIV/AIDS, and other life-limiting disease conditions may not be noticed and dealt with during the early stages of admission period, thereby giving rise to a more complex situation than the disease condition itself [46]. Besides, interpersonal and family relationships can affect chronic disease management outcomes. Uncontrollable pain or other symptoms have such an impact on the psyche that the family may have to watch the loved person change into a self-centered individual, always irritable and demanding attention, perhaps oblivious to the suffering of others. There is described evidence that palliative care, provided concurrently with disease-modifying treatment early in the course of a cancer diagnosis, can improve quality of life, length of survival, symptom burden, mood and utilization of health services [47]. We need to work to develop understanding handshakes rather than handoffs among oncology and palliative care partners, to identify upstream norms for palliative care engagement. Normalizing palliative care upstream, during the active treatment phase, allows time for the optimal management of symptoms and patient-initiated discussion of fears regarding potential future outcomes, when it is not yet a crisis [48]. These discussions can empower the patient and family to ask questions or express worries that they might otherwise not talk about. Upstream co-management also shows the patient and family that their providers are partners, that they do not face abandonment by their oncology provider and that palliative care is an additional, supportive element of their comprehensive cancer treatment plan.

There is therefore a psychosocial dimension to the work of all involved in palliative care and understanding this will strengthen the practice of any professional working in this area. [49]. Psychosocial care, as defined by the National Council for Hospice and Specialist Palliative Care Services, is care concerned with the psychological and emotional well-being of the patients, their family and care providers. These include issues of self-esteem, insight into an adaptation to the illness and its consequences, communication, social functioning and relationships. It is a form of care that encourages patients to express their feelings about the disease while at the same time providing ways by which the psychological and emotional well-being of such patients and their caregivers are improved [50, 51].

In prior studies, psychological distresses in people with LLD are often equated with psychiatric disorders [52]. Rather than labelling the distress endorsed among people with LLD along existing psychiatric nomenclature, it would be relevant to define their distress in terms of an internalizing/externalizing problem as previously defined in the context of children. Although most studies have originated from Euro-American populations [53], data from non-Western societies have suggested a high frequency of internalizing/externalizing problems in people with LLD. There are some reports of individuals with LLD with internalizing/externalizing problems from countries with predominantly Muslim populations but it not clear whether the manifestations of such internalization/ externalization are similar to those reported in Euro-American populations [54,5]. Studies are therefore warranted to shed light on the phenomenology and the magnitude of internalizing/externalizing problems in people with LLD in Oman [56, 57].

If further scrutiny would indeed suggest that Omanis tend to express their internalizing/externalizing problems as somatic distress rather than as cognitive or emotional problems, this would have implications in applying the results of Western research into psychological therapy of its population [58]. By definition, Western psychotherapeutic interventions are designed to uncover mental conflicts. In a society (such as in rural Oman) where misfortunes are misconceived to be attributed to external factors such as envy or evil eye, the standard psychotherapeutic approaches that seek to uncover intrapsychic conflicts would have no heuristic value. The effort should be therefore geared towards devising psychological interventions that resonate with the socio-cultural teaching. If comprehensive palliative care will ever rise in Oman, then any attempt to address unmet psychological needs should be geared towards incorporating socio-cultural teaching [59, 60].

Although good psychiatric care is a core principle of palliative care, palliative medicine training programs may not address the application of psychiatric interventions. It is through this lens that Macleod probe the fragmented relationship between psychiatr and palliative medicine in contemporary health care. Psychiatry can ameliorate distressing physical symptoms in people with terminal illness, for example, psychodynamic intervention seems more applicable when addressing end- of-life issues. This is curious, given evidence that cognitive behavioral approaches to symptom management in palliative care may be useful adjuncts to somatic interventions. Caring for patients with a terminal illness and their families require the skills of many professionals working together as a team. It is often the psychosocial issues surrounding patients and families that cause professionals even greater difficulty than the physical symptoms. The issues of psychosocial assessment, treatment, care, and support of palliative care patients differs from the care of patients with early treatable cancer as time is short compared to terminally ill patients where the emphasis differs both from a patient and carer perspective [61].

Informing a patient of the diagnosis of his condition has become an art. Barriers to effective communication between the physician and his patient where breaking bad news is concerned, include superstition, cultural beliefs, misconceptions, social problems and ignorance. There may be a conflict among healthcare professionals (physicians, nurses, social workers, psychological counsellors) on whose role it is to assist the patient with psychological, emotional, spiritual, and social concerns and thus a large number of the patients' needs remain unmet [62]. For clinicians to avoid the creation of depression in patients with terminal illness, they should apply well-established principles of communication and counselling when breaking bad news, give the individual the information in the manner he desires and allow for the open expression of emotions. Therefore, members of the multidisciplinary team must arm themselves with good communication skills. Compassion and empathy should be their watchword. They should also keep themselves from dismissing anxiety and depression as understandable, thereby denying many of essential treatment. Involvement of specialized palliative care nurses and social workers to give supportive psychotherapy as well as the involvement of family members and religious leaders can help in the care process. Finally, all procedures in palliative care should aim at ensuring the patient lives a life as comfortable as possible until death [63].

Stigmatization affects people with LLD self-worth and dignity which in turn affects their interpersonal relationships, giving rise to withdrawal from family and community. It can prevent affected patients from seeking appropriate medical care and therefore must be dealt with. At the point a diagnosis is made, stigma should be identified and psychological counselling instituted along with treatments for the primary condition. Respect, empathy, symptom control, companionship and encouraging life review are essential ingredients in the process of maintaining or restoring dignity [64]. Without them, palliative care would be incomplete. To achieve all of them for many would be an impossible task for the isolated professional. Hence team work is essential. The social worker should organize family support groups, to get the patient and his family in contact with similar patients and their families. Such a forum would encourage an increase in medical knowledge on the disease condition, allow the exchange of experiences, as well as promote good interpersonal and family relationships. In addition, social worker and other members of the multidisciplinary team should encourage open communication among family members as this will allow the patient to express his fears and concerns about his condition. Advocacy is important as it will bring awareness of the condition to the society. This can be achieved through the dissemination of medical information via social media, patients' retreats and the organization of workshops and seminars [65].

THE ROLE OF NON-ALLOPATHIC HEALING SYSTEM IN MUSLIM SOCIETIES

With the preponderance of non-communicable diseases, the traditional non-allopathic healing system appears to be the most accessible for a significant number of the population in countries in transition [66]. Unlike biomedical care, non-allopathic approaches to health are based on conceptual practices that are compatible with spiritual and socio-cultural teachings. Traditional beliefs and social taboos among the rural societies are often attributed to external supernatural forces such as "jinn," "hassad" (an evil eye that represents extreme envy) or "sihr" (sorcery). In the collective society as in Oman, socio-cultural patterning tends to 'encourage' externalization of the source of mishaps. Thus, an individual with sickness, disability or LDD are likely to be perceived as a victim of these supernatural forces not only to the afflicted individual but also the family or clan. Complementary therapies are widely sought by patients and families and the evidence base is slowly growing. A comprehensive review of such therapies include herbal and homeopathic medicines [30, 67].

Although complementary and alternative medicine (CAM) has been replaced by biomedical care, it increasingly gained momentum in individuals with LLD and it has made its entrance into palliative care [68, 69]. In practice, complementary medicine is used together with biomedical care. Integrative medicine, such as acupuncture is also one of the growing forms of treatments [70]. The traditional healing system is frequently sought as a choice for individuals with LLD and their families and for that matter as a form of palliative care. Due to spiritual and cultural observance, it is likely that the Omani people will be more compliant with those non-allopathic healing systems that have an organic link to the society such as manipulative and body-based as well as biologically based practices that fall under Graeco-Arab (Islamic) medicine or Unani Tibb as well as Prophetic Medicine known as al-Tibb al-Nabawi, [71]. The underlying belief of Unani Tibb, as well as al-Tibb al-Nabawi, tend to pervade socio-cultural teaching in Oman relevant for matters related to health and sickness in traditional Arab-Islamic society [72]. More studies are therefore warranted and efficacy of such types of traditional healing would require examinations and, of course, the potential of the adverse effect of drug interactions.

RESPONSE TO DEATH AND DYING IN SOCIETIES IN TRANSITION

Care of the dying patient has become a specialized discipline within the medical field. By implication, any discussion of palliative care requires a discussion on death. This is not limited to individuals with LLD but also to their families, caretakers and social support network as well. Therefore, coping with impending death and loss is important to be considered in palliative settings.

Pain is one of the most prevalent symptoms near the end of life. Unrelieved pain can be a source of great distress for patients and families and exacerbate other symptoms. Therefore, the adequate management of pain at the end of life is imperative. Although opioid analgesics are the standard of care for treating moderate to severe pain in patients with advanced illness, the false fear that opioids induce respiratory depression and hasten death is a major barrier to their use at the end of life. However, both effects are uncommon when opioids are given at appropriate doses [73]. I had the privilege of chairing the hospital Grievance Committee of our hospital for several years when one of the cases of a terminally ill young adult cancer patient was submitted to us. The husband actually filed a complaint against the treating doctors and nurses for leaving his wife on her death bed, in severe distress from the immense pain. They failed to answer to her screams and calls for help and none of the caregivers went to talk or prepared the patient and the family. The pain medication given to the patient if any, was not adequate to calm her down. It was therefore a torturing experience to the patient as well as her husband and the rest of the family, to watch their loved one undergoing such intense suffering.

Clinicians who care for the chronically ill and for those at the end of life should therefore acquire competency in pain management. As death approaches, a patient's symptoms may require more aggressive palliation. As comfort measures intensify, so should the support be provided to the dying patient's family. After the patient's death, then palliative care should focus primarily on bereavement and support of the family [74, 75].

In Islam, life is described as a temporary transit to the eternal afterlife, where one will reap the rewards of their faith and good deeds they performed during their lifetime. This belief system is assumed to facilitate the acceptance of impending death. Despite such teaching there are several studies on the prevalence of death anxiety among the Arab/Islamic population. These studies generally support the view that death anxiety is also common in such populations [76]. Some studies have suggested that religiosity has little bearing on mitigating death anxiety. This would imply that studies are needed to shed light on mortality awareness among dying patients in Oman [77, 78].

Besides death anxiety, some data have emerged from an Arab/Islamic population on the issue of mourning, grief and bereavement or grief work. Islam teaches that death, as well as all other life events, are a result of God's will, and excessive grieving is equivalent to questioning Divine will [79]. Despite this, Muslim societies vary in the expression of grief. In some countries of North Africa such as Egypt, screaming, yelling, chest beating and other expressions of intense sadness is socially accepted, although this goes against the teaching of Islam. In contrast, majority mourn in a more subdued manner. However, some communities in southern Oman and Bali, express their emotions through cheers and laughter. Examples of grief work suggest that the Arab/Islamic population harbour diverse views on issues pertinent to awareness of mortality [80]. Instead, it suggests that diversity as well as broader similarities are shared among the people of the region. It is unclear whether such socio-cultural factors lead to better or worse coping with impending death. More studies are therefore warranted to examine 'grief work' among Omanis.

There is evidence to suggest that grief-work involving relinquishing the bond with deceased as postulated in western psychological literature may not be the same in some other populations as exemplified by reaction to personality changes due to LLD or untimely death

[81]. Instead, the death or personality changes in parts of rural Oman is equated with a belief known as *mu ghayeb* where a person in question is alleged to have been 'stolen' by a magician. The belief assumes that the sick or dead has been ensorcelled [82]. The consequence of this belief is hoping for the eventual return of the stolen person to her family. *Mu ghayeb* belief in Oman therefore is inconsistent with religion of Islam and dissent the view in western psychological literature that suggest that severing the bond with the deceased is essential in coping with loss.

PROMOTING RESEARCH

The goal of palliative care is to achieve the highest quality of life for patients and their families by providing care and bereavement support. Consequently, the outcome of care should be measured in terms of the extent to which this goal is achieved. Sound evidence to guide palliative care practice decisions is therefore essential [83].

Currently palliative care has a poorly developed research base, but the need to improve this is increasingly recognised. One of the reasons for the lack of research and the variable quality of the research that is undertaken is the difficulty of conducting research with very ill and bereaved people. The field provides a rich and challenging set of research questions. There are many complex medical, ethical and psychosocial issues to consider. These challenges are unique to and significant in palliative care setting. Difficulties arise with recruiting and retaining study participants whose health is declining and who are approaching death as well as identifying and meaningfully engage family members/caregivers. The culture of many hospice and palliative care programs is resistant to research.

There is therefore a challenge of engaging clinicians in a sector where there has not traditionally been a research culture. Problems exist in building collaborative research teams as well as conducting research across the range of perspectives that reflect the multidisciplinary nature of palliative care provision. In addition, the predominance of investigator-led over pharmaceutical company-led research in palliative care limits financing opportunities for researchers.

It is therefore seen that there is a paucity of good end-of-life care research in palliative care which is plagued by poorly designed and executed studies, that can produce unclear or erroneous conclusions. The implementation of evidence into practice should form a continuum throughout the evaluation stages to reveal understanding on the process of intervention delivery, the context and the intended outcome(s) [84]. Standard and well-established research methods may need to be adapted to work in this context. Essential to an evidence-based approach to palliative care is therefore well-designed research to answer important questions relating to issues affecting palliative care patients and their families, friends and caregivers. There is therefore a wide scope for research and to better train motivated hospice and palliative care professionals to conduct quality research [85].

An overarching principle of Patient Centred Outcome Research (PCOR) is to "meaningfully engage" patients and their family members/caregivers. The question here is how can we effectively enable people to let us know what is most important to them at the end of their lives? Terminally ill patients should have as much choice and control as possible over their care and there is an obvious need to espouse PCOR as it can provide people with a "voice" to describe their experiences across the continuum of care (thereby enabling healthcare professionals to address their unmet needs). More solid high-quality evidence is needed regarding how PCOR may result in an improvement in the quality of care of patients with advanced disease. To achieve this there is a need to select reliable and valid outcome measures and determine which ones are appropriate for meeting the complex needs of palliative care populations based on scientifically rigorous criteria. The creation of an international exchange and collaboration network between organisations may possess the potential to further develop the concept of PCOR in palliative care and improve the quality of care for people with advanced and terminal illness [86].

Outcome research in palliative care represents a new dimension of clinical research that need to be investigated. The limits in outcome research are not well defined in nursing research or in palliative care dimension, but it should be properly linked to evidence based practice. Literature review of studies measuring outcomes of palliative care services in different ways suggests that identifying high-quality, effective and appropriate palliative care services are a long way away. Quality of life (QoL) is a concept relevant to the discipline of nursing. There is no single QoL instrument serving as the definitive outcome measure for all aspects of nursing research in oncology and palliative care. Reliable and validated instruments are necessary and all those involved, need to have confidence in the findings of a tool and this tool must be applied in a reliable manner in the setting it is used in. Services must pay greater attention to the requirements of standards in palliative care and form networks between partners in the health care system to evaluate care and identify best practice. Developing standards that apply to all services and evaluating those aspects of palliative care which are still unevaluated should have priority. There is an apparent requirement for prospective studies to accurately record symptoms in random samples of the patient populations. Without these studies the assessment of need to manage these symptoms and the suffering will be open to inaccuracies [87].

The research or study may be done as an academic requirement for the educational course as a thesis or dissertation, or for individual interest, or through funding opportunity. It may be done for making a presentation at a conference and overall for career growth. The first step is identifying the area on which a researcher wants to do a study. Some examples of common broad areas in palliative care that can be related to research topics in reference to Oman are: The impact of family structures as bases for good palliative care practice; Magnitude of internalizing/externalizing problems in LLD patients; Addressing Psychological Needs; Mortality awareness and Grief Work; Traditional Healing Practices; Evaluating Care and identifying Best Practice to develop standards of palliative care.

Conclusion

Ever since the original concept of total pain, with its physical, emotional, social and spiritual components, the demands of palliative care have been met by expanding expertise [63]. Palliative care is a team effort and its impact is unique in that it results from a combination of skills. It includes every approach that assists patients and their families to find their own strengths for a journey that is unique to each person. 'Helping people discover life while losing it, is the day to day stuff of palliative care.' – David Oliviere [14]. Healthcare workers and caregivers need to understand that patients have individualized requirements for receiving and processing information and various ways of coping with diagnosis. Factors such as age, gender and educational level, cultural and social values may play a role [88]. When patients receive adequate information, they are better equipped to accept the diagnosis and face the prognosis.

Predictions for exponential growth in the incidence and prevalence of LLD will require a change in the culture and the tendency of mainstream health services in developing countries to turn their focus from "curing" disease and prolonging life at all costs to palliative care services. It mandates that all medical providers be competent in the basic skill sets of palliative medicine [9]. Oman should provide training in palliative care to help increase the local capacity in implementing palliative care practice. [89, 90].

However, many challenges exist when providing international education to those who care for people at the end of life. It is well recognized that traditions of the past influence norms and dictate policies and procedures of the present [91]. Oncology nurses can improve access by becoming knowledgeable about generalist palliative care and by advocating for local and national practice change.

Providing outstanding palliative care is not merely practical, but imperative. It enhances quality of care when added to the work done by the oncology team. Pain control is central to palliative care, and presents challenges in itself. Palliative care services should be in line with WHO recommendations. The analgesia ladder, as developed by WHO, includes three steps: namely home care, treatment to relieve pain and psychological and spiritual support. Support for caregivers is an essential part of palliative care, whether they be family members or professional health carers [10].

Although palliative care is still a young discipline in research especially in developing countries, the time is probably ripe for reviewing the palliative approach and looking at the dimension of palliative care with evidence-based tools and outcome-oriented criteria. Our main strategy should be a successful research application for palliative care program's growth and development. Research in different aspects of palliative care is important and requires active researchers to have prior knowledge of local settings and environment. Simple methods of planning and conducting a research in the area of palliative care in Oman need to be explored. Together with clinical practice, we should move towards this new dimension [83, 85].

Current studies demonstrate that integrating palliative care into oncology care improves symptom control, rates of patient and family satisfaction, and quality of end-of-life care. However, for systemwide integration to be successful, stakeholders must be engaged in the program, commitment must be made to quality improvement, an infrastructure must be built to support palliative care screening, assessment, and intervention. In addition, value must be demonstrated using metrics that affect quality, care utilization and patient as well as family and care provider satisfaction [92].

Even though most cancer centers in the developed nations have a palliative care program, for some reasons, palliative care remains limited in scope. An integrated approach for palliative care with oncology care requires a systems-based approach, with agreement between all parties on shared common metrics for value [13]. Despite recommendations and evidence, only a subset of cancer centers and community-based oncology clinics currently implement palliative care into ambulatory disease-focused cancer care. Although inpatient palliative care programs are well established, this is not the case for outpatient palliative care settings. The very nature of the work entails ambivalence and uncertainty, with the results of the interventions less immediate and often intangible. However, development and growth of outpatient palliative care programs are an essential component to providing excellence in cancer care and will be necessary to address the many new cases of advanced cancer anticipated in the next decades. When these needs are addressed, the quality of care improves, costs decrease, and goals are aligned between the medical care provided and the patient and family. However, how best to integrate palliative care into oncology care is still an area of investigation [86, 87].

Palliative care can substantially reduce healthcare costs for advanced cancer patients, and when initiated early, it is a key driver in lowering expenditures, according to a new study.

Palliative Care consultations that focus on improving quality of life, managing pain and defining goals at the outset of treatment for patients with serious or life-threatening illnesses can result in shorter hospital stays and lower costs, a new study concludes.

This chapter addresses some of the issues to be contemplated if palliative care becomes more meaningful when it will be implemented in Oman. The gist of the above discussion hinges on the facts that illness, sickness or disability is more apt to be experienced in a social-cultural context. Therefore, culturally sensitive measures are needed if palliative care will develop in societies in transition as Oman. This implies that the ultimate goal of the palliative care is to improve the quality of life for both the person and their family using an approach gleaned via cultural lenses. The biopsychosocial approach appears to have all essential ingredients relevant for embracing cross-cultural populations as those in Oman. This implies that best practice in palliative care would require equal footing for each aspect of biopsychosocial care. Although Oman has been using the biomedical approach while addressing pain management, what remains to be considered is the psychological and social aspect of palliative care. It is necessary to have a concerted effort to embrace the biopsychosocial factors in palliative care that are designed to provide quality of life for people with life-limiting diseases as well as those approaching end of life from societies in transition such as Oman [95].

Acknowledgments

The Author would like to thank Professor Samir Al-Adawi, from the department of Behavioral Medicine, College of Medicine & Health Sciences, Sultan Qaboos University for his contribution on the psychosocial, cultural and spiritual aspects of the Omani Society.

References

[1] Sandy Macleod, *The Psychiatry Palliative Medicine: The Dying Mind*; By Radcliffe Medical Press Ltd. Oxford UK 2007. ISBN – 10: 1846190924.

[2] R. R. Hajjar, T. Atli, Z. Al-Mandhari, M. Oudrhiri, L. Balducci, and M. Silbermann; Prevalence of aging population in the Middle East and its implications on cancer incidence and care: *Ann Oncol.* 2013 Oct; 24(Suppl 7): vii11–vii24.

[3] *WHO Definition of Palliative Care*. World Health Organization. March 16, 2018 from http://www.who.int/cancer/palliative/definition/en/.

[4] Derick T Wade and Peter W Halligan; Do biomedical models of illness make for good healthcare systems? *BMJ*. 2004 Dec 11; 329(7479): 1398–1401.

[5] Al Lamki Z. Improving Cancer Care for Children in the Developing World: Challenges and Strategies. *Curr Pediatr Rev.* 2017; 13(1):13-23. doi: 10.2174/1573396312666 161230145417.

[6] Walsh D, Aktas A, Hullihen B, Induru RR. What is palliative medicine? motivations and skills. *Am J Hosp Palliat Care*. 2011 Feb;28(1):52-8. doi: 10.1177/1049909 110393724.

[7] Ramchandran K, Tribett E, Dietrich B, Von Roenn J. Integrating Palliative Care Into Oncology: A Way Forward; *Cancer control: journal of the Moffitt Cancer Center*: October 2015 Oct;22(4):386-95.

[8] Al Lamki, ZMN. Cancer Care in Regions/Societies in Transition in the Gulf States: Sultanate of Oman. In, Silbermann M, editor. *Cancer Care in Countries and Societies in Transition: Individualized Care in Focus*. New York: Springer; 2016, pp.337-348.

[9] John E. Hennessy, Beth A. Lown, MD, Lindy Landzaat, DO, Karin Porter-Williamson, MD JE Hennessy, BA Lown, L Landzaat… - *Practical Issues in Palliative and Quality-of-Life Care: J Oncol Pract*. 2013 Mar; 9(2): 78–80).

[10] Lucas: *Palliative Care Issues and Challenges*. WHO 2002.

[11] Clemens KE, Kumar S, Bruera E, Klaschik E, Jaspers B, De Lima L. Palliative care in developing countries: what are the important issues? *Palliat Med.* 2007 Apr; 21(3):173-5.

[12] Anoosha Mehboob: *A Closer Look at the Psychological and Social Aspects of Palliative Care*; April 7, 2016.

[13] Mazanec P, Prince-Paul M. Integrating palliative care into active cancer treatment. *Semin Oncol Nurs*. 2014 Nov;30(4):203.

[14] David Oliviere & Rosalind Hargreaves. *Good Practices in Palliative Care: A Psychosocial Perspective*; Published by Ashgate 1998: ISBS 1857423968; 9781857423969.

[15] Stjernswȟrd J, Foley KM, Ferris FD. The public health strategy for palliative care. *Journal of pain and symptom management*. 2007 May 1;33(5):486-93.

[16] Kristjanson LJ, Aoun S. Palliative care for families: remembering the hidden patients. *Can J Psychiatry*. 2004 Jun; 49(6):359-65.

[17] Ismail M, Hussein S. Population aging and long-term care policies in the Gulf region: a case study of Oman. *J Aging Soc Policy*. 2018 Jun 8. doi: 10.1080/08959420.2018. 1485392.

[18] Asif M. Expect steep rise in cancer cases in Oman. *Times of Oman*. January 31, 2018. Accessed on August 5, 2018 from https://timesofoman.com/article/127357.

[19] World Health Organization. Oman country profile. *Noncommunicable diseases: Campaign for action – meeting the NCD targets*. Accessed on June 24, 2018 from http://www.who.int/beat-ncds/countries/oman/en/.

[20] Nishtar S, Niinistö S, Sirisena M, Vázquez T, Skvortsova V, Rubinstein A, Mogae FG, Mattila P, Ghazizadeh Hashemi SH, Kariuki S, Narro Robles J, Adewole IF, Sarr AD, Gan KY, Piukala SM, Al Owais ARBM, Hargan E, Alleyne G, Alwan A, Bernaert A, Bloomberg M, Dain K, Frieden T, Patel VH, Kennedy A, Kickbusch I; Commissioners

of the WHO Independent High-Level Commission on NCDs. Time to deliver: report of the WHO Independent High-Level Commission on NCDs. *Lancet.* 2018 May 31. pii: S0140-6736(18)31258-3.doi:10.1016/S0140-6736(18)31258-3.

[21] Al Mukrashi F. Aids patients living in the dark in Oman. *Gulf News.* Accessed on August 6, 2018 from http://gulfnews.com/news/gulf/oman/aids-patients-living-in-the-dark-in-oman-1.1951612.

[22] Islam MM. The practice of consanguineous marriage in Oman: prevalence, trends and determinants. *J Biosoc Sci.* 2012 Sep;44(5):57194.doi:10.1017/S0021932012000016.

[23] Al-Riyami AA, Suleiman AJ, Afifi M, Al-Lamki ZM, Daar S. A community-based study of common hereditary blood disorders in Oman. *East Mediterr Health J.* 2001 Nov;7(6):1004-11.

[24] Alkindi S, Al Zadjali S, Al Madhani A, Daar S, Al Haddabi H, Al Abri Q, Gravell D, Berbar T, Pravin S, Pathare A, Krishnamoorthy R. Forecasting hemoglobinopathy burden through neonatal screening in Omani neonates. *Hemoglobin.* 2010 Apr 1; 34(2):135-44.

[25] L. Violan C, Foguet-Boreu Q, Flores-Mateo G1, Salisbury C, Blom J, Freitag M, Glynn L. Muth C, Valderas JM; Prevalence, determinants and patterns of multimorbidity in primary care: a systematic review of observational studies. *PLoS One.* 2014 Jul 21; 9(7): e102149. doi: 10.1371/journal.pone.0102149.

[26] Al-Sinawi H, Al-Alawi M, Al-Lawati R, Al-Harrasi A, Al-Shafaee M, Al-Adawi S. Emerging burden of frail young and elderly persons in Oman: For whom the bell tolls? *Sultan Qaboos Univ Med J.* 2012 May; 12(2):169-76.

[27] *Health System Profile: Oman- Regional Health System Observatory.* WHO; 2006.

[28] Al-Mandhari A, Alsiyabi H, Al Rabhi S, Al-Adawi SSH, Al-Adawi, S. Oman: Paradigm Change: Healthy Villages to Meet Tomorrow's Health Needs. In, Braithwaite J, Mannion R, Matsuyama Y, Shekelle PG, Whittaker S, Al-Adawi S (Editors), *Healthcare Systems: Future Predictions for Global Care.* Florida, CRC Press Taylor & Francis Group, 2018, pp.319-325.

[29] Alshishtawy MM. Four decades of progress: Evolution of the health system in Oman. *Sultan Qaboos Univ Med J.* 2010 Apr;10(1):12-22.

[30] Al-Lamki Z, Wasifuddin, SM. Palliative care in Oman. In, Michael Silbermann (Editor), *Palliative Care to the Cancer Patient.* New York, Nova Science Publishers, pp. 155-163, 2014.

[31] Al-Mahrezi A1, Al-Mandhari Z2. Palliative Care: Time for Action. *Oman Med J.* 2016 May;31(3):161-3. doi: 10.5001/omj.2016.32.

[32] Ellen S Wright, Biomedical models and healthcare systems: New model will be useful if it alters allocation of resources; *BMJ.* 2005 Feb 19; 330(7488): 419.

[33] Al-Adawi S. Emergence of diseases of affluence in Oman: Where do they feature in the health research agenda? *Sultan Qaboos Univ Med J.* 2006 Dec; 6(2):3-9.

[34] C. Patricia Mazzotta. Biomedical approaches to care and their influence on point of care nurses: a scoping review; *Journal of Nursing Education and Practice* 2016, Vol. 6 No. 8.

[35] Al-Barwani TA; Albeelyb TS. The Omani Family: Strengths and Challenges. *Marriage & Family Review.* Volume 41, Issue 1 & 2, 2007, Pages 119 – 142.

[36] Ramadan E. Sustainable urbanization in the Arabian Gulf region: problems and challenges. *Arts and Social Sciences Journal.* 2015; 6(2):1-4.

[37] Silbermann M (Editor). *Cancer Care in Countries and Societies in Transition: Individualized Care in Focus.* New York: Springer; 2016.

[38] Zeinah GF1, Al-Kindi SG, Hassan AA.Middle East experience in palliative care. *Am J Hosp Palliat Care.* 2013 Feb; 30(1):94-9. doi: 10.1177/1049909112439619.

[39] Mols F1, Husson O, Roukema JA, van de Poll-Franse LV. Depressive symptoms are a risk factor for all-cause mortality: results from a prospective population-based study among 3,080 cancer survivors from the PROFILES registry. *J Cancer Surviv.* 2013 Sep; 7 (3): 484-92. doi: 10.1007/s11764-013-0286-6.

[40] Mitchell AJ, Ferguson DW, Gill J, Paul J, Symonds P. Depression and anxiety in long-term cancer survivors compared with spouses and healthy controls: a systematic review and meta-analysis. *Lancet Oncol.* 2013 Jul;14(8):721-32. doi: 10.1016/S1470- 2045 (13)70244-4.

[41] Tonia C Onyeka. Psychosocial Issues in Palliative Care: A Review of Five Cases. *Indian J Palliat Care.* 2010 Sep-Dec; 16(3): 123–128. doi: 10.4103/0973-1075.73642

[42] Lueboonthavatchai P. Prevalence and psychosocial factors of anxiety and depression in breast cancer patients. *J Med Assoc Thai.* 2007 Oct;90(10):2164-74.

[43] Yang YL1, Liu L, Wang Y, Wu H, Yang XS, Wang JN, Wang L.. The prevalence of depression and anxiety among Chinese adults with cancer: a systematic review and meta-analysis. *BMC Cancer.* 2013 Aug 22;13:393. doi: 10.1186/1471-2407-13-393.

[44] Mhaidat NM, Ai-Sweedan SA, Alzoubi KH, Alazzam SI, Banihani MN, Yasin MO, Massadeh MM.. Prevalence of depression among relatives of cancer patients in Jordan: a cross-sectional survey. *Palliat Support Care.* 2011 Mar;9(1):25-9. doi: 10.1017/S 1478951510000519.

[45] Shaheen Al Ahwal M, Al Zaben F, Khalifa DA, Sehlo MG, Ahmad RG, Koenig HG. Depression in patients with colorectal cancer in Saudi Arabia. *Psychooncology.* 2015 Sep;24(9):1043-50. doi: 10.1002/pon.3706.

[46] Noorani NH, Montagnini M. Recognizing depression in palliative care patients. *J Palliat Med.* 2007 Apr;10(2):458-64.

[47] Jocham HR1, Dassen T, Widdershoven G, Halfens R; Review Quality of life in palliative care cancer patients: a literature review: *J Clin Nurs.* 2006 Sep;15(9):1188-95.

[48] Sprangers MA, Aaronson NK. The role of health care providers and significant others in evaluating the quality of life of patients with chronic disease: a review. *J Clin Epidemiol.* 1992 Jul;45(7):743-60..

[49] Engel GL. The clinical application of the biopsychosocial model. *J Med Philos.* 1981 May;6(2):101-23.

[50] Mari Lloyd-Williams (Editor): *Psychosocial Issues in Palliative Care: A community-based approach for life limiting illness* 3rd Edition, Published: 22nd May 2018; ISBN-978-019880667 ISBN-10: 0198806671.

[51] I Tanchel. *Psychosocial issues in palliative care,* 2003 https://www.ajol.info/index. php/cme/article/viewFile/43891/2741.

[52] Durkin I, Kearney M, O'siorain L. *Psychiatric disorder in a palliative care unit Palliat* Med. 2003 Mar;17(2):212-8.

[53] Marjolein F. van Wijk-Herbrink, David P. Bernstein, Nick J. Broers, Jeffrey Roelofs, Marleen M. Rijkeboer, andArnoud Arntz. Internalizing and Externalizing Behaviors

Share a Common Predictor: the Effects of Early Maladaptive Schemas Are Mediated by Coping Responses and Schema Modes; *Abnorm Child Psychol.* 2018; 46(5): 907–920.

[54] Abou Kassm S, Hlais S, Khater C, Chehade I, Haddad R, Chahine J, Yazbeck M, Abi Warde R, Naja W. Depression and religiosity and their correlates in Lebanese breast cancer patients. *Psycho-Oncology.* 2018 Jan 1;27(1):99-105.

[55] Goldblatt H, Cohen M, Azaiza F. Expression of emotions related to the experience of cancer in younger and older Arab breast cancer survivors. *Ethn Health.* 2016 Dec;21(6):564-77. doi: 10.1080/13557858.2016.1143089.

[56] Al Lawati J, Al Lawati N, Al Siddiqui M, Antony SX, Al Naamani A, Martin RG, Kolbe R, Theodorsson T, Osman Y, Al Hussaini AA, Al Adawi S. Psychological morbidity in primary healthcare in Oman: A preliminary study. *Journal for Scientific Research: Medical Sciences* 2000, 2, 105–10.

[57] Chand SP, Koul R, Al Hussaini AA. Conversion and dissociative disorders in the Sultanate of Oman. *J Am Acad Child Adolesc Psychiatry.* 2001 Aug; 40(8):869-70.

[58] Dwairy M, Van Sickle TD. Western psychotherapy in traditional Arabic societies. *Clin Psychol Rev.* 1996 Jan 1; 16(3):231-49.

[59] Nathan A Boucher, Ejaz A Siddiqui, Harold G Koenig; Supporting Muslim Patients During Advanced Illness: *Perm J.* 2017; 21: 16-190.

[60] Ibbotson T, Maguire P, Selby P, Priestman T, Wallace L. Screening for anxiety and depression in cancer patients: the effects of disease and treatment. *Eur J Cancer.* 1994;30A(1):37-40.

[61] Stiefel F, Die Trill M, Berney A, Olarte JM, Razavi A. Depression in palliative care: a pragmatic report from the Expert Working Group of the European Association for Palliative Care. *Support Care Cancer.* 2001 Oct;9(7):477-88.

[62] Al-Adawi SH, Martin RG, Al-Salmi A, Ghassani H. Zar: group distress and healing. *Mental Health, Religion & Culture.* 2001 May 1;4(1):47-61.

[63] Malloy P, Paice J, Coyle N, Coyne P, Smith T, Ferrell B. *Promoting palliative care worldwide through international nursing education; J Transcult Nurs.* 2014 Oct;25(4): 410-7. doi: 10.1177/1043659614523993. Epub 2014 Mar 4.

[64] MR Rajagopal: Disease, Dignity and Palliative Care; *Indian J Palliat Care.* 2010 May-Aug; 16(2): 59–60. doi: 10.4103/0973-1075.68400.

[65] Mīrsk JL, Cutchin MP, la Cour K. Identity and home: Understanding the experience of people with advanced cancer. *Health & Place.* 2018 May 31;51:11-8.

[66] World Health Organization. *National Policy on Traditional Medicine and Regulation of Herbal Medicines: Report of A WHO Global Survey.* Accessed on June 21, 2018 from http://apps.who.int/medicinedocs/en/d/Js7916e/.

[67] Al-Rowais N, Al-Faris E, Mohammad AG, Al-Rukban M, Abdulghani HM. Traditional healers in Riyadh region: reasons and health problems for seeking their advice. A household survey. *J Altern Complement Med.* 2010 Feb;16(2):199-204. doi: 10.1089/acm.2009.0283.

[68] Ben-Arye, E. Integrating complementary medicine in cancer supportive care across the Middle East: challenges and opportunities. In, M. Silbermann (Ed.) *Palliative Care to the Cancer Patient: the Middle East as a Model to Emerging Countries.* Nova Science Publishers, NY; 2014:77–97.

[69] Ben-Arye E, Schiff E, Mutafoglu K, Omran S, Hajjar R, Charalambous H, Dweikat T. Ghrayeb I, Sela GB, Turker I, Hassan A, Hassan E, Popper-Giveon A, Saad B, Nimri

O, Kebudi R, Dagash J, Silbermann M. Integration of complementary medicine in supportive cancer care: survey of health-care providers' perspectives from 16 countries in the Middle East. *Support Care Cancer*. 2015 Sep;23(9):2605-12. doi: 10.1007/s00520-015-2619-7

[70] Kramer S, Irnich D, Lorenzl S. Acupuncture for Symptom Relief in Palliative Care- Study Protocol and Semistandardized Treatment Schemes. *J Acupunct Meridian Stud*. 2017 Aug;10(4):294-302. doi: 10.1016/j.jams.2017.04.004.

[71] Jabin F. A guiding tool in Unani Tibb for maintenance and preservation of health: a review study. Afr J Tradit Complement *Altern Med.* 2011;8(5 Suppl):140-3. doi: 10.4314/ajtcam.v8i5S.7.

[72] Al Asmi A, Al Maniri A, Al-Farsi YM, Burke DT, Al Asfoor FM, Al Busaidi I, Al Breiki MH, Lahiri S, Braidy N, Essa MM, Al-Adawi S. Types and sociodemographic correlates of complementary and alternative medicine (CAM) use among people with epilepsy in Oman. *Epilepsy and Behavior*. 2013 Sep 3. doi:pii: S1525-5050(13)00345-10.1016/j.yebeh.2013.07.022.

[73] Robin B Rome, MSN, FNP-C, Hillary H Luminais, RN, Deborah A. Bourgeois, MN, APRN, ACNS-BC, and Christopher M Blais, Ochsner J. *The Role of Palliative Care at the End of Life*; 2011 Winter; 11(4): 348–352.

[74] Wright AA, Zhang B, Ray A, Mack JW, Trice E, Balboni T, Mitchell SL, Jackson VA, Block SD, Maciejewski PK, Prigerson HG. Associations between end-of-life discussions, patient mental health, medical care near death, and caregiver bereavement adjustment. *JAMA*. 2008 Oct 8;300(14):1665-73.

[75] Allen RS, Carpenter BD, Eichorst MK. The international context of behavioural palliative and end-of-life care revisited. In *Perspectives on Palliative and End-of-Life Care* 2018 Jun 13 (pp. 13-16). Routledge.

[76] Parkes CM, Laungani P, Young W (Editors) (2rd Edition). *Death and Bereavement across Cultures*. London, Routledge, 2015.

[77] Abdel-Khalek A, Lester D. Religiosity and death anxiety: no association in Kuwait. *Psychol Rep*. 2009 Jun;104(3):770-2.

[78] Gatrad AR, Sheikh A. Palliative care for Muslims and issues before death. *Int J Palliat Nurs*. 2002 Nov;8(11):526-31.

[79] Al-Adawi S1, Burjorjee R, al-Issa I. Mu-Ghayeb: a culture-specific response to bereavement in Oman. *Int J Soc Psychiatry*. 1997 Summer;43(2):144-51.

[80] Wikan U. Bereavement and loss in two Muslim communities: Egypt and Bali compared. *Soc Sci Med*. 1988;27(5):451-60.

[81] Klass D, Goss R. The politics of grief and continuing bonds with the dead: the cases of Maoist China and Wahhabi Islam. *Death Stud*. 2003 Nov;27(9):787-811.

[82] Al-Adawi S, Al-Busaidi Z, Al-Adawi S, Burke DT. Families coping with disability due to brain injury in Oman: Attribution to belief in spirit infestation and ensorcellment. *Sage Open*. 2012 Jul 23;2(3):2158244012457400.

[83] Santosh K Chaturvedi: How to Plan Research in Palliative Care; *Indian J Palliat Care*. 2011 Jan; 17(Suppl): S4–S7.

[84] Potts M1, Cartmell KB, Nemeth L, Bhattacharjee G, Qanungo S. A Systematic Review of Palliative Care Intervention Outcomes and Outcome Measures in Low- Resource Countries. *J Pain Symptom Manage*. 2018 May; 55(5):1382-1397.e7. doi: 10.1016/j.jpainsymman.2017.12.487.

[85] Julia M. Addington-Hall (editor), Eduardo Bruera (editor), Irene J. Higginson (editor), Sheila Payne (editor). *Research Methods in Palliative Care*; Publisher: Oxford University Press ISBN 9780198530251.

[86] Thomas J Lynch. *Patient-Centred Outcomes Research in Palliative Care – End of Life Studies Podcast*; University of Glasgow: June 2, 2015

[87] De Palma R, Fortuna D, Hegarty SE, Louis DZ, Melotti RM, Moro ML. Effectiveness of palliative care services: A population-based study of end-of-life care for cancer patients. *Palliat Med*. 2018 Jun 1:269216318778729. doi: 10.1177/0269216318778729.

[88] Saeed F, Hoerger M, Norton SA, Guancial E, Epstein RM, Duberstein PR. Preference for Palliative Care in Cancer Patients: Are Men and Women Alike? *J Pain Symptom Manage*. 2018 Mar 23.

[89] Al-Zadjali M, Al Sinawi F, Al Touby S, Al Busaidi M, Al Jardani F. Palliative Care Nursing in Oman; Moving towards Palliative Care Nursing. *Journal of Palliative Care Medicine* 2015, S5:003. doi:10.4172/2165-7386.1000S5003.

[90] Arthur G. Lipman, Editor: *Pain Management for Primary Care Clinicians*; 2004 PharmD.

[91] Kübler-Ross E. *On death and dying: What the dying have to teach doctors, nurses, clergy and their own families*. New York, Taylor & Francis; 2009.

[92] Adelman RD, Tmanova LL, Delgado D, Dion S, Lachs MS. Caregiver burden: a clinical review. *JAMA*. 2014 Mar 12; 311(10):1052-60.

[93] Pamela Stitzlein Davies, Maryjo Prince-Paul. Palliative Care in the Outpatient Cancer Center Current Trends: *Journal of Hospice and Palliative Nursing* December 14(8):506-513.

[94] Miličević N. The hospice movement: history and current worldwide situation. *Arch Oncol*. 2002; 10(1):29-31.

[95] Carl B. Becker, Elizabeth Clark, Lynne A DeSpelder, Diana Wilkie: A call to action: An IWG Charter for a Public Health Approach to Dying, Death, And Loss. *OMEGA- J Death Dying*; Dec 2014.

BIOGRAPHICAL SKETCH

Zakiya Al Lamki

Zakiya Al Lamki graduated with MD from Cairo University in 1979. She subsequently received her postgraduate training at the Institute of Child Health in London and later enhanced her experience in the subspecialty of pediatric hematology and oncology at the M.D. Anderson Cancer Center and Texas Children's Cancer Centre (TCCC) in U.S.A. She attended as a visiting Professor for six weeks at the Centre of Genomics and Policy at the McGill University. She holds Fellowships of the Royal College of Physicians and Child Health in London; (FRCP FRCPCH) as well as the Royal College of Physicians of (Ireland).

Dr. Al Lamki was a pioneer in the establishment of the Department of Child Health at the Sultan Qaboos University which she headed from 1995 to 2005. She was a founder of the Pediatric Hematology and Oncology services at the Institution. Over the years, she took a leading role in the multi-dimensional activities of the Department including Clinical,

Academic Research. She organized several international conferences and training courses, fund raising and patients support. She was one of the early teachers who taught the next generation of pediatricians in the country.

She established links in clinical education, training programs and research with many renowned institutions abroad. One of her joint projects in collaboration with TCCC was amongst the first strategic projects, funded by His Majesty's Research Grants. Apart from the scientific and training goals, this project accomplished important improvements in genetic diagnosis and clinical practice related to Childhood Leukemia in Oman as well as the transfer of molecular diagnostics and data management practices. The hospital based comprehensive childhood cancer registry she built, underpins current and future research projects.

Dr. Al Lamki has successfully achieved International recognition in bringing Oman to various international and regional professional bodies and scientific organizations. Besides, she serves as a Temporary Advisor of WHO's Data, Safety and Monitoring Board in childhood vaccine trials and collaborates closely with regional scientific bodies such as the Middle East Childhood Cancer Alliance (MECCA) in studies on the genetics and behavior of Childhood Cancer in the region.

She was honored with the National Award for outstanding contribution to the Welfare of Omani Society and received the Gulf Cooperation Council (GCC) Scientific Award for Excellent Services. Her goal and interest remain in capacity-building; including training others to carry on research and clinical activities.

Part V. Far East

In: Palliative Care
Editor: Michael Silbermann

ISBN: 978-1-53616-199-1
© 2019 Nova Science Publishers, Inc.

Chapter 21

PALLIATIVE CARE NURSING IN JAPAN: PRACTICE AND RESEARCH

Tomoko Majima[*], *PhD* *and Tomoko Otsuka*
Chiba University Graduate School of Nursing, Chiba, Japan

ABSTRACT

Cancer incidence in Japan, which has been the leading cause of death since 1981, has consistently increased. The Cancer Professional Infrastructure Promotion Plan has improved interprofessional education for patient-centered care. In the Japanese payment system for medical services, a fee for new systems has been collected for activities of certified nurse specialists and certified nurses involved in cancer care. Community health-care systems are tasked with providing comprehensive medical care and social services, while visiting nurses play a central role in collaboration with care professionals. A survey conducted for visiting nurses in Japan compared those who had or had not received further education after acquiring a registered nurse's license. This comparison showed that advanced care planning and palliative care were performed more frequently by those with further education. Furthermore, visiting nurses in the group who had received continuing education were performing professional end-of-life care. In the context of Japanese culture, there is insufficient cooperation with medical and non-medical professionals who conduct complementary alternative medicine.

Keywords: palliative care qualitative research, certified nurse specialist, advanced care planning, visiting nursing

---

[*] Corresponding Author's E-mail: tmajima61@outlook.com.

BACKGROUND

The total population of Japan is 126.93 million, with those aged 65 or over years numbering 34.59 million, and the aging rate is 27.3% [1]. The rate in Japan was the world's highest in 2005, and is expected to remain high in the future. Since the World Health Organization (WHO) advocated healthy life in 2000, there has been growing interest not only in extending life expectancy but also in extending the period of healthy life.

According to WHO World Health Statistics 2016, Japan's life expectancy was 83.7 years. However, the Ministry of Health, Labor and Welfare of Japan indicated the difference between average and healthy life expectancy in 2016 was large (healthy life, 72.14 year for men and 74.79 years for women) [2] (Figure 1).

The government is considering a policy to extend healthy lives by more than three years by 2040, when the aged population is expected to peak. Despite this, from 2025, the demand for medical and nursing care is expected to increase further due to population increase of those aged 75 years or older. The government aims to build a system to enable people to continue living in their community until life's end, even if they require care. A comprehensive system including prevention of illness, medical and nursing care in hospitals, and a visiting nurse system that includes end-of-life care in the community is necessary. Visiting nurses must play a central role in promoting collaboration among medical caregivers.

Cancer prevalence has consistently increased among Japanese, and was the leading cause of death since 1981. Of total deaths in 2016, the percentage of cancer patients was 28.5%, and approximately one in every 3.5 deaths was due to cancer [3]. The government is therefore examining gene mutations in cancer patients and promoting "cancer genome medicine," which administers optimal therapeutic drugs, and employs preventive measures for frail people whose muscular strength and cognitive ability are weakened, aiming to extend a healthy life span.

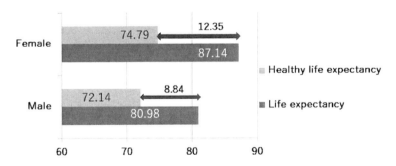

Figure 1. Difference between the average life expectancy and healthy life expectancy.

TRENDS IN PALLIATIVE CARE MEASURES AND MEDICAL TREATMENT FEES OF ADVANCED PRACTICAL NURSES

As a policy for educating medical personnel on cancer patients, the Cabinet approved the Third Basic Plan to Promote Cancer Control Programs. This plan shows the direction of cancer research, human resource development, cancer education, and promoting wellness [4].

Table 1. Nursing professions involved with cancer care

	Particular Field
Certified Nurse Specialist*	Cancer Nursing
	Psychiatric Mental Health Nursing
Certified Nurse**	Cancer Pain Management Nursing
	Cancer Chemotherapy Nursing
	Radiation Therapy Nursing
	Breast Cancer Nursing
	Palliative Care
	Dysphagia Nursing
	Wound, Ostomy and Continence Nursing

*Received an education for two years or more through an accredited graduate school curriculum and is qualified and certified.
**Received at least six months of training and passed the qualification examination.

In the Cancer Professional Infrastructure Promotion Plan, education for multiple relevant occupations is relevant for realizing patient-centered medical care for cancer. The plan will support genomic cancer medicine, childhood cancer, and young cancer patients, and improve support through life stages. In this new system, a health fees for healthcare services will be paid for the activities of certified nurse specialists and certified nurses involved in cancer care (Table 1).

SURVEY OF NURSES IN PALLIATIVE CARE IN JAPAN

In 2008, research on knowledge and difficulties concerning nurses' palliative care provided in hospitals and at home showed that management of patients' psychological symptoms was insufficient. However, further data in 2014 showed improvement [5].

Yet another study showed visiting nurses' challenges. From the results of this survey on December in 2009 on visiting nurses' educational situation and learning needs, 382 visiting nurses in Nagano Prefecture showed learning needs regarding dementia, respiratory care, and home terminal care [6].

Suzuki et al. [7] revealed the high priority of cancer research in cancer nursing in a cross-sectional study of 3,400 members of the Japanese Society of Cancer Nursing. The results found the highest priorities were support for patients' decision-making during discharge at hospitals and palliative care, ethical issues, and improvement of cancer nursing research.

Cancer diagnosis and the transition from curative treatment to terminal care can produce a psychological crisis. The psychological crisis of a cancer patient refers to a condition of strong stress on the mind and body caused by cancer incidence and treatment. Kamma et al. [8] revealed the assistance of nurses with cancer patients in crisis situations in helping them overcome the crisis and promote a process of well-being. They interviewed eight nurses, and analyzed the data qualitatively. They clarified 10 categories of nursing interventions for cancer patients to help overcome their crisis. The preventative categories were: ensuring patients' physical safety and comfort, making the best of their competences, and helping them develop appropriate attitudes for confronting crisis.

Patients who received palliative or end-of-life care may be told by physicians that there is no treatment option, and that the place of care will move from the hospital to the home. At that time, feelings may fluctuate. Sakurai et al. [9] expressed this as *yure*, a Japanese word expressing the anxiety, ambivalence, conflict, and confusion experienced by terminal cancer patients and their families, leading them to reconsider and retract decisions during the process of deciding on and transitioning to end-of-life palliative care. They clarified *yure* in the decision to make the transition to such care among families of terminal cancer patients with six months or less to live.

As a result, *yure* in the families included: being thankful for information provided as a source of help to provide the best care to the patient; being overwhelmed and confused by the large quantity and impact of information, preparation, and devotion required as a family caregiver; loss of caregiver self-confidence when the patient's condition deteriorates; striving to understand the patient's wishes and feelings; and difficulties in maintaining consideration for their intentions. This suggested the need for psychological support in the cognition of patients and families when implementing decision-making changes.

As Japan becomes a super-aged society, a great deal of dying will take place. Because it is necessary to support decision making regarding treatment periods and locales for treatment or recuperation for older cancer patients, advanced care planning is needed. Such an approach upholds patient and family values and shares the goals of treatment and care in this highly stressful situation. Nurses and caregivers need strong communication skills to help support patients and families in decision making.

For this reason, in Japan, many education systems have been developed to improve communication with patients and professionals. Topics include perspectives of life and death, and mutual support systems with patients and professionals.

JAPANESE DATA FROM AN INTERNATIONAL COMPARATIVE STUDY OF PALLIATIVE CARE GIVEN BY VISITING NURSES

This research is an analysis of part of Silbermann's research data conducted in November 2017.

Research Objectives:

This survey clarified the role of visiting nurses, work environments, satisfaction, barriers, and strengths and resources of home care, and support for continuing education.

- Participants' facilities: 13 (in Hokkaido, Tokyo, Kanagawa, Chiba, and Aichi Prefectures)
- Number of participants: 62 questionnaires distributed (collected, 47; collection rate, 75.8%; effective response rate, 100%)
- Background of participants

Average age: 45.3 (27–66, standard deviation, 9.28) years

Years of nursing experience: 18.5 (range, 2–34, standard deviation, 8.29) Gender: female, 45; male, 2.

Employment form: full-time, 74.5%, part-time, 25.5%

Care provision area: rural (fewer than 50,000 people), 4.9%, urban (more than 50,000 people), 85.1% Education: university graduates, 14.9%
Qualification: nurse, 100% (public health nurse: 29.8%, midwife: 0%)

- Results

Results showed collaborative practice with other professions (Figure 2), frequency of providing care (Figure 3), satisfaction with provided care (Figure 4), and barriers to providing care (Figure 5).

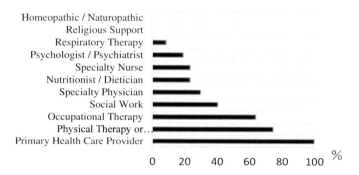

Figure 2. Collaborative profession.

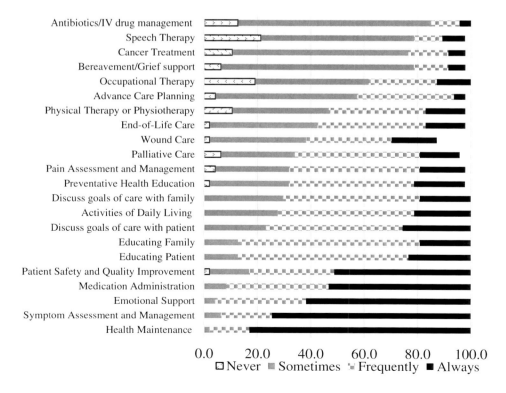

Figure 3. Frequency of provide care.

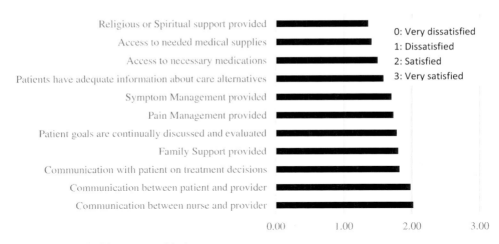

Figure 4. Satisfaction with care provided.

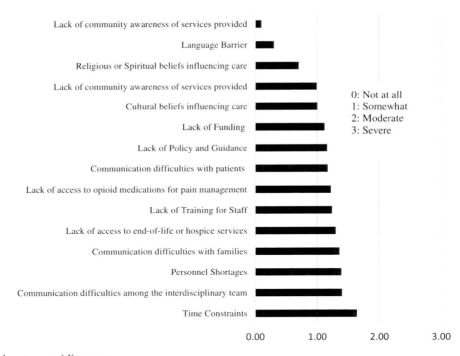

Figure 5. Barriers to providing care.

COMPARISON BETWEEN PRESENCE AND ABSENCE OF CONTINUING EDUCATION

We compared those who had received continuing education (N = 30), and those who had not (N = 17), after acquiring a nursing license. We found that advanced care planning (p = 0.005) and palliative care (p = 0.026) were performed significantly more by those who had received continuing education.

CONCLUSION

A challenge in Japan is limiting medical expenses associated with the growing population of older people. It is also a challenge to enhance these people's quality of life because of the large difference between average and healthy life expectancy.

A policy of new medical education for palliative care has been launched to promote research and human resource development. From an economic standpoint, medical care is shifting from hospitals to communities. Expectations of the roles of advanced nurses are increasing in both, which affects medical fees. Some palliative care research has proposed methods for enhancing the quality of community based palliative care.

Study results of our investigations of palliative care by visiting nurses showed that barriers to care included: accessing services for end-of-life care, introducing opioids, insufficient length of time for providing care, and human resource shortages.

It was also revealed that visiting nurses in the group who received continuing education conducted professional end-of-life care. However, results showed that these nurses had not conducted spiritual support. Recently, many cancer survivors have assumed roles of mutual support through social networking systems and small group meetings.

REFERENCES

[1] http://www.stat.go.jp/data/jinsui/pdf/201807.pdf.
[2] http://www.mhlw.go.jp/file/05-Shingikai-10601000-Daijinkanboukouseikagakuka-Kouseikagakuka/0000166296_6.pdf.
[3] http://www.mhlw.go.jp/toukei/saikin/hw/jinkou/geppo/nengai16/dl/gaikyou28.pdf.
[4] http://www.mhlw.go.jp/file/06-Seisakujouhou-10900000-enkoukyoku/0000196974.pdf.
[5] Yamagishi A, Sato K, Miyashita M, et al. (2014) Changes in quality of care and quality of life of outpatients with advanced cancer after a regional palliative care intervention program. *J Pain Symptom Manage.* 48(4), 602-610.
[6] Karasawa K, Yasuda K, Mikoshiba Y, et al.(2012) *Current Status in-Service Training and Learning Needs of Home-Visiting Nurses in Nagano Prefecture* (2nd Report): Analysis of the Questionnaire Survey of Nursing Staff. Nagano Collage of Nursing. 14, 25-34.
[7] Suzuki K, Hayashi N, Fujita S, et al. (2017) Research Priorities of Oncology Nursing in Japan: The Website Survey by Member of Japanese Society of Cancer Nursing in 2016. *Journal of Japanese Society of Cancer Nursing.* 31, 57-65.
[8] Kamma Y, Sato M, Masujima M, Shibata J, Majima T. (2008) Nursing interventions for cancer patients to help overcome their crisis. *Journal of Chiba Academy of Nursing Science.* 14(2), 20-27.

[9] Sakurai C, Majima T. (2013) 'Yure' in Decisions by Families of Cancer Patients Regarding the Transition to terminal Palliative Care. *Journal of Cultural Nursing Studies.* 5(1), 20-27.

BIOGRAPHICAL SKETCHES

Tomoko Majima, RN, PhD

Professor, Adult Nursing Care, Graduate School of Nursing, Chiba University

E-mail Address: tmajima61@outlook.com

Education:
  1998 Ph.D. Nursing Chiba University, Graduate School of Nursing, JAPAN
  1990 M.S. Nursing Chiba University, Graduate School of Nursing, JAPAN
  1983 B.N. Nursing Chiba University, School of Nursing, JAPAN

Fields of Specialty
  Cardiac Rehabilitation
  End of life care
  Cancer nursing
  Education for Certified nurse specialist (cancer)

A. Publications (selected)

1. Sano M, Majima, T. (2018): Self-Management of Congestive Heart Failure among Elderly Men in Japan, *International Journal of Nursing Practice.* https://doi.org/10.1111/ijn.12653.
2. Kosaka, M, Majima, T. (2016): Nursing intervention to improve flexible coping of postoperative gastric cancer patients receiving ambulatory chemotherapy, *Journal of Graduate School of Nursing Chiba University*, 21(2), 9-16.
3. Majima, T., Sato R et al. (2015): Cognitive changes experienced by nurses who participated in a support program for certified nurse specialists, *Journal of School of Nursing, Chiba University.* (37), 57-64.

B. Conference (International) Selected

1. Majima, T. Sakai, I et al. (2017), Nursing Student Experience of Clinical Interprofessional Education in the Intensive Care Unit. *the 7th Hong Kong International Nursing Forum* (Hong Kong).
2. Otsuka, T, Majima, T. (2016), Cause of stigma cancer patients: A literature Review. *International Conference on Cancer Nursing* (Hong Kong).
3. Majima, T., Yamamoto,T et al.(2016), Comparison of Competency for Interprofessional Collaborative Practice and Job Satisfaction among Medical

Professionals in Intensive Care Units and Operational Rooms at Two Hospital in Japan, *19TH East Asia Forum of Nursing Scholars*, (Japan).

Tomoko Otsuka, (PhD Candidate), RN, MS
Doctor course, Adult Nursing, Graduate School of Nursing, Chiba University

Business Address: 1-8-1, lnohana, Chuo-ku, Chiba 260-8672, JAPAN

Education:
2014 M.S. Nursing Chiba University, Graduate School of Nursing, JAPAN
2007 B.N. Nursing School of Nursing and Rehabilitation Sciences. Showa University, JAPAN

Fields of Specialty: Cancer nursing, Nursing education

Publications Selected:

1. Otsuka T, Makiko N, Shiromaru M, et.al (2018) Student's leaning from operating room observation practice as part of perioperative nursing training. *Sapporo Journal of Health Sciences*, 7, 31-37.
2. Sato K, Otsuka T, Nakamura M, et.al (2018) Investigation into achievement levels and experience frequencies employing nursing skills among students in the final year of nursing study. *Sapporo Journal of Health Sciences*, 7, 50-54.
3. Otsuka T, Ohno T, Majima T (2017) Experience of Women Diagnosed with a Pre-Cancerous Cervical Lesion during the Consultation Period. *Journal of Japanese Society of Cancer Nursing,* 3 I, 21-30.
4. Otsuka T, Makino N, Shiromaru M, et.al (2017) Evaluation of leaning performance based on the taxonomy of education objectives (part I). *Sapporo Journal of Health Sciences*, 6, 35-41.

Conference (International) Selected:

1. Otsuka T, Majima T: Stigma of Japanese women diagnosed with precancerous lesions of the cervix. *International Conference on Cancer Nursing* (ICCN). Auckland, New Zealand. 2018.
2. Otsuka T, Makino N, Shiromaru M, et al.: Student's Leaning from Study Visiting to ICU and ACCEC (Advanced Critical Care & Emergency Center) as Part of Practical Training in Adult Nursing. *20th East Asian Forum of Nursing Scholars* (EAFONS). Hong Kong, China. 2017.
3. Otsuka T, Majima T: *Causes of Stigma in Cancer Patients: A Literature Review*. International Conference on Cancer Nursing (ICCN). Hong Kong, China. 2016.

Part VI. Oceania

In: Palliative Care
Editor: Michael Silbermann

ISBN: 978-1-53616-199-1
© 2019 Nova Science Publishers, Inc.

Chapter 22

THE ROLE AND IMPORTANCE OF RESEARCH IN PROMOTING PALLIATIVE CARE PRACTICE: METHODS AND OUTCOMES

Paul A. Glare[*]

Northern Clinical School, Faculty of Medicine and Health, University of Sydney, Sydney, Australia
Discipline of Pain Medicine, Sydney Medical School, Sydney, Australia
Pain Management Research Institute, Faculty of Medicine, Faculty of Medicine and Health, University of Sydney, Sydney, Australia

ABSTRACT

Palliative care is a relatively new specialty. Becoming established in the Evidence Based Medicine era, there has been a strong argument, even claims of a moral imperative, for the care of incurable patients that is delivered in the name of "palliative care" to be scientifically proven [1]. No doubt some components of palliative care, e.g., the pharmacological management of symptoms, would seem to be amenable to traditional research methods such as randomized controlled trials [2]. The evidence base of palliative care, while under-developed compared to other medical specialties, is growing and has contributed to the better understanding of symptom mechanisms, the limits of old approaches and the benefits of new ones. However, there are many challenges to be faced when undertaking research in palliative care and they question the validity and generalizability of the results. The aim of this chapter is to present some of the principles and challenges of undertaking research in palliative medicine, and how one might go about getting started in research to build their case. Reflecting on the vicissitudes of my own research career, the challenges of studying pain and other symptoms, prognostication, and screening are discussed in detail. Research in the new area of behavioral insights and palliative care is also discussed. Anyone these days who is serious about a research career in palliative care really should enroll in a PhD.

---

[*] Corresponding Author's E-mail: paul.glare@sydney.edu.au.

Keywords: palliative care, research, clinical trials, pain, prognosis, screening, decision-making

INTRODUCTION

Palliative care is a relatively new specialty. Becoming established in the Evidence Based Medicine era, there has been a strong argument, even claims of a moral imperative, for the care of incurable patients that is delivered in the name of "palliative care" to be scientifically proven [1]. No doubt some components of palliative care, e.g., the pharmacological management of symptoms, would seem to be amenable to traditional research methods such as randomized controlled trials [2]. The evidence base of palliative care, while underdeveloped compared to other medical specialties, is growing and has contributed to the better understanding of symptom mechanisms, the limits of old approaches and the benefits of new ones. However, there are many challenges to be faced when undertaking research in palliative care and they question the validity and generalizability of the results. Others would argue there is a moral obligation to relieve suffering [3] – as Gandhi said, *"a society is judged by how it cares for its most vulnerable."* Some have even gone so far as to say there is no place for research in palliative care on the grounds it is inappropriate and unethical [4]. Certainly, these days if you are dealing with hard-headed administrators while trying to build a palliative care program in your hospital you will need to make a persuasive business case that demonstrates the benefits of palliative care for the institution. The results of research will be part of that business case. The aim of this chapter is to present some of the principles and challenges of undertaking research in palliative medicine, and how one might go about getting started in research to build their case.

PRINCIPLES OF PALLIATIVE CARE RESEARCH

There are three key issues to keep in mind when designing palliative care research. The first is that palliative care is not a disease or a diagnosis but a philosophy of care of patients with various diagnoses. Various groups beginning with the World Health Organization (WHO) in 1990 have defined palliative care and what kind of activities should be done under this rubric [5]. These activities can be studied in clinical trials and in fact have been shown to be efficacious in improving the construct known as quality of life, [6] but ultimately science cannot answer metaphysical questions about ensuring the dignity of humans as they die.

The second issue is related to the first – given that palliative care is not a disease, the term "palliative care patient" does not mean the same as "a cancer patient" or "an AIDS patient", and cannot be used in the inclusion/exclusion criteria of a research study. "Palliative care patient" can be short hand for two different sets of patients – those with diseases that cause the kinds of needs that are best addressed using a palliative care approach, or those who have been referred to a palliative care team.

This leads to the third issue: the distinction between palliative care as a philosophy and palliative care as a medical specialty. Professional organizations such as the National Quality Forum define palliative care as a multidisciplinary approach to specialized medical and nursing care for people with life-limiting illnesses [7]. It focuses on providing relief from the symptoms, pain, physical stress, and mental stress at any stage of illness. The goal is to improve quality of life for both the person and their family. It may be decided by a hospital or other organization that this specialized, multidisciplinary care is best organized as Service and the impact of Palliative Care Services can be studied. But the relief of symptoms and other distress, the making of difficult decisions, and the support of the patient and family involves many other people, including non-professionals.

Notwithstanding these caveats pose some unique challenges for study design and analysis, there is a growing evidence base for the interventions undertaken in the name of palliative care which forms the body of knowledge of the medical specialty of Hospice & Palliative Medicine. This evidence can be used to advance the case for a new palliative care program. The evidence base includes studies of interventions for pain management, the control of other symptoms, and the impact of palliative care as a more complex intervention on outcomes such as quality of life, health care utilization, cost and survival.

This research has largely followed the standard research cycle (see Figure), with the exception that most hypotheses are generated from case reports, surveys, or the transfer of existing ideas from other fields, rather than from innovative preclinical research. Unlike disease-based disciplines such as oncology and immunology, there has been very little preclinical biomedical research undertaken in the name of Palliative Medicine with the aim of identifying novel mechanisms and pathways for which novel druggable targets could discovered and new molecules developed to be tested in translational research that would transform the lives of patients with progressive eventually fatal illnesses. Certainly many clinical trials have been undertaken in palliative care but they have been almost entirely studies of new formulations of old drugs (e.g., sustained release opioids and TIRF's), [8] studies of current formulations of old drugs for "off-label" use (e.g., haloperidol for chronic nausea of advanced disease), [9] or even studies of current formulations of old drugs for which little evidence exists – as is currently the case with medicinal cannabis [5] A small number of new molecules have come along, such as nerve growth factor antibody and naloxegol, [10, 11] with the early Phase clinical trials of both in first decade of this century. Some have appeared promising but failed to be approved (e.g., the ghrelin inhibitor, anamorelin, for anorexia cachexia) [12]. However, these agents (perhaps with the exception of anamorelin) were not developed specifically by palliative care scientists or for patients with eventually fatal illnesses, if for no other reason than palliative care is too small of a pharmaceutical market to justify the R&D costs.

To be sure, there are laboratories that are undertaking preclinical research that is of direct relevance to symptom management of patients with advanced disease, such as the Mantyh lab in Arizona that is studying pain from bone metastases, [13] or the Golub lab at the Broad institute (Cambridge MA) which is researching the genomics of cachexia (http://grantome.com/grant/NIH/R01-CA190101-01). It is well known it takes decades and millions of dollars for new molecules to make it to the pharmaceutical market but hopefully one day labs such as these will produce a wonder drug.

Prognostication is another topic that has been within the bailiwick of palliative care research, and is easy to study as the outcome event is common and objective. In the early days (1980's), in the USA interest in prognostication was driven by the legal requirement for clinicians to document a prognosis of < 6 months for hospice eligibility – with harsh penalties for under-estimating survival – but in Europe and elsewhere it was driven by a desire to improve communication with patients and families about what to expect and as a technical pre-requisite for good clinical decision making in patients with progressive, eventually fatal illnesses. Advances in statistical computing enabled predictive models to be developed, but the date of death is affected by many variables so the models have failed to achieve better predictive accuracy than the clinical intuition of experienced clinicians [14]. Predicting death also raises ethical concerns for some people. For these reasons, the models have not been widely taken up or tested as decision aids. As we move into the age of 'big data' and machine learning, better models will be possible and prognostication may make a research renaissance.

In recent years there has been a surge in research on health care utilization, impact on informal caregivers and spirituality at the end of life [15-17]. This may reflect changes in the WHO definition of palliative care early this century [18]. Originally focused on incurable cancer and pain management, [5] the current definition now emphasizes "early identification and impeccable assessment and treatment of pain and other problems, physical, psychosocial and spiritual". Studies such as the RCT of early palliative care in lung cancer have evaluated the hypothesis that combining palliative care with cancer treatment is more effective than cancer treatment alone [15]. These studies have evaluated palliative care as a complex intervention, and primarily psychosocial rather than biomedical. Others have obtained similar results, [19, 20] the data have been synthesized, [6] and guidelines developed by groups such as the American Society of Clinical Oncology and the National Comprehensive Cancer Network [21, 22]. The guidelines provide recommendations for oncologists on the "what, when, and how" of palliative care. Implementation studies complete the research cycle for this question, but to date, surveys indicate that implementation in the clinical setting is limited, and improving this is challenging [23]. This generates more questions, and the research cycle is renewed.

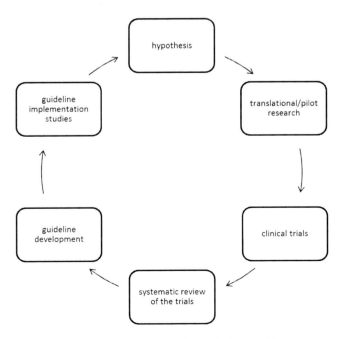

Figure 1. Research cycle to establish a new treatment for a clinical problem.

The intellectual cycle of research (see Figure 1) is essentially the same in palliative care as in other clinical research, and so too are the other components of the research endeavor. The highly productive Australian Palliative Care Clinical Studies Collaborative (PaCCSC) has confirmed that to successfully conduct research that changes practice, there are many other operational considerations to allow for. These include (https://www.uts.edu.au/research-and-teaching/our-research/IMPACCT/paccsc/what-paccsc): [24]

- developing a research group,
- building research capacity, including mentoring junior researchers and supervising research students;
- developing expertise in grant writing;
- obtaining funding and spending it effectively;
- protocol writing;
- dealing with IRB's and other governance issues;
- providing good project management (recruiting and hiring research staff; timely collection, analysis and interpretation of data; report writing),
- closure of the grant,
- dissemination of results,
- data management,
- dealing with any IP issues.

But even when all these components are done carefully, palliative care research, especially clinical trials, is notoriously difficult to do because of problems with recruitment and attrition.

PUTTING IT INTO PRACTICE: MY PERSONAL RESEARCH CAREER

Having trained in a university teaching hospital in which participation in research and teaching were the norm, I have been raised to believe that clinicians from the Palliative Care Service should do the same. While I have done research on various topics, I would review for 4 which inform the objectives of this chapter.

Pain and Other Symptoms: Scientifically Feasible but Methodologically Difficult; Clinically Relevant

Cancer Pain
My career began shortly after the WHO launched its Cancer Pain Relief program. In that era, understanding and studying the neuropharmacology of pain and other symptom control was prioritized. The pharmacologic management of difficult symptoms was the unique biomedical expertise we could bring to the clinical setting. On becoming the Australian equivalent of Board-certified in internal medicine and palliative medicine, I travelled to the USA to undertake a 2 year research fellowship under the supervision of T. Declan Walsh MD at the Cleveland Clinic. My main project there was completely biomedical and preclinical.

Working in the Applied Clinical Pharmacology lab of the Biochemistry Department, my project aimed to develop a simplified method for measuring morphine and metabolites in plasma utilizing a high-sensitivity fluorimeter. Tthe objective was to have simpler alternative for therapeutic drug monitoring than electrochemical detection which in those days was cumbersome to use. This project was completed despite a number of scientific difficulties e.g., the native fluorescence of morphine was hard to detect with the equipment, [25]. But in the end it was biologically futile as it became increasingly clear there was no correlation, with the possible exception of methadone, between peripheral blood levels of opioids and their clinical effects or side effects. We did manage to advance science: using the fluorimeter, we detected normorphine in the plasma of a patient on a very high dose morphine infusion who had the same kind of neurotoxicity caused by norpethidine [26]. During the research fellowship, I did also undertake some clinical studies in cancer pain, including the first-ever dose-ranging study of oxycodone showing that it could be safely titrated like morphine [27]. (Perhaps this is not something to boast about in the opioid crisis).

This era was also the height of the AIDS epidemic and on returning to Sydney from Cleveland my first post as junior faculty member of the Palliative Care Service involved caring for patients dying of AIDS. I undertook some research documenting the characteristics of AIDS pain and how to apply the principles of palliative care to people with HIV [28]. Fortunately, HAART therapy was developed a short time later and the need for palliative care for this disease disappeared virtually overnight. I was involved in recruiting patients with cancer pain to industry-sponsored clinical trials and this led to establishing the Sydney Palliative Care Clinical Trial Group some 25 years ago which was the forerunner of the previously mentioned PaCCSC. With the support of funding by the makers of a once-daily sustained release morphine formulation, we wrote an investigator-initiated protocol for a double blind placebo controlled RCT to evaluate the effects of time of day (a.m. vs. p.m.) of administration. We quickly recruited 45 people with opioid-responsive pain on stable doses of analgesics and advanced cancer from five regional palliative care programs around Australia (The results found only small differences between morning and evening dosing and unlikely to be clinically significant for most) [29]. PaCCSC has gone on to undertake other multicenter pain studies, most notably an RCT of ketamine for malignant neuropathic pain involving 180 participants. [30]. This study found little difference between ketamine and the control arm but much worse side effects in the intervention group. It was concluded ketamine does not have net clinical benefit when used as an adjunct to opioids and standard coanalgesics in cancer pain. Assuming these results were valid, it was shown that if this low value care were to be adopted, there would be substantial savings to the Australian health system [31]. A subsequent survey of Australian palliative care found two-thirds of respondents reported practice change as a result of this study but the others remained convinced of the benefit of the drug from their own observations and would require additional evidence [32]. This highlights the problem of clinical research where patient self-report of symptoms are the primary outcome. Placebo and nocebo effects are powerful and are difficult to control for during data collection even with blinding; this needs to be taken into account when interpreting these results.

Chronic Nausea in Advanced Cancer

I obtained funding from Australia's National Health and Medical Research Council to develop a clinical practice guideline for managing chronic nausea in advanced cancer. We undertook a survey of the oncology ward at the University teaching hospital which showed that, like cancer pain, it was an under-treated problem [33]. We assembled an interdisciplinary team including palliative care specialists, oncologists, family physicians, nurses, pharmacists, house staff and consumer representative. We reviewed the data and found that, while the data base was thin, [34] we felt there was enough information to proceed, based on what was known of the neuropharmacology of the emetic pathway and the descriptive data e.g., "clinical pictures," [35, 36] to design a guideline that incorporated two decision aids – a diagnostic tool to identify the clinical picture, and a treatment tool to direct selection of antiemetics. We undertook a study of implementing the guideline which was based on academic detailing of the junior medical staff who were treating the patients. Academic detailing involved delivery of a power point presentation regarding the emetic pathway and how to use the tools. The results were disappointing, and we have not attempted to publish them. During 3 implementation periods only a minority of patients were included on the pathway. When followed, the treatment was not very effective and one patient developed severe extrapyramidal symptoms from haloperidol. The biggest barrier was that the oncologist disagreed with the treatment tool and frequently over-ruled the algorithm. Subsequently PaCCSC has utilized its strong infrastructure to definitively study this guideline-driven approach to nausea management in 185 patients under the care of 8 palliative care teams across Australia and New Zealand [37]. It found an etiology-based, guideline-directed approach to antiemetic therapy may offer more rapid benefit, but is no better than single agent treatment with haloperidol at 72 h.

Prognostication

In developing a research framework for decision making in palliative care, it seemed that prognostication was an important "technical pre-requisite." This was not about hospice eligibility but about whether a treatment option was appropriate or not (i.e., live long enough but not too long). This appeared relevant to patients, families and clinicians and had been identified through research as important [38]. But surveys had also shown contemporary physicians are not trained to prognosticate and avoid doing it, [39] and I confirmed in a meta-analysis that they are not very good at it [40]. Unlike undertaking RCT however, research in prognosis seemed eminently doable: consent was easy, there was no intervention, the event rate was high and follow up complete. In lieu of a PhD, I undertook a Master of Medicine in Clinical Epidemiology with the objective of learning how to do survival analysis. It was easy to validate existing models developed in other populations and settings, and I began with validating the Palliative Prognostic Score, developed in Italian home hospice patients, in hospitalized Australian oncology patients [41]. Subsequently, I took the so-called NRF model that had been developed in Canadian cancer patients having palliative RT as outpatients and validated it in ambulatory cancer patients attending a pain & palliative care clinic [42]. We obtained very similar predictions from this simple system, which uses only site of cancer, site of metastases, and performance status to categorize patients in to 3 different, clinically relevant, prognostic groups with median survivals of approximately less than 3, 6 and greater than 12 months. I personally continue to use this tool when making major decisions with patients with advanced cancer in my clinical practice but I am not aware of its use elsewhere.

Increasing Access: Screening for Palliative Care Need

As the benefits of early palliative care become clearer and more palliative care programs are set up, the next question to answer is: Are the patients who need palliative care getting access to it? From 2008-2016 I was Chief of the Pain and Palliative Care Service at Memorial Sloan Kettering Cancer Center (MSKCC) in New York, and this became a locally relevant question for us as the Press-Gainey satisfaction survey indicated that there were several floors in the hospital where satisfaction with pain relief was not hitting the benchmark targets and this was seen as a sentinel for poor palliative care.

The NCCN Clinical Practice Guideline for Palliative Care recommends screening all patients for palliative care (PC) needs at the first visit with their oncologist at subsequent, clinically relevant times. Furthermore it is recommends to call a PC consult when certain referral criteria are met. While these guidelines had been in existence for some years, [22] no one had published data on implementing them or evaluating them for their clinical utility. I modified the palliative care screening tool presented in the CAPC book "A Guide to Building a Hospital Palliative Care Program" so that it was specific for a cancer population [43] because it draws on the indicators of palliative care need outlined in the NCCN guideline. My modified tool gave a score from 0 to 13, and we used 5 as a cut point for indicating the need for a palliative care referral.

At MSKCC, the Gastrointestinal Oncology Service (GIOS) was the busiest admitting unit in the Department of Medicine with a daily census of approximately 40. It was one of the floors missing the pain satisfaction benchmark. The referral rate to the Pain & Palliative Care Service on that floor was low, so it provided an excellent quality improvement project to evaluate the feasibility of implementing the screening and referral components of the NCCN Guidelines in patients admitted to the GIOS. Because the GIOS is so busy, it is split into two teams. They are essentially the same and the division is purely to make the workload manageable, with a daily census of 20 each. This enabled us to design a prospective, quasi-randomized, comparative study of the tool, funded by the Mayday Foundation [44]. All patients admitted under Team A were screened with the Tool, while those admitted to Team B received standard care, being referred to the palliative care when the on-service oncologist considered it necessary. Those with a high score would receive automatic palliative care consult. We presented the idea to the 20 GI oncologists and 90% of them were happy for their patients to be approached. Floor nurses performed the initial screening of all patients admitted to the 2 teams-Team A and Team B-of the GIOS on one floor of Memorial Hospital for 3 months. In addition, only the patients admitted to Team A were evaluated according to the referral criteria, triggering a PC consult if results were positive. Nurses were surveyed regarding satisfaction with and the acceptability of screening. During the study period, 229 patients, representing 90% of total admissions were screened. Of them, 169 (73%) screened positive. Of the Team A admissions, 72 (64%) met the referral criteria. More consults occurred for patients in Team A (47 vs 15; P=.001). In 30% of the referral criteria-triggered consults, the PC needs were manageable by the primary team. Nurses reported screening to be easy and quick (<5 minutes per patient) but only somewhat helpful. Being unfamiliar with many patients and families, floor nurses often felt unable to screen them accurately for some issues.

We concluded that screening was feasible, increased access to PC, but that given several items (performance status, comorbid conditions, severity of distress) were subjective there were concerns about accuracy. Likewise, there was uncertainty about the usefulness. Not only from the nurses but the palliative care team as well, for the tool indicated a consult in 64% patients yet almost half of them were for problems evinced to be manageable by the primary team. We concluded that the criteria were perhaps too sensitive for the inpatient environment of a comprehensive cancer center. It was felt that more evaluation was needed before widespread implementation could be recommended. There was also some hesitation on the part of palliative care staff that the tool could generate professional conflict.

Subsequently we did a validation study of the tool using the data collected in the primary study [45]. Content validity was assessed by a panel of local PC experts. Construct and criterion validities were evaluated using data obtained from a previous study of guideline-based screening and referral. Content validity of the tool was high, with eight of the tool's 11 items rated as 'essential'. Patients who were closer to death had significantly higher scores, indicating its construct validity. Scores were also higher in patients who were identified as needing a consult and in those who had worse pain and other symptoms, indicating its criterion validity. Using a score of ≥ 5 as the trigger, approximately one third of hospitalized patients in the previous study would have been referred to a PC specialist, twice as many as occurred when the attending oncologist relied on his or her clinical judgment. Thus, the tool seems to be a valid method for identifying patients with cancer with complex PC needs who would benefit from a PC consult. Reliability testing, external validation, and demonstration of the utility of the tool as a decision aid all await confirmation.

We also evaluated the tool in the ambulatory practice of one of the GI oncologists [46]. All patients attending clinic during a 3-week period were screened by the office practice nurse (OPN). There were 152 clinic visits by 125 individual patients during the surveillance period; 119 were screened. Median age was 61 years; half were male. Eighty percent had colorectal cancer, and two thirds had advanced disease. Screening took approximately 3 to 5 minutes per patient, so would add considerably to the clinic workload. Depending on the palliative care definition used, between 7% and 17% of patients screened positive; all met the NCCN referral criteria. Psychosocial distress was commoner than physical symptoms. The maximum screening score was 8. A cut point of 5 had the best predictive value for specialist referral, and would result in 13% patients having PC consultations. Given the workload of screening, it was decided the benefits of implementing routine screening need to be carefully evaluated.

Although outpatient specialty palliative-care clinics improve outcomes of such patients, [15, 20] there is no consensus on who should be referred or the optimal timing for referral. We validated the screening tool in this population. In response to this issue, I participated in a Delphi study to develop consensus on a list of criteria for referral of patients with advanced cancer at secondary or tertiary care hospitals to outpatient palliative care [47] 60 international experts (26 from North America, 19 from Asia, 11 from Europe and myself from Australia) on palliative cancer care rated 39 needs-based criteria and 22 time-based criteria in three iterative rounds. Nearly all experts responded in each round. Consensus was defined by an a priori agreement of 70% or more. Panelists reached consensus on 11 major criteria for referral: severe physical symptoms, severe emotional symptoms, request for hastened death, spiritual or existential crisis, assistance with decision making or care planning, patient request for referral, delirium, spinal cord compression, brain or leptomeningeal metastases, within 3 months of advanced cancer diagnosis for patients with median survival of 1 year or less, and progressive disease despite second-line therapy. Consensus was also reached on 36 minor criteria for specialist palliative-care referral. These criteria, if validated, could provide guidance for identification of patients suitable for outpatient specialty palliative care.

Despite having published research showing the tool was valid and effective, it has not widely adopted at MSKCC. And it is not a matter of timing either: as was the case with the nausea guideline a decade earlier, introduction of a screening tool is not sufficient to change behavior so that it is implemented.. Other approaches are needed. These may include: having automated mechanisms to make screening facile; developing algorithms for assessment and intervention; addressing barriers such as branding of palliative medicine; educating staff in primary palliative care skills such as pain management and therapeutic communication [48].

Behavioral Insights: Nudging Patients towards Palliative Care

Even if patients are correctly identified as needing palliative care in a timely manner, they have to agree to it. The advent of EBM rightly moved decision making away from the old paternalistic "doctor-knows-best" approach towards the shared decision making process that now prevails. But this change is problematic if the MD abrogates their part in decision making and sees their role as simply presenting the evidence and executing the treatment. It is well known that people are prone to cognitive biases which can lead to suboptimal decision making in any aspect of life. This is particularly so when the stakes and emotions are high as is the case with medical decision making about a life limiting illness [49, 50]. In particular, Prospect Theory has shown that people are not rational decision makers but display a number of irrational characteristics when making choices, including being loss averse and discounting future losses [51].

After more than 25 years of clinical practice and seeing what research can and can't offer, I have become most interested in helping my patients make the right decision – one that is in their objective best interests. This is not easy when there are multiple options, none of them ideal, and the outcomes are uncertain. I have been collaborating with a social psychologist to help progress knowledge in this field. How the message is framed is very important. In advertising, most messages are framed positively (buy this car for a better ride/performance/safety). However, health care messages seem to be most effective if they are loss framed (if you don't stop smoking/have a mammogram/consent to surgery, you will be worse off than if you do these things). So how you present information is very important [52]. A classic study of choosing surgery vs. radiotherapy showed that preferences for one modality or the other reverse valence (from preferred to not preferred) depending on how the outcome data is presented [53]. Understanding this phenomenon and its implications are important for every clinician [54].

We have been interested to apply a pair of theoretical constructs regarding people's motivation to choose a particular way of acting, called Regulatory Focus Theory and Regulatory Fit Theory, [55, 56] to end-of-life decision making. In a nutshell, Regulatory Focus Theory posits that when people are pursuing a goal they have an intrinsic tendency (based on personality, culture, and social factors) to eagerly seek gains ("promotion" focus) or to vigilantly avoid losses ("prevention" focus). People from Western cultures tend to be more promotion focused, while people from Eastern cultures tend to be more prevention-focused. While Regulatory Focus is a trait, it is situational and can be manipulated (see below). Regulatory Fit Theory predicts that a strategy for pursuing the goal will fit ("feel right") if it is consistent with the person's Regulatory Focus. 'Fit' strategies are motivating, while 'Non-fit' strategies are demotivating.

In the case of someone with cancer, Regulatory Focus theory would predict a patient with a Promotion focus will eagerly obtain lots of 'second opinions' and try lots of different treatments in seeking to prolong their life, while a Prevention focused person will be diligent in finding the best oncologist and then stick very closely to the prescribed treatment plan to avoid it not working. Travelling to another city to enroll in a new Phase I clinical trial would be a feel right for a Promotion patient; adhering to conventional chemotherapy recommended by the world's best oncologist would feel right for a Prevention patient. A corollary to the motivating power of Regulatory Fit is the demotivation associated with non-fit strategies. For example, introducing an unemployed high school drop-out to a lazy middle school student is likely to be effective in getting them to study.

We sought to apply Non-Fit as a solution to overly-aggressive care at the end of life. Advanced cancer patients with limited options for further treatment are often reluctant to enroll in hospice, and these negative emotions can be strong to the point that they reject the option out of hand. We studied whether a Non-Fit statement was helpful in reducing these negative emotions and make the patient more open to considering hospice. We presented participants with a scenario of a hypothetical patient with advanced cancer weighing up the options of pursuing further treatment or forgoing it in favor of hospice. They were given evidence based data on the likely outcomes of both options and asked them to state their attitude towards hospice. After they recorded their attitude performed a writing task that primed towards one regulatory focus or the other. Next they read statements about hospice care that either fit or not with their induced regulatory focus at that moment. The participants were randomized to one of four 'conditions' (promotion or prevention focus, with fit or non-fit statements about hospice).

Firstly we carried out this experiment in healthy volunteers who completed the survey anonymously on line [57]. Subsequently we carried it out in patients at MSKCC [58]. In both cases, we found that many participants were initially negative in their attitude towards hospice. The greatest change in attitude occurred in patients who were given non-fit statements, and consistent with our hypothesis that non-fit statements are demotivating, the direction of the attitude change was towards amelioration i.e., a de-intensification of their negativity, making them less likely to reject a hospice recommendation out of hand. Having shown this effect, a simple communication strategy could be developed to help people be open minded about treatment options they originally consider to be undesirable.

CONCLUSION

Developing a palliative care program isn't easy. To achieve the goal of a setting up and maintaining an adequately resourced team that is utilized to provide a service to patients and families who need it requires a different skill set than those that you need as a health care provider and a palliative care clinician. To achieve this objective requires one to be an entrepreneur, politician, negotiator, diplomat, advocate and salesman. Whether or not you consider yourself to be capable in these roles, you can go into meetings with administrators much more confidently if you are armed with facts. These will be facts about patient volumes, diagnosis codes, symptoms cores, length of stay, disposition status and satisfaction surveys. But it will also include being across the latest research evidence in palliative care which demonstrates what can be done to improve the quality of the care of patients with progressive, eventually fatal illnesses, (even if implementing these changes is extremely difficult). These data will be even more effective if they are generated locally or at least generalizable and transferrable to your setting. Understanding the research cycle and the principles of research are important for all palliative care clinicians. Even if not actively participating in research, one also needs to understand how to appraise the research literature. Similarly, these days anyone who is serious about a research career in palliative care really should enroll in a PhD.

REFERENCES

[1] Glimelius B, Ekstrom K, Hoffman K, et al. Randomized comparison between chemotherapy plus best supportive care with best supportive care in advanced gastric cancer. *Ann Oncol* 1997;8:163-8.

[2] White C, Hardy JR, Glare P. Principles of palliative medicine research. In: Walsh D, ed. *Palliative Medicine*. Philadelphia: Saunders Elsevier; 2009:136-43.

[3] Randall FM. Ethical issues in palliative care. *Acta Anaesthesiol Scand* 1999;43:954-6.

[4] de Raeve L. Ethical issues in palliative care research. *Palliative medicine* 1994;8:298-305.

[5] *Cancer pain relief and palliative care: report of a WHO Expert Committee*. Geneva: World Health Organization; 1990.

[6] Davis MP, Temel JS, Balboni T, Glare P. A review of the trials which examine early integration of outpatient and home palliative care for patients with serious illnesses. *Ann Palliat Med* 2015;4:99-121.

[7] Altilio T, Otis-Green S, Dahlin CM. Applying the National Quality Forum Preferred Practices for Palliative and Hospice Care: a social work perspective. *J Soc Work End Life Palliat Care* 2008;4:3-16.

[8] Wiffen PJ, Wee B, Moore RA. Oral morphine for cancer pain. *Cochrane Database Syst Rev* 2016;4:CD003868.

[9] Hardy JR, O'Shea A, White C, Gilshenan K, Welch L, Douglas C. The efficacy of haloperidol in the management of nausea and vomiting in patients with cancer. *J Pain Symptom Manage* 2010;40:111-6.

[10] Jimenez-Andrade JM, Ghilardi JR, Castaneda-Corral G, Kuskowski MA, Mantyh PW. Preventive or late administration of anti-NGF therapy attenuates tumor-induced nerve sprouting, neuroma formation, and cancer pain. *Pain* 2011;152:2564-74.

[11] Tack J, Lappalainen J, Diva U, Tummala R, Sostek M. Efficacy and safety of naloxegol in patients with opioid-induced constipation and laxative-inadequate response. *United European Gastroenterol J* 2015;3:471-80.

[12] Dalton JA, Keefe FJ, Carlson J, Youngblood R. Tailoring cognitive-behavioral treatment for cancer pain. *Pain Manag Nurs* 2004;5:3-18.

[13] Mantyh PW. Bone cancer pain: from mechanism to therapy. *Curr Opin Support Palliat Care* 2014;8:83-90.

[14] Gwilliam B, Keeley V, Todd C, et al. Development of prognosis in palliative care study (PiPS) predictor models to improve prognostication in advanced cancer: prospective cohort study. *BMJ* 2011;343:d4920.

[15] Temel JS, Greer JA, Muzikansky A, et al. Early palliative care for patients with metastatic non-small-cell lung cancer. *N Engl J Med* 2010;363:733-42.

[16] Balboni MJ, Sullivan A, Amobi A, et al. Why is spiritual care infrequent at the end of life? Spiritual care perceptions among patients, nurses, and physicians and the role of training. *J Clin Oncol* 2013;31:461-7.

[17] Balboni TA, Vanderwerker LC, Block SD, et al. Religiousness and spiritual support among advanced cancer patients and associations with end-of-life treatment preferences and quality of life. *J Clin Oncol* 2007;25:555-60.

[18] Sepulveda C, Marlin A, Yoshida T, Ullrich A. Palliative Care: the World Health Organization's global perspective. *J Pain Symptom Manage* 2002;24:91-6.

[19] Bakitas M, Lyons KD, Hegel MT, et al. The project ENABLE II randomized controlled trial to improve palliative care for rural patients with advanced cancer: baseline findings, methodological challenges, and solutions. *Palliat Support Care* 2009;7:75-86.

[20] Zimmermann C, Swami N, Krzyzanowska M, et al. Early palliative care for patients with advanced cancer: a cluster-randomised controlled trial. *Lancet* 2014;383:1721-30.

[21] Ferrell BR, Temel JS, Temin S, et al. Integration of Palliative Care Into Standard Oncology Care: American Society of Clinical Oncology Clinical Practice Guideline Update. *J Clin Oncol* 2017;35:96-112.

[22] Levy MH, Back A, Benedetti C, et al. NCCN clinical practice guidelines in oncology: palliative care. *J Natl Compr Canc Netw* 2009;7:436-73.

[23] Isenberg SR, Aslakson RA, Smith TJ. Implementing Evidence-Based Palliative Care Programs and Policy for Cancer Patients: Epidemiologic and Policy Implications of the 2016 American Society of Clinical Oncology Clinical Practice Guideline Update. *Epidemiol Rev* 2017;39:123-31.

[24] Shelby-James TM, Hardy J, Agar M, et al. Designing and conducting randomized controlled trials in palliative care: A summary of discussions from the 2010 clinical research forum of the Australian Palliative Care Clinical Studies Collaborative. *Palliative medicine* 2012;26:1042-7.

[25] Glare PA, Walsh TD, Pippenger CE. A simple, rapid method for the simultaneous determination of morphine and its principal metabolites in plasma using high-performance liquid chromatography and fluorometric detection. *Ther Drug Monit* 1991;13:226-32.

[26] Glare PA, Walsh TD, Pippenger CE. Normorphine, a neurotoxic metabolite? *Lancet* 1990;335:725-6.

[27] Glare PA, Walsh TD. Dose-ranging study of oxycodone for chronic pain in advanced cancer. *J Clin Oncol* 1993;11:973-8.

[28] Glare PA. Palliative care in acquired immunodeficiency syndrome (AIDS): problems and practicalities. *Ann Acad Med Singapore* 1994;23:235-43.

[29] Currow DC, Plummer JL, Cooney NJ, Gorman D, Glare PA. A randomized, double-blind, multi-site, crossover, placebo-controlled equivalence study of morning versus evening once-daily sustained-release morphine sulfate in people with pain from advanced cancer. *J Pain Symptom Manage* 2007;34:17-23.

[30] Hardy J, Quinn S, Fazekas B, et al. Randomized, double-blind, placebo-controlled study to assess the efficacy and toxicity of subcutaneous ketamine in the management of cancer pain. *J Clin Oncol* 2012;30:3611-7.

[31] McCaffrey N, Hardy J, Fazekas B, et al. Potential economic impact on hospitalisations of the Palliative Care Clinical Studies Collaborative (PaCCSC) ketamine randomised controlled trial. *Aust Health Rev* 2016;40:100-5.

[32] Hardy JR, Spruyt O, Quinn SJ, Devilee LR, Currow DC. Implementing practice change in chronic cancer pain management: clinician response to a phase III study of ketamine. *Intern Med J* 2014;44:586-91.

[33] Greaves J, Glare P, Kristjanson LJ, Stockler M, Tattersall MH. Undertreatment of nausea and other symptoms in hospitalized cancer patients. *Support Care Cancer* 2009;17:461-4.

[34] Glare P, Pereira G, Kristjanson LJ, Stockler M, Tattersall M. Systematic review of the efficacy of antiemetics in the treatment of nausea in patients with far-advanced cancer. *Support Care Cancer* 2004;12:432-40.

[35] Grunberg SM, Hesketh PJ. Control of chemotherapy-induced emesis. *N Engl J Med* 1993;329:1790-6.

[36] Bentley A, Boyd K. Use of clinical pictures in the management of nausea and vomiting: a prospective audit. *Palliative Medicine* 2001;15:247-53.

[37] Hardy J, Skerman H, Glare P, et al. A randomized open-label study of guideline-driven antiemetic therapy versus single agent antiemetic therapy in patients with advanced cancer and nausea not related to anticancer treatment. *BMC Cancer* 2018;18:510.

[38] Strang P. Existential consequences of unrelieved cancer pain. *Palliative medicine* 1997;11:299-305.

[39] Christakis NA, Iwashyna TJ. Attitude and self-reported practice regarding prognostication in a national sample of internists. *Arch Intern Med* 1998;158:2389-95.

[40] Glare P, Virik K, Jones M, et al. A systematic review of physicians' survival predictions in terminally ill cancer patients. *BMJ* 2003;327:195-8.

[41] Glare PA, Eychmueller S, McMahon P. Diagnostic accuracy of the palliative prognostic score in hospitalized patients with advanced cancer. *J Clin Oncol* 2004;22:4823-8.

[42] Glare P, Shariff I, Thaler HT. External validation of the number of risk factors score in a palliative care outpatient clinic at a comprehensive cancer center. *Journal of Palliative Medicine* 2014;17:797-802.

[43] Meier DE, Sieger CE. *A Guide to Building a Hospital Palliative Care Program.* New York: Center To Advance Palliative Care; 2004.

[44] Glare P, Plakovic K, Schloms A, et al. Study using the NCCN guidelines for palliative care to screen patients for palliative care needs and referral to palliative care specialists. *J Natl Compr Canc Netw* 2013;11:1087-96.

[45] Glare PA, Chow K. Validation of a Simple Screening Tool for Identifying Unmet Palliative Care Needs in Patients With Cancer. *J Oncol Pract* 2015;11:e81-6.

[46] Glare PA, Semple D, Stabler SM, Saltz LB. Palliative care in the outpatient oncology setting: evaluation of a practical set of referral criteria. *J Oncol Pract* 2011;7:366-70.

[47] Hui D, Mori M, Watanabe SM, et al. Referral criteria for outpatient specialty palliative cancer care: an international consensus. *Lancet Oncol* 2016;17:e552-e9.

[48] Ramchandran K, Winget M, Tribett EL, Anderson B, Morris A, Blayney DW. Is screening enough? Implications of a pilot utilizing standard screening criteria for early palliative referral. *Journal of Clinical Oncology* 2015;33:119.

[49] Khatcheressian J, Harrington SB, Lyckholm LJ, Smith TJ. 'Futile care': what to do when your patient insists on chemotherapy that likely won't help. *Oncology* (Williston Park) 2008;22:881-8; discussion 93, 96, 98.

[50] Quill TE, Arnold R, Back AL. Discussing treatment preferences with patients who want "everything." *Ann Intern Med* 2009;151:345-9.

[51] Verma AA, Razak F, Detsky AS. Understanding choice: why physicians should learn prospect theory. *JAMA* 2014;311:571-2.

[52] Rothman AJ, Salovey P. Shaping perceptions to motivate healthy behavior: the role of message framing. *Psychol Bull* 1997;121:3-19.

[53] McNeil BJ, Pauker SG, Sox HC, Jr., Tversky A. On the elicitation of preferences for alternative therapies. *N Engl J Med* 1982;306:1259-62.

[54] Fridman I, Epstein AS, Higgins ET. Appropriate Use of Psychology in Patient-Physician Communication: Influencing Wisely. *JAMA Oncol* 2015;1:725-6.

[55] Higgins ET, Silberman I. Development of Regulatory Focus: Promotion and Prevention as Ways of Living. In: Heckhausen J, Dweck CS, eds. *Motivation and Self-Regulation across the Life Span.* New York: Cambridge University Press 1998: 78-113.

[56] Avnet T, Higgins ET. How regulatory fit affects value in consumer choices and opinions. *J Marketing Res* 2006;18:1-10.

[57] Fridman I, Scherr KA, Glare PA, Higgins ET. Using a Non-Fit Message Helps to De-Intensify Negative Reactions to Tough Advice. *Pers Soc Psychol Bull* 2016;42:1025-44.

[58] Fridman I, Glare PA, Stabler SM, et al. Information Framing Reduces Initial Negative Attitudes in Cancer Patients' Decisions about Hospice Care. *J Pain Symptom Manage* 2018;55:1540-5.

BIOGRAPHICAL SKETCH

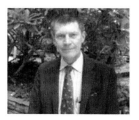

Professor Paul Glare, MBBS, FRACP, FFPM ANZCA, FAChPM RACP, MA Applied Ethics (Healthcare), MMed (Clin Epidemiol)

Pain physician

- Chair in Pain Medicine, Sydney Medical School, University of Sydney- Northern Clinical School

- Head, Discipline of Pain Medicine, Sydney Medical School
- Director, Pain Management & Research Institute, Faculty of Medicine, University of Sydney

Prior to his current appointments, Paul was Chief of the Pain & Palliative Care Service, Memorial Sloan Kettering Cancer Center in New York from 2008 to 2016, with an affiliated appointment as Professor of Medicine at Weill Cornell Medical College.

After graduating from University of Sydney's Medical School in 1981, Professor Glare undertook physician training at Royal Prince Alfred Hospital during which time he developed an interest in cancer pain and palliative care. Subsequently, he spent 2 years as a research fellow (working on opioid pharmacology in cancer pain) at the Cleveland Clinic, Ohio USA before returning to Sydney in 1991 as staff specialist in palliative care until he moved to New York in 2008. He was made a Foundation Fellow of the Faculty of Pain Medicine in 2000. He is also a Fellow of the Chapter of Palliative Medicine of the RACP.

His two current research interests are pain in cancer survivors, and the decision architecture of pain management, in particular tapering of opioids.

COUNTRIES REPRESENTED IN THIS VOLUME

Australia
Cyprus
France
Israel
Italy
Japan
Poland
Portugal
Qatar
Spain
Sultanate of Oman
United Arab Emirates
United Kingdom
United States of America

ABOUT THE EDITOR

Prof. Michael Silbermann
Executive Director, Technion – Israel Institute of Technology, Haifa, Israel

In the past decade Prof. Silbermann has focused his activities in promoting palliative care in the Middle East. The latter included basic and advanced courses in palliative care to physicians, nurses, pharmacists and social workers working in major hospitals as well as in primary health care centers in the community. These educational and training activities intended to make palliative care recognized as a new medical specialty as any other specialty practiced nowadays in the developed world. Since in the Middle East hospices, as known in North America, Western Europe and Australia, are not as yet in operation, special efforts are directed in the promotion of palliative care services in communities. In order to initiate regional research activity, we have started with regional surveys about the needs for palliative care services, needs for spiritual care and requirements for integrative modalities of care. Concomitantly, scientists and clinicians in the region collaborate in publishing academic work in the international literature.

LIST OF CONTRIBUTORS

NORTH AMERICA

United States

Professor Lodovico Balducci, MD
Medical Oncologist and Geriatrician
Director, International Relations
Moffitt Cancer Center
Tampa, FL, US
lodovico.balducci@moffitt.org

Kye Y. Kim, MD
Professor, Department of Psychiatry and Behavioral Medicine
Virginia Tech Carilion School of Medicine
Geriatric Psychiatrist, Carilion Clinic Center for Healthy Aging
Roanoke, VA, US
kykim@carilionclinic.org

Phyllis Whitehead, PhD, APRN/CNS, ACHPN, RN-BC
Department of Internal Medicine
Carilion Clinic & Virginia Tech Carilion School of Medicine
Roanoke, Virginia, US

Senaida Keating, MD
Department of Internal Medicine
Carilion Clinic & Virginia Tech Carilion School of Medicine
Roanoke, Virginia, US

Shereen Gamaluddin, MD
Department of Internal Medicine
Carilion Clinic & Virginia Tech Carilion School of Medicine
Roanoke, Virginia, US

Dr. Jeannine Brant, PhD, APRN, AOCN
Oncology Clinical Nurse Specialist Research Scientist
Billings Clinic Inpatient Cancer Care
Billings, MT, US
jbrant@billingsclinic.org

Dr. Regina M. Fink, RN, PhD, AOCN, CHPN, FAAN
University of Colorado
College of Nursing and School of Medicine
Aurora, Colorado, US
regina.fink@ucdenver.edu; reginamfink@aol.com

Egidio Del Fabbro, MD
Assoc. Prof. & Palliative Care Endowed Chair
Director, Palliative Care Program
Division of Hematology, Oncology & Palliative Care
Virginia Commonwealth University
Richmond, VA, US
egidio.delfabbro@vcuhealth.org

J. Brian Cassel, PhD
Virginia Commonwealth University
Richmond, VA, US

Emily Lu, MD
Icahn School of Medicine at Mount Sinai
New York, NY, US
lu.emily@mssm.edu

Craig D. Blinderman, MD, MA, FAAHPM
Director, Adult Palliative Care Service
Assoc. Prof. Department of Medicine
Columbia University Medical Center
New York, NY, US
cdb21@cumc.columbia.edu

Lidia Schapira, MD
Director, Cancer survivorship Program at Stanford Cancer Institute
Professor, Stanford University School of Medicine
Stanford, CA, US
schapira@stanford.edu

Karl Lorenz, MD, MSHS
Section Chief, VA Palo Alto – Stanford Palliative Care Programs
Stanford University School of Medicine
Director, VA Palliative Care Quality Improvement Resource Center (QuIRC)

Palo Alto, CA, US
Kalorenz@stanford.edu, Karl.lorenz@va.gov

WESTERN EUROPE

Spain

Professor Amparo Oliver, PhD
Professor in Methodology in Behavioral Sciences
Faculty of Psychology
Universitat de Valencia
Valencia, Spain
Amparo.oliver@uv.es

Dr. Laura Galiana, PhD
Assoc. Prof. in Quantitative Methods Applied to Behavioral Sciences
Faculty of Psychology
University of Valencia
Valencia, Spain
laura.galiana@uv.es

Noemí Sansó, RN, MSC, PhD
Assoc. Prof., Department of Nursing & Physiotherapy
University of Balearic Island
Palma de Mallorca, Spain

Juan Manuel Gavala, RN, MSC
Director of Nursing, Hospital Son Espases
Palma de Mallorca, Spain

Paz Fernández-Ortega, PhD, MSc, RN
Nursing Research Coordinator, Department Salut Pública
Materno-infantil, Escola Infermeria UB
Despatx 300, Spain
mpax2001@gmail.com

Julio C. de la Torre-Montero, PhD
San Juan de Dios School of Nursing and Physical Therapy
Comillas Pontifical University
Madrid, Spain

Portugal

Manuel Luis Vila Capelas, PhD
Portuguese Catholic University
Institute of Health Sciences
Center for Interdisciplinary Research in Health
Portuguese Observatory for Palliative Care
Lisbon, Portugal
manuelluis.capelas@gmail.com

Silvia Patricia Coelho, PhD
Portuguese Catholic University
Institute of Health Sciences
Portuguese Observatory for Palliative Care
Oporto, Portugal

Tania Sofia Afonso, MsPC, PhD Candidate
Portuguese Catholic University
Institute of Health Sciences
Portuguese Observatory for Palliative Care
Lisbon, Portugal

United Kingdom

Professor Richard Harding
Cicely Saunders Institute
King's College, London, UK
richard.harding@kcl.ac.uk

Kennedy Nkhoma, MD
Cicely Saunders Institute
King's College, London, UK
kennedy.nkhoma@kcl.ac.uk

Ping Guo, MD
Cicely Saunders Institute
King's College, London, UK
ping.guo@kcl.ac.uk

Eve Namisango
Cicely Saunders Institute
King's College, London, UK
& African Palliative Care Association
Kampala, Uganda

Dr. Stephen R. Connor, PhD
Executive Director
Worldwide Hospice Palliative Care Alliance
London, UK
sconnor@thewhpca.org

Dr. Angelos P. Kassianos
Department of Applied Health Research
UCI, London, UK

Italy

Simone Cheli DPsy
School of Human Health Sciences
University of Florence
Florence, Italy
Simone.cheli@unifi.it

France

Rana Istambouly, MHM, MSc (Pall)., PhD (candidate)
PalliaMed Consultancy
Paris, France
Rana.313@hotmail.com

EASTERN EUROPE

Poland

Professor Zbigniw (Ben) Zylicz, MD, PhD
Institute of Experimental & Clinical Medicine
University of Rzeszów
Rzeszow, Poland
z.zylicz@ru.edu.pl

Aleksandra Kotlínska-Lemieszek, MD, PhD
Chair, Dept. Palliative Medicine
Karol Marcinkowski University of Medical Sciences
Poznan, Poland

MIDDLE EAST

Cyprus

Dr. Haris Charalambous, BM, MRCP, FRCR
Senior Consultant, Bank of Cyprus Oncology Centre
Nicosia, Cyprus
haris.charalambous@bococ.org.cy

Israel

Professor Miri Cohen, PhD
Head, School of Social Work
Faculty of Health Sciences
Haifa University
Haifa, Israel
mcohen2@univ.haifa.ac.il

Adi Ivzari Erel, MD
The Ruth and Bruce Rappaport Faculty of Medicine
Technion – Israel Institute of Technology, Haifa, Israel

Lee Greenblatt Kimron, PhD
Ariel University
Department of Social Work
Ariel, Israel

Professor Elon Eisenberg, MD
Pain Research Unit, Institute of Pain Medicine
Rambam Health Care Campus
Haifa, Israel
E_eisenberg@rambam.health.gov.il

Sultanate of Oman

Zakiya M.N. Al-Lamki, FRCP, FRCPcH
Department of Child Health, Haematology/Oncology Unit
College of Medicine and Health Sciences, Sultan Qaboos University
Muscat, Sultanate of Oman
Zakiya.allamki@gmail.com

Qatar

Dr. Azar Naveen Saleem
National Center for Cancer Care and Research
Hamad Medical Corporation
Doha, Qatar
azarnavin@gmail.com

Dr. Azza Adel Hassan, MD
National Center for Cancer Care & Research
Hamad Medical Corporation
Doha, Qatar
newazza@gmail.com

United Arab Emirates

Tahani Al Dweikat, RN, BSN, EMHCA, OCN
Head Nurse, Oncology/Hematology Unit
Sheikh Khalifa Medical City
Abu Dhabi, United Arab Emirates
tahanidweikat@live.com

FAR EAST

Japan

Prof. Tomoko Majima, RN., PHN., Ph.D.
Chiba University Graduate School of Nursing
Adult Nursing
Chiba, Japan
tmajima@faculty.chiba-u.jp

Tomoko Otsuka, RN., PHN., Ph.D. candidate
Chiba University Graduate School of Nursing
Chiba, Japan
t-otsuka@chiba-u.jp

OCEANIA

Australia

Paul A. Glare, MBBS, FFPMANZCA
Director, Pain Management Research Institute

University of Sydney & Royal North Shore Hospital
NSW, Australia
paul.glare@sydney.edu.au

INDEX

A

access, xv, 3, 4, 5, 6, 7, 8, 19, 30, 31, 45, 49, 50, 51, 52, 54, 55, 64, 66, 67, 72, 83, 84, 87, 89, 92, 102, 103, 113, 134, 135, 136, 137, 138, 139, 141, 142, 152, 157, 158, 160, 163, 164, 170, 176, 180, 181, 182, 183, 185, 205, 279, 295, 326
accessibility, 3, 8, 9, 50, 54, 87, 98, 100, 102, 139, 144, 145, 164, 285
acupuncture, 171, 291
adaptation, 126, 138, 170, 241, 258, 259, 260, 289
adjustment, 91, 99, 165, 241, 257, 258, 259, 301
administrators, 47, 62, 71, 320, 329
adults, xiv, 6, 65, 76, 78, 79, 89, 91, 107, 134, 135, 154, 185, 223, 231, 232, 235, 236, 269, 272, 299
advance care planning (ACP), 35, 39, 51, 53, 61, 63, 64, 67, 69, 70, 72, 73, 77, 80, 99, 173, 181, 222
advanced cancer, xii, 21, 35, 38, 48, 51, 57, 74, 75, 77, 84, 87, 90, 91, 92, 93, 103, 107, 108, 126, 130, 131, 143, 152, 196, 198, 201, 202, 204, 212, 213, 218, 219, 221, 222, 223, 224, 227, 228, 233, 236, 240, 251, 253, 258, 259, 260, 261, 269, 270, 272, 273, 283, 296,300, 313, 324, 325, 327, 329, 331, 332
advanced cancer patient, 126, 143, 236, 240, 253, 261, 283, 296, 331
advancements, xv, 58, 221
adverse effects, 192, 193
adverse event, 168, 284
advocacy, 47, 56, 99, 133, 137, 145
affective disorder, 3, 4
affluence, 284, 298
Africa, 49, 50, 54, 134, 136, 137, 138, 139, 141, 142, 143, 144, 145, 149, 152, 153
age, xiv, xxii, 4, 8, 18, 59, 60, 62, 63, 65, 66, 68, 70, 79, 119, 135, 171, 179, 245, 252, 269, 295, 310, 322, 327
ageing population, 134, 283
agencies, 136, 269

aggressiveness, 201, 202, 203, 209, 210, 223
aging population, xvi, 58, 89, 296
Ahmedzai, Sam, 193
AIDS, 55, 75, 77, 140, 142, 144, 146, 149, 154, 159, 286, 320, 324, 331
Aleksandra Kotlińska-Lemieszek. She and Prof. J. Łuczak, 194
alternative, xix, 15, 26, 30, 100, 107, 165, 177, 214, 231, 275, 276, 279, 280, 281, 284, 291, 301, 307, 324, 333
alternative medicine, 276, 279, 280, 281, 291, 301, 307
ambivalence, 17, 248, 296, 310
ambulatory, 71, 140, 145, 149, 198, 275, 276, 295, 314, 325, 327
analgesic, 37, 49, 55, 224, 227, 228, 230, 232, 236
anorexia, 168, 321
antiemetics, 325, 332
anti-inflammatory drugs, 232, 235
anxiety, xiv, 59, 70, 71, 91, 113, 114, 115, 117, 118, 119, 120, 123, 124, 125, 126, 130, 171, 202, 210, 211, 212, 219, 240, 243, 244, 245, 246, 258, 259, 288, 290, 292, 299, 300, 301, 310
appetite, 59, 93, 233, 268
appointments, 205, 214, 215, 334
Asia, 71, 109, 138, 165, 223, 327
assessment, 14, 16, 21, 31, 37, 38, 42, 60, 67, 69, 72, 82, 85, 99, 100, 108, 143, 157, 161, 183, 185, 197, 198, 203, 207, 215, 216, 236, 249, 262, 266, 269, 270, 271, 280, 284, 290, 294, 295, 322, 328
assessment tools, 67, 100
attitudes, 6, 30, 43, 68, 113, 114, 115, 120, 136, 161, 168, 170, 171, 224, 275, 309
audit, xii, 139, 144, 150, 332
autonomy, 175, 176, 179, 181, 183, 287
avoidance, 51, 90, 114, 129, 185
awareness, 8, 30, 31, 60, 73, 88, 100, 120, 137, 168, 209, 252, 265, 267, 285, 288, 291, 292, 294

348 Index

B

barriers, ix, xii, xiv, xvi, 7, 9, 30, 31, 33, 47, 48, 49, 54, 58, 64, 65, 67, 68, 80, 101, 133, 137, 138, 139, 144, 159, 160, 167, 168, 169, 172, 173, 183, 275, 276, 277, 278, 279, 280, 281, 290, 310, 311, 312, 313, 328
behaviors, 6, 45
Belgium, 206, 212, 220
benchmarking, 92, 101
benchmarks, 87, 177
beneficial effect, 19, 269
beneficiaries, 93, 165, 222
benefits, 5, 10, 14, 15, 19, 30, 31, 48, 61, 64, 73, 85, 126, 137, 140, 148, 168, 171, 176, 177, 180, 182, 201, 202, 265, 266, 269, 319, 320, 326, 327
benign, 16, 18, 19
bias, xii, 7, 70, 127, 128, 170, 216, 217, 232, 266, 271
bilateral, 27, 34
blood, 20, 298
bone, 227, 232, 236, 321
bone pain, 227, 232
Botswana, 48, 141
bottom-up, 191, 192, 193, 195, 232
bottom-up research, 191, 192, 195
bowel, 220, 268
brain, 301, 327
breast cancer, xxi, 13, 14, 15, 21, 23, 43, 46, 55, 92, 143, 144, 230, 250, 260, 299, 300
breathlessness, 154, 194, 197
burn, 257, 262
burnout, 55, 114, 117, 118, 119
Buss, Tomasz, 194, 197, 198

C

cachexia, xvii, 88, 321
cancer care, xvi, 45, 58, 92, 119, 126, 142, 144, 219, 222, 234, 235, 269, 275, 278, 280, 295, 301, 307, 309, 327, 332
candidates, 158, 219
cannabinoids, 227, 233, 234, 236, 237
cannabis, 233, 234, 235, 236, 321
capacity building, 134, 141
carcinoma, 203
cardiovascular disease, 6, 135, 179
care model, 7, 138, 143, 176, 180, 185, 195, 205, 269
caregivers, xv, xxii, 19, 50, 51, 52, 54, 88, 98, 100, 102, 107, 109, 114, 124, 126, 136, 138, 139, 140, 143, 147, 150, 169, 176, 177, 180, 181, 183, 185, 205, 228, 267, 270, 271, 289, 292, 293, 295, 310, 322
caregiving, xiii, xiv, xvi, 169
case study, 49, 297
castration, 233, 235
CBD, 233, 235
certificate, 49, 104, 152, 158
certification, 40, 42, 273
certified nurse specialist, 307, 309, 314
challenges, xi, xii, xiv, xvi, xvii, 6, 8, 16, 17, 19, 43, 50, 51, 53, 54, 57, 58, 64, 67, 68, 70, 74, 83, 84, 88, 99, 100, 124, 127, 129, 135, 136, 137, 139, 140, 142, 143, 147, 148, 157, 158, 169, 173, 180, 185, 186, 216, 231, 266, 268, 272, 275, 276, 277, 293, 295, 297, 298, 300, 309, 319, 320, 321, 331
chemotherapy, 4, 15, 21, 26, 27, 34, 35, 40, 41, 85, 90, 91, 92, 202, 209, 211, 218, 222, 224, 227, 228, 232, 233, 235, 244, 276, 278, 279, 309, 314, 329, 330, 332, 333
childhood, xxii, 17, 45, 256, 303, 309
childhood cancer, 303, 309
children, xv, xxi, 13, 15, 16, 17, 18, 20, 48, 116, 117, 118, 134, 135, 149, 158, 184, 245, 257, 286, 288, 289
China, 133, 135, 142, 146, 147, 148, 152, 301, 315
Christianity, 249, 253
chronic diseases (CDs), 5, 14, 54, 58, 65, 74, 170, 176, 179, 180, 181, 182, 183, 184, 186, 187
chronic illness, 59, 62, 136, 146, 177, 185, 267, 284
chronic kidney (CKD), 57, 58, 59, 60, 61, 62, 63, 64, 65, 66, 67, 68, 69, 70, 72, 73, 74, 75, 76, 77, 78, 79, 80, 81
chronic obstructive pulmonary disease, 65, 75, 77, 197
citizens, 45, 169
classification, 127, 147, 182
climate, 99, 179
clinical judgment, 235, 327
clinical trials, xii, 14, 21, 39, 51, 83, 85, 86, 90, 139, 147, 170, 173, 204, 219, 224, 229, 267, 269, 275, 320, 321, 323, 324
cognition, 234, 288, 310
cognitive impairment, 65, 271
collaboration, 8, 10, 30, 36, 41, 53, 136, 176, 276, 294, 303, 307, 308
collaborative research groups, 83, 86
colon cancer, 15, 65
color, iv, 54
colorectal cancer, 299, 327
commercial, 4, 33
common symptoms, 45, 159
communication, xi, xxii, 7, 11, 19, 31, 35, 51, 52, 56, 61, 63, 67, 68, 70, 71, 72, 73, 74, 81, 82, 88, 102,

108, 109, 114, 124, 126, 131, 137, 138, 151, 154, 171, 173, 201, 202, 203, 209, 212, 247, 249, 262, 269, 277, 280, 284, 288, 289, 290, 291, 310, 322, 328, 329, 333
communication skills, 51, 63, 67, 70, 71, 72, 74, 154, 262, 290, 310
comorbidity, 21, 61, 65
compassion, 17, 19, 52, 53, 91, 99, 114, 118, 120, 129
competence with death, 113, 117
complement, 21, 285
complementary, 229, 275, 276, 277, 278, 279, 280, 281, 291, 300, 301, 307
complexity, 6, 14, 60, 86, 98, 99, 129, 130, 147, 168, 177, 242, 252, 257
compliance, 215, 216
complications, xii, 26, 66, 73, 168, 178, 179
compression, 196, 197, 327
conception, 182, 253
conference, 13, 42, 204, 294
conflict, 128, 202, 253, 290, 310, 327
congruence, 71, 97
consensus, 61, 64, 99, 106, 132, 170, 206, 229, 235, 240, 268, 327, 332
consent, 280, 288, 325, 328
conserving, 21, 130
constipation, 85, 90, 168, 171, 269, 272, 330
construct validity, 139, 327
consumption, 141, 142, 163
content analysis, 239, 247
control group, 5, 84, 140, 204, 207, 208, 217, 221
controlled substances, 160, 164
controlled trials, 27, 28, 67, 84, 88, 93, 124, 126, 127, 146, 193, 194, 203, 204, 210, 213, 229, 230, 231, 232, 233, 234, 266, 277, 319, 320, 331
conversations, 6, 18, 51, 64, 66, 67, 68, 70, 72, 73, 77, 253, 256
cooperation, 86, 158, 307
coordination, 8, 45, 51, 99, 100, 109, 137, 181, 182
COPD, 146, 173, 194
coping strategies, xii, 114, 242, 253
correlation, 217, 223, 233, 245, 254, 270, 324
costs, xi, 14, 45, 48, 49, 55, 60, 62, 84, 85, 90, 97, 98, 99, 100, 102, 107, 108, 138, 147, 157, 158, 162, 163, 165, 177, 181, 182, 185, 195, 265, 266, 284, 295, 296, 321
cough, 194, 198
counseling, 127, 257
critique, 25, 29, 30, 31, 32
cultural diversity, 275
culture, xi, xiii, xv, 25, 26, 33, 48, 52, 53, 67, 68, 139, 170, 195, 242, 247, 252, 257, 286, 293, 295, 301, 307, 328

cure, xi, 4, 16, 53, 137, 252, 283, 284, 286
curricula, 37, 63, 71, 73, 118, 161
curriculum, xxii, 74, 309
Cyprus, 201, 224, 225, 335, 344

D

daily living, 18, 158, 246
data analysis, 29, 39
data collection, 29, 39, 92, 247, 324
data gathering, 267, 268
database, 277, 279
deaths, 5, 6, 51, 53, 62, 134, 135, 158, 178, 179, 182, 240, 253, 254, 308
decision makers, 7, 328
decision-making, 61, 66, 67, 70, 71, 73, 81, 82, 99, 103, 124, 176, 177, 206, 228, 288, 309, 310, 320
decision-making process, 61, 66, 73, 103, 124, 176, 177
deficiencies, 63, 87, 180, 219, 221, 267
delirium, 85, 327
dementia, 65, 66, 81, 91, 309
demographic transition, 175, 176, 178
denial, 250, 252, 253, 256
Denmark, 104, 205, 210, 220
depression, xiv, 3, 4, 7, 10, 14, 59, 60, 67, 69, 71, 75, 76, 77, 80, 85, 91, 124, 125, 126, 129, 130, 131, 192, 202, 207, 208, 210, 211, 212, 213, 219, 222, 240, 242, 243, 244, 245, 246, 259, 260, 261, 269, 286, 288, 290, 292, 299, 300
depressive symptoms, 76, 84, 171, 208, 209
depth, 63, 74, 153, 168, 170, 183, 239, 242, 247, 252
despair, 126, 179
detection, 5, 181, 324, 331
developed countries, xvi, 89, 176, 220, 266, 268
developed nations, 87, 268, 295
developing countries, xiii, xiv, xv, xix, xxi, 53, 82, 134, 141, 143, 179, 220, 284, 285, 295, 297
dialysis, 4, 58, 59, 60, 61, 62, 63, 64, 65, 66, 67, 68, 69, 70, 71, 72, 73, 74, 75, 76, 77, 78, 79, 80, 81
dignity, 121, 126, 138, 177, 179, 183, 257, 290, 320
directives, 6, 10, 61, 91, 267
disability, 65, 179, 266, 286, 287, 291, 296, 301
disappointment, 18, 192
discomfort, 14, 19, 66, 176, 177, 178, 268
disease progression, 66, 72, 79
diseases, xvi, 4, 5, 9, 49, 58, 61, 62, 65, 89, 114, 134, 136, 141, 153, 154, 155, 158, 170, 176, 178, 179, 181, 182, 183, 184, 240, 242, 262, 265, 266, 284, 286, 291, 296, 297, 298, 320
disorder, 91, 163, 262, 299
distress, xiii, 11, 14, 17, 19, 48, 51, 57, 71, 82, 85, 88, 119, 125, 126, 181, 183, 202, 207, 211, 219,

241, 250, 251, 259, 261, 268, 269, 270, 271, 285, 288, 289, 292, 300, 321, 326, 327
distribution, xiv, 160, 168, 198, 228
diversity, xiv, 130, 139, 220, 275, 292
Do Not Attempt to Resuscitate (DNAR), 267
docetaxel, 15, 235
doctors, 20, 51, 154, 191, 193, 195, 205, 244, 269, 292, 302
Doha, 265, 273, 345
drug interaction, 194, 198, 291
drugs, 49, 55, 138, 168, 171, 178, 193, 194, 195, 198, 231, 236, 278, 285, 308, 321
dyspnea, 59, 85, 90

E

early palliative care, viii, 51, 82, 83, 84, 176, 180, 181, 201, 202, 222, 223, 269, 322, 326
Easter, 6, 9
Eastern Europe, viii, 165, 189, 343
economic status, 245, 247
editors, 55, 104, 105, 106, 267
education, xv, xvii, xxii, 7, 32, 35, 37, 39, 40, 41, 42, 43, 45, 55, 56, 60, 63, 64, 70, 71, 81, 100, 102, 108, 118, 121, 124, 127, 130, 134, 137, 138, 145, 146, 147, 150, 160, 161, 163, 169, 175, 194, 205, 244, 246, 249, 261, 262, 272, 273, 278, 279, 284, 285, 295, 298, 300, 303, 307, 308, 309, 310, 311, 312, 313, 314, 315
Egypt, 265, 273, 292, 301
e-health, 97, 102, 182
elderly population, 79, 158, 284
eligibility criteria, 220, 271
embedded, 57, 58, 68, 69, 71, 74, 129
emergency, 69, 72, 99, 100, 101, 102, 107, 117, 162, 181, 182, 209
emotional distress, xii, xiv, 117, 239, 243, 250, 268
emotional well-being, 242, 289
empathy, 17, 71, 114, 119, 290
employment, 15, 50
end of life (EoL), viii, xii, xv, xvi, xvii, 3, 10, 11, 32, 37, 50, 51, 54, 57, 59, 61, 62, 63, 64, 67, 70, 71, 72, 76, 77, 82, 85, 91, 92, 98, 101, 104, 107, 108, 116, 121, 135, 138, 142, 148, 153, 159, 165, 167, 168, 173, 179, 181, 182, 201, 202, 207, 209, 222, 223, 234,239, 240, 242, 243, 246, 247, 249, 250, 251, 252, 253, 254, 255, 257, 259, 261, 262, 265, 266, 267, 268, 269, 270, 272, 273, 280, 284, 292, 295, 296, 301, 302, 322, 329, 331
end stage renal disease (ESRD), 58, 59, 60, 61, 62, 63, 64, 65, 66, 67, 70, 75, 76, 77, 78, 79, 80, 81, 86
endocrine, 219, 220

Engels, Yvonne, 104, 193
England, 67, 71, 80, 103
enrollment, xiii, 69, 79, 89
epidemic, 136, 181, 324
epidemiological transition, 176, 184, 185
epidemiology, 134, 222
equipment, 163, 324
equity, 100, 121, 182
ethical issues, xii, xiv, 99, 309
ethics, 11, 82, 138, 171, 177
Europe, 77, 86, 105, 139, 193, 221, 280, 321, 327
evidence, xi, xii, xiii, xv, xix, xxii, 25, 26, 27, 28, 29, 30, 31, 32, 33, 34, 35, 44, 45, 51, 73, 75, 77, 84, 87, 88, 89, 91, 98, 107, 114, 115, 118, 123, 124, 125, 126, 127, 129, 130, 133, 134, 135, 137, 138, 139, 140, 143, 144, 151, 155, 162, 163, 164, 167, 168, 170, 176, 180, 193, 195, 213, 217, 219, 220, 222, 227, 228, 229, 230, 231, 232, 233, 234, 235, 266, 268, 269, 272, 275, 276, 277, 278, 279, 289, 290, 291, 292, 293, 294, 295, 319, 320, 321, 324, 328, 329, 330
evidence-based, 7, 25, 26, 33, 34, 37, 125, 169, 236, 331
evidence-based practice, 25, 32, 33, 34, 35, 124, 272, 275, 276, 277, 279, 294
evil, 289, 291
evolution, 43, 126, 129, 137, 179, 180, 182
exclusion, 29, 202, 203, 229, 320
expenditures, 162, 296
expertise, xi, 30, 35, 72, 194, 202, 203, 205, 221, 228, 267, 285, 294, 323
exposure, 52, 63, 72, 114, 119, 120, 140

F

factor analysis, 113, 115, 117
faith, xii, 16, 18, 19, 20, 136, 240, 247, 249, 253, 292
families, xii, xx, 48, 50, 52, 53, 56, 57, 58, 61, 62, 64, 66, 68, 72, 73, 77, 84, 85, 102, 103, 108, 114, 118, 124, 126, 137, 138, 139, 144, 146, 153, 154, 160, 162, 165, 168, 169, 171, 176, 181, 202, 262, 265, 266, 267, 268, 269, 284, 285, 287, 290, 291, 292, 293, 294, 297, 302, 310, 322, 325, 326, 329
family life, 17, 286
family members, xxii, 7, 71, 85, 89, 114, 168, 175, 179, 255, 262, 268, 269, 271, 285, 288, 290, 291, 293, 295
family physician, 262, 325
family relationships, 285, 288, 289, 290
family therapy, 126, 128
fantasy, 248, 252
fatigue, 59, 72, 85, 88, 90, 91, 93, 114, 118, 120, 125, 131, 168, 194, 197, 198, 209, 219, 260, 277

fear, 16, 53, 113, 114, 119, 142, 179, 195, 250, 253, 286, 291, 288, 289, 292
feelings, xxi, 14, 114, 117, 124, 241, 250, 251, 253, 289, 310
fellowship, 11, 12, 36, 63, 71, 72, 78, 81, 82, 93, 145, 224, 237, 279, 302, 323
financial, 31, 33, 50, 101, 135, 162, 182, 192, 193, 194, 277, 285
financial support, 192, 193, 194
Finlay, Ilora, 193
fluid, 66, 196, 197
food, 49, 171
formation, 271, 330
fragility, 7, 179, 252
France, viii, 175, 176, 181, 182, 183, 184, 187, 281, 335, 343
freedom, 20, 270
friendship, xx, 171
funding, xii, 40, 83, 84, 85, 86, 93, 97, 100, 136, 195, 268, 269, 279, 294, 323, 324
future research, 8, 29, 129, 266, 271

G

general practitioner, 98, 155
generalizability, 67, 69, 217, 220, 319, 320
gerontology, 262, 263
global, viii, xix, xxi, 11, 32, 39, 41, 42, 47, 48, 49, 54, 55, 56, 67, 74, 135, 136, 137, 142, 143, 144, 146, 147, 149, 150, 153, 154, 157, 158, 163, 164, 165, 179, 180, 182, 183, 184, 185, 203, 259, 261, 298, 300, 331
goal-concordant, 58, 61, 64, 72, 73
goals, xi, 6, 16, 45, 51, 55, 61, 64, 66, 69, 71, 72, 85, 87, 101, 169, 176, 181, 202, 205, 206, 223, 241, 252, 284, 296, 303, 310
God, 18, 20, 171, 240, 249, 250, 253, 270, 292
governance, 280, 323
governments, xiii, 86, 137, 193
Grądalski, Tomasz, 194
grants, 35, 86, 224, 263
growth, 67, 157, 158, 232, 258, 262, 266, 277, 283, 286, 294, 295, 296
guidance, xix, xx, 61, 66, 72, 99, 141, 151, 221, 260, 328
guidelines, xii, xv, 8, 27, 31, 61, 65, 84, 87, 88, 123, 124, 127, 139, 140, 141, 160, 193, 194, 195, 205, 206, 221, 230, 278, 322, 326, 331, 332

H

head and neck cancer, 26, 27

healing, 158, 178, 179, 183, 278, 280, 284, 288, 291, 300
health care, 5, 7, 16, 18, 30, 38, 39, 40, 44, 45, 49, 51, 67, 83, 86, 93, 97, 98, 100, 102, 103, 133, 134, 135, 136, 138, 139, 159, 160, 161, 162, 163, 169, 202, 214, 220, 221, 263, 265, 266, 268, 271, 278, 280, 284, 285, 286, 288, 290, 294, 295, 299, 321, 322, 328, 329, 337
health care costs, 97, 100, 162, 265, 266
health care professionals, 16, 18, 38, 39, 49, 98, 102, 103, 138, 139, 202, 214, 221, 278, 280, 284
health care system, 67, 83, 133, 135, 159, 160, 161, 163, 271, 284, 287, 288, 294
health problems, 284, 286, 300
health services, 6, 60, 103, 136, 181, 211, 243, 262, 267, 289, 295
healthcare system, 8, 60, 67, 159, 176, 177, 180, 182, 183, 184, 283, 286, 297, 298
health-related quality of life (HRQoL), 21, 59, 60, 64, 67, 72, 74, 201, 202, 203, 207, 208, 210, 211, 212, 213, 216, 217, 218, 219, 220, 223
heart disease, 66, 75, 77
heart failure, 58, 62, 65, 73, 82, 88, 92, 102, 108, 142, 148, 150, 152, 155, 314
hematology, 119, 281, 302
hemodialysis, 59, 63, 65, 66, 74, 75, 76, 77, 79, 80
herbal medicine, 278, 280
heterogeneity, 83
heterogeneity of health systems and clinical models, 83
high school, 15, 329
history, 8, 13, 16, 17, 19, 40, 81, 82, 90, 191, 249, 267, 302
HIV, 134, 135, 136, 139, 140, 143, 144, 145, 146, 148, 149, 150, 152, 153, 154, 160, 285, 286, 288, 324
holistic care, 49, 177, 201
home care services, 163, 205
home palliative care, vii, 97, 102, 107, 165
home palliative care team, 97, 98, 103
homeostasis, xii, 128
homes, 37, 98, 102, 262
Hong Kong, 69, 80, 103, 314, 315
hospice, xi, xv, xvi, xvii, 4, 7, 10, 11, 32, 36, 37, 39, 42, 49, 50, 54, 56, 58, 62, 63, 64, 70, 77, 79, 80, 81, 82, 84, 87, 89, 92, 93, 104, 105, 106, 108, 109, 110, 115, 118, 120, 130, 136, 139, 141, 142, 143, 145, 147, 148, 150, 157, 158, 164, 165, 173, 181, 184, 185, 191, 192, 193, 194, 196, 203, 209, 221, 223, 239, 243, 246, 249, 259, 262, 265, 267, 268, 269, 270, 273, 280, 284, 289, 293, 302, 321, 325, 329, 330, 333, 343

hospice care, xv, xvi, xvii, 4, 42, 62, 64, 70, 89, 106, 158, 164, 173, 203, 246, 262, 265, 267, 284, 329, 330, 333
hospital death, 101, 107
hospitalization, 66, 76, 77, 88, 101, 206
host, 159, 228
human, 14, 17, 18, 20, 21, 48, 97, 98, 102, 111, 117, 126, 128, 129, 134, 141, 162, 181, 183, 240, 241, 252, 258, 260, 308, 313
human existence, 240, 252
human experience, 17, 18, 126
human resource development, 308, 313
human resources, 97, 98, 102, 162
human right, 102, 134, 141, 181
husband, 15, 16, 17, 19, 292
hypothesis, 287, 322, 329

I

ideal, 50, 88, 328
identification, 72, 98, 99, 100, 101, 104, 266, 284, 322, 328
identity, xiv, 71, 254, 287
illness trajectory, 64, 65, 72, 135
improvements, 44, 69, 87, 99, 140, 208, 219, 303
impulses, 193
in transition, 42, 130, 284, 286, 287, 288, 291, 296
incidence, xiv, 4, 79, 134, 135, 284, 286, 295, 296, 307, 309
income, ix, xi, xiv, 50, 133, 134, 135, 138, 143, 144, 146, 155, 158, 162, 165, 284, 286
independence, 79, 286, 288
India, 55, 133, 135, 136, 138, 142
individuals, 7, 8, 9, 10, 16, 19, 51, 53, 58, 60, 81, 99, 131, 133, 134, 136, 228, 242, 248, 251, 252, 255, 286, 287, 288, 289, 291
induction, 27, 34, 214
induction chemotherapy, 27, 34
industrialized countries, 287
industry, 193, 195, 324
infancy, 136, 138, 285
infection, 65, 277, 278
informed consent, 116, 243, 287
infrastructure, 51, 87, 295, 325
ingredients, 33, 152, 290, 296
inhibitor, 193, 321
initiation, 59, 61, 63, 65, 66, 71, 76, 79
injections, 231, 233
injury, iv, 65, 158, 301
inpatient, xiii, 51, 62, 70, 85, 89, 90, 101, 109, 143, 147, 223, 269, 275, 276, 295, 327, 340
institutions, 8, 64, 85, 86, 89, 169, 192, 205, 277, 279, 303

integration, xxii, 6, 7, 8, 20, 21, 26, 50, 51, 57, 58, 81, 82, 83, 86, 90, 133, 134, 135, 136, 137, 139, 159, 168, 177, 181, 195, 203, 204, 207, 221, 222, 223, 224, 255, 275, 277, 280, 285, 295, 330
integrity, 240, 288
intensive care unit, 171, 209
internalizing, 289, 294
interpersonal relations, 171, 290
interpersonal relationships, 171, 290
intervention, 5, 14, 26, 28, 35, 38, 39, 68, 69, 70, 74, 80, 81, 83, 84, 88, 90, 99, 100, 110, 118, 120, 121, 131, 132, 140, 150, 152, 154, 168, 177, 180, 185, 201, 202, 203, 204, 205, 210, 212, 213, 214, 215, 216, 217, 218, 219, 220, 221, 222, 223, 228, 229, 254, 260, 288, 290, 293, 295, 313, 314, 321, 322, 324, 325, 328
investment, 48, 138, 169
Iowa, 32, 34
Ireland, xv, xvii, 235, 302
Islam, 249, 253, 278, 292, 293, 298, 301
Islamic middle-income country, ix, 284
isolation, 102, 139
Israel, v, xvi, 82, 90, 227, 233, 237, 239, 243, 257, 258, 260, 261, 262, 263, 335, 337, 344
issues, xi, xii, xiv, xvi, xxi, xxii, 6, 32, 45, 61, 63, 64, 70, 85, 99, 106, 110, 115, 124, 133, 136, 138, 165, 201, 202, 213, 218, 219, 221, 242, 247, 248, 249, 252, 253, 261, 266, 277, 284, 289, 290, 292, 293, 296, 297, 299, 301, 320, 323, 326, 330
Italy, 23, 103, 123, 205, 210, 220, 335, 343

J

Japan, ix, 102, 107, 307, 308, 309, 310, 313, 314, 315, 335, 345
Jassem, Ewa, 194, 198
Jews, 244, 246, 257
Jordan, xxi, 34, 133, 136, 143, 299
journal club, 25, 30, 31
justification, 51, 268

K

Kaasa, Stein, 92, 170, 173, 193, 198
Kenya, 136, 140, 141, 143, 144, 145, 146, 149, 154
ketamine, 194, 198, 324, 332
kidney, 57, 58, 59, 60, 61, 62, 63, 64, 65, 66, 67, 68, 69, 70, 72, 73, 74, 75, 76, 77, 78, 79, 80, 81, 141, 179
Klepstad, Pål, 193, 198
Krajnik, Małgorzata, 192, 194, 196, 197, 198

L

landmark clinical trials, 83
languages, 37, 138, 139, 148, 204
Latinos, 35, 38, 39
laws, 141, 183
leadership, 44, 56, 99, 137, 163, 281
learning, 8, 47, 52, 54, 70, 72, 73, 123, 138, 153, 193, 247, 256, 257, 309, 325
legislation, 152, 183
lens, 58, 290
Leppert, Wojciech, 193, 196
level of education, 249, 278
levels of evidence, 25, 28, 127, 229, 230
Lichodziejewska-Niemierko, Monika, 194, 198
life course, 98, 184
life expectancy, 4, 17, 59, 61, 179, 286, 308, 313
light, 29, 32, 126, 242, 243, 246, 256, 288, 289, 292
liver, 15, 278
local authorities, 47, 136, 163
longitudinal study, 78, 259
love, 17, 20, 175, 251, 257
low and middle income countries, viii, 133, 134, 135, 137
low income countries, 134
Łuczak, Jacek, 193
Łuczak, Prof. J., 193
lung cancer, 52, 74, 82, 84, 90, 185, 197, 208, 211, 216, 218, 222, 223, 252, 260, 267, 322, 331
lung disease, 194, 252
lymph, 196, 197
lymphedema, 196, 197

M

magnitude, 59, 135, 213, 234, 266, 286, 289
major depression, 3, 4
majority, xxi, 5, 6, 14, 59, 63, 67, 88, 97, 134, 135, 182, 228, 230, 251, 270, 277, 284, 292
malignancy, 65, 104, 210, 234, 266
malnutrition, 65, 135
management, xv, xvi, 3, 4, 5, 9, 11, 16, 19, 27, 28, 30, 34, 38, 42, 44, 51, 54, 57, 58, 59, 60, 63, 64, 65, 67, 68, 69, 70, 72, 73, 74, 75, 76, 78, 79, 80, 81, 82, 85, 91, 93, 99, 124, 138, 140, 141, 146, 147, 148, 167, 169, 170, 176, 177, 178, 180, 181, 182, 183, 186, 196, 201, 202, 205, 214, 219, 221, 234, 235, 237, 269, 270, 277, 281, 284, 288, 290, 292, 297, 303, 309, 319, 320, 321, 323, 325, 330, 332
mapping, 137, 148
marijuana, 233, 236
marriage, 286, 298
mass, 31, 48, 84, 231
mastectomy, 14, 15, 21, 228
materials, 72, 137, 248
matter, iv, 90, 175, 183, 185, 233, 247, 272, 291, 328
meaning-focused coping, 240, 241, 242
measurement, 21, 29, 68, 91, 101, 106, 115, 116, 120, 133, 134, 139, 144, 147, 149, 150, 153, 155, 157, 158, 159, 161, 162, 163, 173, 186, 258, 260, 271, 275, 276
media, 53, 185, 277, 291
median, 161, 325, 327
Medicaid, 4, 165, 184
medical, xii, xiv, xxii, 5, 6, 7, 8, 11, 12, 13, 14, 15, 16, 17, 37, 39, 48, 51, 53, 55, 56, 61, 78, 80, 81, 82, 91, 93, 109, 135, 161, 165, 177, 178, 180, 182, 184, 192, 194, 195, 205, 206, 212, 214, 215, 217, 224, 228, 229, 230, 233, 234, 235, 236, 252, 254, 258, 262, 269, 276, 277, 285, 287, 288, 290, 291, 293, 295, 296, 301, 307, 308, 309, 313, 319, 320, 321, 325, 328, 337
medical care, 5, 14, 91, 165, 180, 254, 269, 290, 296, 301, 307, 308, 309, 313
Medicare, 4, 62, 76, 89, 93, 158, 184, 222
medication, 6, 37, 50, 231, 233, 268, 292
medicine, xiii, 7, 9, 11, 14, 21, 33, 48, 49, 51, 53, 56, 67, 83, 86, 93, 107, 135, 160, 161, 175, 176, 177, 178, 179, 180, 181, 182, 191, 192, 193, 195, 228, 229, 232, 234, 235, 236, 252, 262, 265, 266, 267, 268, 269, 270, 271, 275, 276, 278, 280, 284, 290, 291, 295, 297, 300, 301, 308, 309, 319, 320, 323, 328, 330, 331, 332
menopause, 15, 17
mental health, 6, 7, 8, 9, 45, 91, 165, 285, 288, 301
mental health professionals, 9
mental illness, 3, 4, 5, 7, 8, 9, 10, 11
mental state, 8, 288
mentor, 35, 39
mentoring, 86, 98, 161, 323
mentorship, xix, 30, 44, 87, 141
messages, 17, 328
meta-analysis, xvi, 28, 75, 76, 80, 88, 91, 124, 127, 130, 131, 213, 217, 223, 234, 236, 237, 269, 299, 325
metabolism, 193, 231, 278
metabolites, 324, 331
metastatic cancer, 51, 126, 202, 203, 222, 244, 259
metastatic disease, 218, 233
methadone, 163, 324
methodology, 29, 127, 159, 266, 277
Middle East, v, viii, xix, xxi, 36, 38, 40, 41, 42, 133, 136, 139, 147, 199, 273, 276, 278, 280, 284, 288, 296, 299, 300, 301, 303, 337, 344

middle income countries, 162, 165
minorities, 152, 171
misconceptions, 72, 137, 290
mission, 48, 49, 52, 53, 99
model, viii, xiii, 7, 22, 32, 33, 34, 43, 44, 48, 49, 50, 51, 57, 58, 64, 67, 68, 69, 70, 71, 73, 74, 78, 83, 84, 85, 87, 88, 89, 99, 100, 106, 116, 117, 118, 121, 126, 129, 130, 136, 138, 139, 151, 155, 157, 158, 159, 160, 161, 163, 172, 175, 176, 177, 178, 180, 182, 183, 184, 185, 195, 196, 201, 202, 204, 205, 213, 214, 221, 240, 241, 242, 246, 250, 258, 269, 283, 284, 285, 287, 288, 297, 298, 299, 300, 322, 325, 331
Modlińska, Aleksandra, 194
molecules, 232, 321
momentum, 83, 291
Montana, 39, 40, 41, 43, 45
moral imperative, 319, 320
morbidity, 179, 284, 300
morphine, 49, 52, 90, 141, 142, 160, 163, 194, 197, 230, 231, 236, 324, 330, 331
mortality, 3, 4, 5, 6, 7, 26, 49, 59, 60, 65, 70, 76, 77, 78, 79, 158, 159, 163, 179, 202, 292, 299
mortality rate, 3, 4, 7, 49
motivation, 50, 175, 242, 286, 328
multidimensional, 75, 100, 120
music, 144, 170
Muslims, 257, 301
mutations, 218, 308

N

narrative, 13, 17, 18, 19, 20, 21, 22, 82, 126, 127, 128, 130, 280
National Institutes of Health, v, 76, 86
nausea, 85, 192, 209, 210, 219, 233, 288, 321, 324, 328, 330, 332
need assessment, 157
negative effects, 114, 251
negative emotions, 241, 329
neoplasm, 203
nephrology, 57, 58, 60, 61, 63, 64, 65, 66, 67, 68, 69, 70, 71, 72, 73, 74, 76, 77, 78, 79, 80, 81, 194
nerve, 228, 232, 236, 321, 330
nerve growth factor, 232, 321
Netherlands, 103, 193, 194
networking, 31, 35, 100
neuropathic pain, 85, 88, 194, 196, 237, 324
neuropathy, 90, 227, 228, 232, 235, 236
neuropharmacology, 323, 325
New England, 174, 185
New Zealand, 159, 280, 315, 325
Nigeria, 49, 108

non-dialysis care, 59, 65, 66, 68
non-transmissible diseases (NTDs), 176, 179, 180, 181
North Africa, 147, 292
North America, vii, xxii, 1, 159, 185, 269, 327, 337, 339
NSAIDs, 227, 231, 232, 235
nurses, xi, xiii, xix, 20, 35, 39, 41, 43, 44, 49, 51, 69, 70, 71, 74, 99, 113, 116, 117, 118, 119, 140, 161, 169, 193, 195, 205, 206, 214, 215, 270, 275, 276, 277, 279, 285, 290, 292, 295, 298, 302, 307, 308, 309, 310, 313, 314, 325, 326, 327, 331, 337
nursing, xvii, 7, 15, 34, 35, 37, 42, 61, 84, 85, 86, 98, 110, 119, 161, 184, 195, 294, 300, 307, 308, 309, 310, 312, 314, 315, 321
nursing care, 35, 308, 321
nursing home, 37, 61, 85, 98
nutrition, 62, 167, 171

O

obstacles, 123, 268
Oceania, ix, 317, 345
oncology supportive care, 58, 69
opioids, 7, 50, 53, 54, 91, 134, 137, 138, 139, 141, 144, 145, 152, 160, 163, 194, 198, 227, 230, 231, 232, 234, 236, 237, 292, 313, 321, 324, 334
opportunities, xi, xvi, 6, 43, 48, 50, 51, 72, 108, 136, 152, 169, 248, 257, 279, 293, 300
optimism, 19, 260
organization of services, 97
organizational culture, 33, 52, 53
organize, 267, 290
outcomes, vii, viii, ix, xiii, xiv, xvi, 3, 8, 9, 25, 26, 27, 30, 31, 33, 34, 37, 38, 43, 44, 45, 58, 60, 63, 65, 68, 69, 71, 73, 74, 75, 76, 80, 83, 86, 87, 88, 89, 90, 91, 92, 93, 97, 99, 100, 101, 102, 103, 106, 107, 109, 116, 125, 133, 134, 138, 139, 140, 141, 142, 143, 144, 149, 151, 153, 155, 157, 158, 161, 162, 163, 165, 173, 204, 213, 216, 218, 219, 220, 221, 222, 223, 230, 232, 265, 266, 267, 271, 276, 289, 294, 301, 302, 319, 321, 327, 328, 329
outpatient, xiii, 40, 51, 69, 80, 81, 84, 85, 87, 88, 91, 107, 108, 109, 146, 153, 173, 202, 206, 223, 224, 270, 272, 275, 295, 302, 313, 325, 327, 330, 332
outreach, 35, 107
ovarian cancer, 218, 223
overlay, 139, 141

P

P2X4, 193, 196

Index

paclitaxel, 15, 236
pain care, 42, 43
pain management, xxi, 11, 37, 39, 42, 48, 60, 82, 134, 139, 140, 152, 224, 227, 228, 236, 276, 283, 292, 296, 321, 322, 328, 332, 334
palliative care medicine, 191, 267, 271, 302
palliative care qualitative research, 307
palliative medicine in practice, 195
pancreatic cancer, 210, 216
parallel, 176, 235, 247
parents, 52, 184, 257, 286
parotid, 27, 34
paroxetine, 192, 193, 196
participants, xi, 29, 30, 31, 85, 115, 216, 230, 231, 239, 243, 244, 245, 246, 247, 248, 249, 250, 251, 252, 253, 254, 255, 269, 270, 293, 310, 324, 329
patient care, 25, 26, 30, 33, 62, 98, 99, 100, 120, 195, 265, 269, 271, 275, 277, 279, 281, 287
patient recruitment, 139
peace, 16, 17, 18, 19, 270, 287
pediatric nurses, viii, 113, 116, 117, 118
peer review, 35, 165, 204, 222, 224, 225
peripheral neuropathy, 90, 232, 235
permission, iv, 160
permit, 168, 177
personal autonomy, 14, 180
personality, 3, 4, 292, 328
personality disorder, 3, 4
pharmaceutical, xi, 149, 171, 193, 293, 321
pharmacology, 194, 195, 334
Philadelphia, 34, 330
physical health, 7, 286
physical therapy, 197, 206
physicians, xi, xiii, xix, xxi, 51, 61, 70, 71, 85, 89, 91, 99, 161, 169, 202, 206, 214, 215, 221, 265, 266, 270, 273, 276, 277, 279, 285, 288, 290, 310, 325, 331, 332, 333, 337
pilot study, 37, 60, 69, 70, 76, 77, 118, 236, 258, 260
placebo, 28, 90, 93, 192, 194, 229, 231, 233, 234, 235, 236, 266, 324, 331, 332
platform, 30, 45, 86, 138, 151
platinum, 218, 223
playing, 65, 171, 260
Poland, viii, 191, 193, 195, 196, 335, 343
policy, 50, 56, 67, 100, 134, 137, 139, 141, 144, 145, 148, 151, 154, 157, 158, 160, 163, 184, 221, 285, 288, 308, 313
policy makers, 53, 137, 221, 285
polypharmacy and drug interactions, 194
population, xiv, xv, 3, 4, 5, 6, 9, 14, 26, 27, 28, 31, 47, 49, 50, 51, 59, 60, 62, 64, 65, 77, 89, 98, 100, 103, 104, 133, 135, 136, 140, 151, 152, 155, 158, 163, 168, 170, 178, 179, 181, 184, 186, 204, 229, 230, 233, 235, 240, 266, 267, 268, 270, 271, 277, 284, 286, 287, 289, 291, 292, 299, 302, 308, 313, 326, 327
Portugal, 97, 103, 110, 111, 335, 342
practices and research, 284
predictive accuracy, 322
premature death, 3, 6, 286
preparation, iv, 249, 253, 270, 310
preparedness, 63, 71, 72
preservation, 14, 301
President, 41, 237, 281
prevention, 8, 26, 27, 34, 38, 41, 225, 235, 236, 266, 284, 286, 308, 328, 329
principles, xii, 57, 64, 68, 72, 74, 99, 100, 106, 161, 290, 319, 320, 324, 330
prior knowledge, 295
professionals, xii, xv, xix, xxii, 7, 9, 15, 25, 33, 35, 37, 38, 47, 50, 51, 53, 56, 98, 99, 100, 113, 114, 115, 117, 118, 119, 120, 126, 132, 136, 137, 139, 141, 143, 145, 147, 168, 169, 171, 177, 181, 182, 203, 204, 243, 254, 268, 280, 285, 290, 293, 294, 307, 310, 321
prognosis, 5, 51, 58, 61, 63, 65, 66, 67, 72, 79, 85, 118, 135, 154, 158, 180, 192, 202, 209, 210, 211, 212, 213, 218, 223, 243, 244, 295, 320, 321, 325, 331
prognostic tools, 65, 79
prognostication, 64, 65, 67, 72, 319, 321, 325, 331, 332
project, 45, 53, 108, 138, 140, 146, 147, 303, 323, 326, 331
prophylaxis, 26, 30
prostate cancer, 224, 233, 235
pruritus, 59, 192, 193, 196
psychiatric disorders, 124, 289
psychiatry, 7, 8, 10, 12
psychological distress, 25, 254, 261, 270, 285, 288, 289
psychologist, 165, 206, 215, 328
psychology, 21, 161, 260, 261
psychometric properties, 43, 101, 113, 115, 117, 118, 139
psychosocial factors, 75, 299
psychosocial interventions, 124, 125, 127, 128, 129
psychotherapy, 126, 127, 128, 129, 259, 260, 290, 300
public health, 41, 45, 82, 99, 100, 104, 105, 106, 134, 136, 137, 140, 142, 143, 145, 150, 157, 159, 161, 163, 164, 179, 180, 181, 182, 185, 284, 286, 297, 302, 311
publishing, xx, 50, 168, 193, 279, 337

Q

qualitative, 8, 13, 17, 20, 21, 27, 28, 29, 30, 34, 35, 37, 39, 45, 46, 50, 55, 61, 66, 75, 77, 80, 88, 103, 108, 109, 119, 143, 146, 147, 151, 153, 154, 159, 167, 168, 172, 173, 198, 203, 239, 240, 242, 246, 247, 250, 251, 252, 253, 259, 260, 261, 280
qualitative research, 13, 17, 30, 50, 75, 168, 173, 242, 247, 259, 307
quality improvement, 35, 38, 42, 97, 100, 101, 103, 144, 150, 295, 326
quality of life (QoL), vii, xv, xvi, xxi, 3, 4, 5, 8, 11, 13, 14, 16, 19, 20, 21, 22, 26, 33, 35, 44, 46, 48, 58, 59, 64, 66, 68, 69, 72, 75, 77, 82, 83, 84, 87, 90, 92, 98, 99, 101, 102, 103, 114, 118, 120, 121, 125, 138, 139, 140, 143, 151, 153, 162, 169, 171, 173, 176, 177, 186, 187, 197, 201, 202, 203, 207, 212, 219, 239, 240, 242, 243, 244, 245, 246, 250, 251, 254, 259, 261, 263, 266, 267, 268, 269, 270, 277, 283, 284, 285, 286, 289, 293, 294, 296, 299, 313, 320, 321, 331
quantitative, 8, 13, 21, 28, 29, 30, 35, 39, 45, 88, 120, 146, 167, 168, 239, 240, 242, 243, 246, 247, 251, 341
quantitative research, 168, 247
questionnaire, 5, 13, 16, 17, 92, 115, 116, 208, 243, 250, 259, 277

R

Radbruch, Lukas, 91, 104, 105, 106, 153, 154, 155, 164, 193, 236
radiation, 26, 27, 228, 230, 309
radiation therapy, 26, 27, 228, 230
radiotherapy, 27, 34, 244, 328
randomized controlled trials (RCTs), 27, 67, 84, 88, 124, 126, 127, 203, 204, 210, 213, 229, 230, 231, 232, 233, 234, 266, 277, 319, 320, 331
rating scale, 269, 270
reactions, 119, 285
reading, 30, 248
reality, 28, 241, 248, 252, 260
receptor, 193, 194, 196, 197, 233
recognition, 20, 57, 58, 59, 100, 248, 265, 269, 285, 303
recommendations, iv, xxii, 6, 32, 51, 61, 77, 100, 127, 196, 228, 230, 235, 279, 295, 322
reconstruction, 15, 258
recruiting, xi, 220, 293, 323, 324
reform, 180, 184, 195
refugees, 133, 136, 143
regions of the world, 48, 54

regression, 245, 246
rehabilitation, 151, 154
relatives, 114, 171, 210, 257, 299
relevance, 69, 139, 283, 287, 321
reliability, 29, 113, 115, 116, 117, 118, 243, 327
relief, xv, 47, 49, 50, 51, 135, 137, 138, 140, 142, 143, 154, 158, 159, 160, 170, 196, 221, 233, 266, 283, 284, 321, 326, 330
religion, 15, 19, 20, 22, 170, 247, 249, 253, 278, 287, 293
religiosity, 19, 20, 246, 253, 270, 292, 300
religious beliefs, 19, 241, 278
religiousness, 239, 261
remission, 15, 16
renaissance, 129, 322
renal impairment, 194, 198
renal replacement therapy, 66, 78, 79
renal supportive care, vii, 57, 58, 63, 64, 68, 70, 71, 72, 73, 74, 78
requirement, 294, 321
requirements, 50, 294, 295, 337
research funding, 139, 268
research institutes, 191
researchers, xi, xiv, 5, 28, 35, 37, 50, 53, 86, 87, 88, 89, 115, 138, 140, 168, 191, 193, 194, 195, 221, 231, 251, 266, 268, 271, 293, 295, 323
residential, 98, 104
resistance, 47, 218, 287
resource utilization, 62, 70, 76
resources, xiii, 26, 31, 32, 48, 54, 56, 58, 68, 70, 86, 89, 97, 98, 99, 100, 101, 107, 128, 135, 137, 139, 142, 192, 221, 234, 277, 286, 298, 310
response, 13, 15, 45, 71, 111, 136, 139, 183, 191, 198, 217, 218, 220, 234, 284, 301, 310, 327, 330, 332
restrictions, 108, 205
rights, iv, 183, 228
risk factors, 66, 79, 332
roots, 53, 171
rules, 129, 193, 255, 268
Rwanda, 49, 55, 136, 141

S

sacraments, 13, 18, 20, 21
safety, 44, 102, 164, 227, 228, 233, 235, 236, 278, 309, 328, 330
Saudi Arabia, 278, 279, 280, 281, 299
Saunders, Cicely, 133, 137, 138, 140, 141, 145, 147, 148, 150, 151, 184, 193, 265, 267, 272, 330, 342
savings, 102, 163, 164, 324
schizophrenia, 3, 4, 5, 7
scholarship, 141, 150

school, xxii, 37, 39, 161, 309, 329
science, xv, 21, 22, 31, 41, 44, 89, 130, 138, 139, 174, 176, 192, 228, 252, 320, 324
scope, xix, 10, 16, 17, 26, 32, 86, 88, 135, 288, 293, 295
screening, 6, 19, 43, 87, 92, 181, 202, 204, 225, 295, 298, 300, 319, 320, 326, 327, 328, 332, 333
security, 109, 126, 249, 251
selective serotonin reuptake inhibitor, 193
self-efficacy, 120, 211
self-worth, 45, 290
sensations, 170, 180
serendipity, 193
serotonin, 193, 196
serotonin reuptake inhibitors, 193
service provider, 133, 136, 279
service provision, viii, 133, 134, 135, 137
services, iv, xi, xiii, xv, xix, 5, 7, 9, 43, 49, 50, 51, 53, 62, 70, 72, 80, 84, 86, 87, 89, 91, 97, 98, 99, 100, 106, 107, 109, 115, 116, 117, 118, 134, 135, 136, 137, 138, 139, 141, 149, 155, 159, 161, 162, 163, 165, 170, 178, 182, 185, 195, 202, 205, 206, 220, 221, 268, 269, 281, 284, 294, 295, 302, 307, 309, 313, 337
severe and persistent mental illness, vii, 3, 4, 9, 10
sex, 125, 153
sexuality, 167, 171
shape, 6, 126, 127, 221, 259
shared decision-making, 61, 63, 64, 66, 72, 73, 77, 99
shortage, xiii, 49, 89, 93, 138, 160, 195
shortness of breath, 60, 160
showing, 59, 115, 202, 213, 324, 328
side effects, xvi, 3, 4, 6, 85, 171, 180, 233, 276, 277, 288, 324
signs, 176, 177
Sinai, 57, 81, 340
skills training, 81, 219
sleep disturbance, 76, 270
smoking, 233, 328
Sobański, Piotr, 193
social network, 143, 252, 287, 313
social problems, 240, 290
social support, 19, 21, 60, 64, 242, 269, 291
social workers, xi, xix, 62, 69, 70, 71, 74, 98, 161, 169, 205, 206, 214, 270, 285, 290, 337
society, xiv, 20, 21, 99, 100, 103, 195, 222, 242, 257, 283, 287, 289, 291, 310, 320
socioeconomic status, 135, 278
solution, 20, 183, 233, 329
solutions, xix, 45, 47, 48, 53, 55, 99, 195, 331
Sopata, Maciej, 193, 233, 236

South Africa, 49, 93, 102, 107, 136, 140, 141, 154, 155
South Asia, 138, 143
Spain, 103, 113, 117, 121, 158, 167, 168, 171, 172, 335, 341
specialists, 8, 47, 48, 63, 71, 89, 140, 169, 171, 181, 205, 206, 219, 307, 309, 314, 325, 332
specialization, 157, 160, 161
specialized palliative care, 51, 105, 161, 169, 201, 203, 223, 224, 290
spiritual care, 98, 123, 285, 331, 337
spirituality, xii, 13, 18, 19, 20, 22, 119, 120, 128, 138, 167, 170, 171, 172, 173, 253, 258, 270, 273, 322
squamous cell, 27, 34
St. John of God, 171
staffing, 50, 85
stakeholders, 31, 99, 276, 277, 295
standard deviation, 117, 244, 310
standardization, 89, 123, 127, 129
state, xii, 41, 65, 66, 73, 93, 136, 142, 143, 149, 193, 245, 253, 329
states, 65, 66, 70, 83, 88, 129, 179, 181
statistics, 29, 116, 117, 257, 281
stigma, 6, 8, 288, 290, 314
strategic planning, 56, 106
streptococci, 27, 34
stress, xiv, 60, 114, 119, 181, 240, 241, 258, 260, 262, 263, 309, 321
stressful life events, 257, 260
stroke, 109, 158
structure, 69, 71, 83, 84, 85, 100, 101, 113, 115, 116, 242
subgroups, 60, 70, 72
subjective well-being, 251, 260
sub-Saharan Africa, 49, 55, 134, 137, 139, 140, 143, 144, 146, 149, 150, 165
subspecialty, xxii, 51, 57, 58, 74, 302
substance abuse, 82, 137
substance use, 5, 6
suffering, vii, xi, xii, xvi, xxi, 16, 26, 33, 47, 48, 50, 51, 52, 88, 99, 100, 114, 118, 126, 128, 129, 130, 134, 135, 137, 157, 158, 159, 162, 176, 178, 179, 182, 183, 194, 202, 240, 242, 251, 252, 258, 259, 261, 262, 266, 271, 283, 284, 288, 289, 292, 294, 320
suicide, 5, 6, 183, 192
sulfate, 231, 331
supervision, 148, 323
supportive care, 58, 64, 68, 69, 70, 71, 73, 75, 76, 77, 79, 82, 119, 120, 130, 145, 173, 219, 223, 224, 259, 273, 280
surrogates, 70, 80

survival, 14, 43, 58, 59, 62, 65, 66, 67, 73, 75, 76, 79, 84, 86, 131, 175, 183, 201, 202, 203, 210, 211, 212, 213, 218, 233, 251, 267, 269, 289, 321, 325, 327, 332
survivors, xvi, 21, 45, 46, 227, 262, 299, 300, 313, 334
Switzerland, 42, 193
symptom assessment, 60, 67, 69, 72, 82, 87, 209, 269, 272
symptom burden, 58, 59, 60, 63, 67, 68, 70, 72, 74, 76, 85, 153, 216, 221, 289
symptom management, xvi, 3, 4, 9, 10, 11, 37, 38, 40, 44, 58, 60, 63, 64, 67, 68, 69, 72, 73, 80, 93, 119, 120, 124, 138, 140, 141, 142, 143, 144, 146, 152, 154, 164, 165, 169, 173, 178, 185, 196, 197, 198, 202, 205, 214, 219, 221, 259, 269, 270, 277, 280, 284, 290, 297, 321
symptoms, xii, xiii, xvi, 3, 4, 5, 7, 8, 16, 25, 26, 33, 35, 51, 59, 60, 63, 64, 66, 67, 68, 69, 72, 75, 76, 77, 78, 84, 85, 88, 93, 100, 109, 110, 124, 125, 138, 140, 141, 159, 167, 168, 170, 171, 176, 178, 180, 183, 201, 202, 206, 207, 209, 211, 212, 216, 219, 220, 221, 233, 234, 240, 242, 243, 244, 245, 251, 268, 269, 271, 276, 277, 285, 288, 290, 292, 294, 299, 309, 319, 320, 321, 323, 324, 325, 327, 330, 332
syndrome, 118, 148, 228, 278
synthesis, 32, 148, 154, 186, 187, 193, 260

T

Tanzania, 49, 137, 141, 142
Task Force, 11, 77, 91, 93, 99, 106, 110, 155, 268
taxonomy, 280, 315
team members, 30, 35, 50, 70, 169
teams, xi, xix, 32, 33, 37, 61, 64, 70, 71, 85, 90, 97, 98, 99, 102, 107, 124, 128, 136, 139, 165, 167, 168, 169, 203, 216, 221, 267, 269, 271, 293, 325, 326
techniques, 68, 72, 74, 126, 128, 168, 285
telephone, 84, 108, 109, 205, 214, 215, 216, 243
terminal care, 203, 266, 267, 309
terminal illness, 7, 130, 248, 257, 259, 267, 283, 285, 288, 290, 294
terminally ill, 49, 104, 106, 117, 129, 195, 198, 259, 290, 292, 332
testing, 21, 35, 36, 45, 124, 150, 161, 162, 232, 327
therapeutic effect, 52, 233
therapeutic interventions, 28, 93
therapy, 26, 46, 53, 63, 66, 73, 79, 127, 128, 131, 140, 144, 153, 177, 193, 197, 202, 218, 219, 220, 221, 223, 242, 255, 276, 278, 279, 289, 324, 325, 327, 330, 332

thoughts, 117, 124, 175, 255
threats, xii, 241
toll-like receptor, 193, 196
top-down, viii, 191, 192, 232
top-down research, 191
traditional therapies, 275, 276
traditions, 283, 287, 295
trainees, 63, 64, 71, 72, 119
training, xv, xix, xxi, 10, 11, 12, 19, 35, 39, 42, 49, 50, 51, 52, 63, 67, 68, 70, 71, 72, 74, 78, 81, 89, 99, 100, 102, 106, 111, 115, 117, 118, 119, 120, 124, 136, 137, 139, 140, 141, 145, 148, 161, 163, 168, 169, 203, 205, 214, 219, 220, 221, 224, 275, 279, 284, 285, 290, 295, 302, 303, 309, 313, 315, 331, 334, 337
training programs, xix, 72, 118, 290, 303
trajectory, xix, xxi, 7, 58, 64, 65, 66, 67, 72, 78, 92, 119, 124, 129, 135, 158, 180, 213, 218, 283, 284, 285
transformation, 33, 42
translating research into practice, 25, 30
translation, xxii, 58, 139, 148, 167
transplant, 60, 76
transplantation, 27, 34, 64
trauma, 17, 45, 241, 262
treatment, xii, xiii, xv, xix, 3, 4, 5, 6, 7, 13, 14, 15, 16, 17, 19, 21, 26, 27, 34, 48, 51, 54, 58, 59, 60, 61, 62, 64, 66, 67, 69, 72, 73, 79, 84, 87, 104, 114, 124, 125, 131, 135, 141, 145, 146, 152, 160, 163, 170, 171, 177, 178, 180, 181, 182, 194, 196, 198, 202, 206, 207, 208, 219, 224, 227, 228, 229, 230, 231, 232, 233, 234, 235, 236, 237, 239, 240, 243, 244, 247, 249, 251, 254, 257, 260, 261, 266, 268, 269, 270, 275, 276, 277, 278, 280, 284, 285, 288, 289, 290, 295, 296, 297, 300, 309, 310, 322, 325, 328, 329, 330, 331, 332, 333
trials, viii, xii, xiii, xiv, xv, xvii, 14, 27, 28, 34, 39, 68, 69, 73, 74, 80, 84, 85, 86, 87, 90, 91, 93, 108, 115, 123, 125, 131, 132, 140, 144, 146, 152, 154, 165, 192, 193, 194, 196, 197, 201, 202, 203, 204, 205, 207, 213, 214, 215, 216, 217, 218, 219, 220, 221, 222, 223, 224, 229, 232, 233, 234, 236, 259, 260, 268, 269, 303, 321, 329, 330, 331, 332
triggers, 70, 72, 288
tuberculosis, 134, 154
tumor, 203, 228, 232, 236, 261, 269, 330
tumours, 194, 219, 220
Twycross, Robert, 193, 196, 198

U

uniform, 63, 213
United Kingdom, xxii, 335, 342

United Nations, 134, 163, 179
United States, xix, 41, 47, 51, 53, 58, 62, 66, 67, 71, 73, 74, 76, 77, 80, 85, 86, 87, 89, 102, 158, 164, 168, 267, 269, 278, 281, 335, 339
universities, 161, 169, 191, 192, 193
urban, 60, 66, 143, 144, 149, 311
urbanization, 287, 298

V

Valencia, 113, 120, 341
validation, 91, 119, 120, 128, 138, 143, 147, 148, 150, 272, 327, 332
validity, 29, 113, 115, 116, 117, 118, 127, 139, 140, 177, 217, 259, 266, 319, 320, 327
variables, xii, 29, 118, 168, 244, 245, 246, 251, 252, 322
vision, 49, 99, 139, 172, 182, 183, 192
visiting nursing, 307
Vissers, Kris, 108, 109, 193
vomiting, 192, 209, 210, 330, 332

W

war, 162, 178, 262
Washington, 55, 93, 106, 130, 258
water, 15, 49, 278
weakness, 254, 277
web, 108, 186

welfare, 14, 121, 243, 288
well-being, 22, 45, 60, 125, 144, 175, 183, 195, 233, 242, 251, 253, 258, 260, 261, 280, 286, 289, 309
Western countries, 124, 136, 288
Western Europe, vii, 95, 159, 220, 337, 341
White Paper, 91, 106, 155, 205
withdrawal, 60, 66, 71, 77, 290
workers, 50, 118, 119, 120, 153, 254, 285, 290, 295
workforce, 52, 93, 161
workload, 277, 326, 327
World Health Organization (WHO), 5, 6, 32, 49, 56, 104, 105, 106, 134, 135, 136, 137, 141, 142, 150, 151, 157, 158, 159, 160, 163, 164, 165, 179, 180, 181, 184, 201, 205, 210, 211, 212, 221, 227, 230, 231, 236, 257, 266, 272, 276, 281, 284, 295, 297, 298, 300, 303, 308, 320, 322, 323, 330, 331
worldwide, xxi, xxii, 50, 89, 157, 158, 165, 179, 191, 240, 254, 268, 276, 278, 279, 300, 302

Y

yield, 27, 69, 228, 232, 233, 251
young people, xv, 149, 191, 193, 195

Z

Zbigniew, (Ben) Zylicz, viii, 191, 193, 196, 198, 343
Zimbabwe, 136, 140, 141, 153

Related Nova Publications

OXIDATIVE STRESS AND ANTIOXIDANT DEFENSE: BIOMEDICAL VALUE IN HEALTH AND DISEASES

EDITORS: Md. Sahab Uddin and Aman B. Upaganlawar

SERIES: New Developments in Medical Research

BOOK DESCRIPTION: *Oxidative Stress and Antioxidant Defense: Biomedical Value in Health and Diseases* represent current findings on the impact of oxidative stress in the pathogenesis of diseases and underlying mechanisms of antioxidants influencing health and disease processes.

HARDCOVER ISBN: 978-1-53615-687-4
RETAIL PRICE: $310

AN ESSENTIAL GUIDE TO ASTAXANTHIN: DIETARY SOURCES, PROPERTIES AND HEALTH BENEFITS

EDITOR: Paul A. Melborne

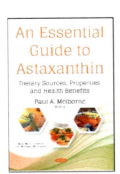

SERIES: New Developments in Medical Research

BOOK DESCRIPTION: *An Essential Guide to Astaxanthin: Dietary Sources, Properties and Health Benefits* begins with a review of published studies regarding the efficacy and application of natural astaxanthin in aquaculture and human health, respectively.

SOFTCOVER ISBN: 978-1-53615-571-6
RETAIL PRICE: $82

To see a complete list of Nova publications, please visit our website at www.novapublishers.com

Related Nova Publications

SENSORY INTEGRATION: DEVELOPMENT, DISORDERS AND TREATMENT

AUTHOR: Izabela Bieńkowska, PhD

SERIES: New Developments in Medical Research

BOOK DESCRIPTION: This book attempts to address and answer questions about different types of disorders in particular developmental spheres in children with learning and behavioral problems. It suggests how a child with sensory integration disorders can be helped in therapy and via other means using methods supporting disturbed sensory integration and other methods supporting the child's development.

SOFTCOVER ISBN: 978-1-53615-454-2
RETAIL PRICE: $95

To see a complete list of Nova publications, please visit our website at www.novapublishers.com